Tumour Immunobiology

The Practical Approach Series

SERIES EDITORS

D. RICKWOOD
Department of Biology, University of Essex
Wivenhoe Park, Colchester, Essex CO4 3SQ, UK

B. D. HAMES
Department of Biochemistry and Molecular Biology,
University of Leeds, Leeds LS2 9JT, UK

Affinity Chromatography
Anaerobic Microbiology
Animal Cell Culture (2nd Edition)
Animal Virus Pathogenesis
Antibodies I and II
Biochemical Toxicology
Biological Data Analysis
Biological Membranes
Biomechanics—Materials
Biomechanics—Structures and Systems
Biosensors
Carbohydrate Analysis
Cell–Cell Interactions
Cell Growth and Division
Cellular Calcium
Cellular Neurobiology
Centrifugation (2nd Edition)
Clinical Immunology
Computers in Microbiology
Crystallization of Nucleic Acids and Proteins
Cytokines
The Cytoskeleton
Diagnostic Molecular Pathology I and II
Directed Mutagenesis
DNA Cloning I, II, and III
Drosophila
Electron Microscopy in Biology
Electron Microscopy in Molecular Biology
Electrophysiology
Enzyme Assays
Essential Molecular Biology I and II
Eukaryotic Gene Transcription
Experimental Neuroanatomy
Fermentation
Flow Cytometry
Gel Electrophoresis of Nucleic Acids (2nd Edition)
Gel Electrophoresis of Proteins (2nd Edition)
Genome Analysis
Growth Factors
Haemopoiesis
Histocompatibility Testing
HPLC of Macromolecules
HPLC of Small Molecules
Human Cytogenetics I and II (2nd Edition)
Human Genetic Diseases
Immobilised Cells and Enzymes

In Situ Hybridization
Iodinated Density Gradient Media
Light Microscopy in Biology
Lipid Analysis
Lipid Modification of Proteins
Lipoprotein Analysis
Liposomes
Lymphocytes
Mammalian Cell Biotechnology
Mammalian Development
Medical Bacteriology
Medical Mycology
Microcomputers in Biochemistry
Microcomputers in Biology
Microcomputers in Physiology
Mitochondria
Molecular Genetic Analysis of Populations
Molecular Neurobiology
Molecular Plant Pathology I and II
Monitoring Neuronal Activity
Mutagenicity Testing
Neural Transplantation
Neurochemistry
Neuronal Cell Lines
Nucleic Acid and Protein Sequence Analysis
Nucleic Acid Hybridisation
Nucleic Acids Sequencing
Oligonucleotides and Analogues
Oligonucleotide Synthesis
PCR
Peptide Hormone Action
Peptide Hormone Secretion
Photosynthesis: Energy Transduction
Plant Cell Culture
Plant Molecular Biology
Plasmids
Pollination Ecology
Postimplantation Mammalian Embryos
Preparative Centrifugation
Prostaglandins and Related Substances
Protein Architecture
Protein Engineering
Protein Function
Protein Purification Applications
Protein Purification Methods
Protein Sequencing
Protein Structure
Protein Targeting
Proteolytic Enzymes
Radioisotopes in Biology
Receptor Biochemistry
Receptor–Effector Coupling
Receptor–Ligand Interactions
Ribosomes and Protein Synthesis
RNA Processing
Signal Transduction
Solid Phase Peptide Synthesis
Spectrophotometry and Spectrofluorimetry
Steroid Hormones
Teratocarcinomas and Embryonic Stem Cells
Transcription Factors
Transcription and Translation
Tumour Immunobiology
Virology
Yeast

Tumour Immunobiology

A Practical Approach

Edited by

G. GALLAGHER

University of Glasgow Department of Surgery
Queen Elizabeth Building
Glasgow Royal Infirmary
Glasgow, UK

R. C. REES

Institute for Cancer Studies
The University of Sheffield Medical School
Sheffield, UK

and

C. W. REYNOLDS

Biological Response Modifiers Program
National Cancer Institute
Frederick, USA

IRL PRESS
at
OXFORD UNIVERSITY PRESS
Oxford New York Tokyo

Oxford University Press, Walton Street, Oxford OX2 6DP
Oxford New York Toronto
Delhi Bombay Calcutta Madras Karachi
Kuala Lumpur Singapore Hong Kong Tokyo
Nairobi Dar es Salaam Cape Town
Melbourne Auckland Madrid
and associated companies in
Berlin Ibadan

Oxford is a trade mark of Oxford University Press

A Practical Approach is a registered trade mark
of the Chancellor, Masters, and Scholars of the University of Oxford
trading as Oxford University Press

Published in the United States
by Oxford University Press Inc., New York

A catalogue record for this book is available from the British Library

Library of Congress Cataloging in Publication Data
Tumour immunobiology : a practical approach / edited by G. Gallagher,
R. C. Rees, and C. W. Reynolds.
(Practical approach)
Includes bibliographical references and index.
1. Tumors—Immunological aspects. 2. Tumor antigens.
I. Gallagher, G. II. Rees, Robert C. III. Reynolds, Craig W.
IV. Series: Practical approach series.
[DNLM: 1. Neoplasms—immunology. QZ 200 T9212]
QR188.6.T863 1993 616.99'4079—dc20 92–49322

ISBN 0–19–963370–3 (Hbk)
ISBN 0–19–963369–X (Pbk)

Typeset by Footnote Graphics, Warminster, Wilts
Printed in Great Britain by Information Press Ltd, Eynsham, Oxon

To the memory of Brian Green

Preface

Tumour immunology has had a long and varied history. Probably the best early example of immunotherapy was the work of Coley, in the first part of this century. His remarkable results from the use of various bacterial extracts for the treatment of advanced tumours may well have been the earliest example of cytokine therapy, but they set the tone for the relationship between cancer clinicians and immunologists that persists today: exciting initial observations that did not bear fruit. For some reason, much more has been expected of cancer immunotherapy than the investigators would ever have claimed and so BCG therapy, the NK cell, interferon, monoclonal antibodies, and LAK-cells have all come and gone. In doing so, each has heightened the scepticism about whether immune manipulation could ever constitute a viable therapeutic option. Even the very idea that the immune system could recognize tumours was condemned as artefactual in the late 1970s, as it became obvious that the murine models then in use were much more antigenic than natural human tumours appeared to be.

Despite past therapeutic failures, it is clear that tumour-associated responses do exist in human cancer (otherwise cytokine-transfected tumours could not confer protection against non-transfected cells); mutated oncogene fragments are obvious tumour-associated antigens (although poor MHC expression on tumours may lead to T-cell anergy). Understanding the mechanisms governing the immune response against cancer has not proved to be a simple task; it has become necessary to consider the complexities of the tumour and its environment so that existing immune responses can be manipulated, or new ones induced. With human cancers in particular, the constant progression to ever-increasing complexity and heterogeneity of the tumour and its metastases must compound the problem.

However, there are instances where immunotherapy of human tumours has been beneficial. In the past decade we have witnessed the application of cytokine therapy to the treatment of incurable tumours and this has rekindled enthusiasm to look at possible mechanisms underlying tumour regression in these cases. It is only with an understanding of these processes at a cellular and molecular level that tumour immunologists will be able to suggest more accurately areas where immunotherapy might be appropriate. Although experimental systems and *in vitro* methods are limited, they are none the less crucial to understanding the effective generation of anticancer immunity in man.

In this publication, we have attempted to compile those techniques and methodologies which have been applied successfully to study cancer immunology. The authors have first-hand experience in the techniques described and have used them successfully in their research.

The book is divided into four broad sections. The first (Chapters 1–11) contains details of how to perform basic, important experiments such as deriving tumour cell-lines, assessing their immunogenicity, and examining the function of those immune cells most usually found in and around tumours. The second (Chapters 12–17) brings out techniques for characterizing and manipulating antibody responses. The third (Chapters 18–21) examines the characterization of cellular responses and a final short section (Chapters 22–24) looks at how all of these procedures can be applied in pre-clinical models.

There is still much to learn about the immune response to cancer and this book does not claim to be a complete armoury of techniques for the researcher interested in anticancer immunity. It does, however, provide carefully defined starting points which provide a solid base upon which individual researchers can build in almost any direction. Current and future developments will add to the list of techniques used, understanding gained, and therapies successfully developed. The 'magic bullet' may be no more, but the 'smart bomb' could be just around the corner . . .

October 1992

G.G.
B.R.
C.R.

Contents

List of contributors xxiv

List of abbreviations xxix

1. Preparation of tumour cell-lines 1

A. P. Wilson

1. Introduction 1

2. Materials required for the preparation of tumour cell-lines 2

3. Collection of clinical material 4

4. Disaggregation of solid tumours 4
Mechanical disaggregation of tumours 5
Disaggregation of tumours by enzyme digestion 6

5. Effusions 8

6. Clean-up procedures 8
Removal of red blood cells and dead cells 8
Preliminary separation of epithelial and stromal cells 9

7. Setting up primary cultures 9

8. Characterization 11

9. Pitfalls and trouble-shooting 13
Cross-line contamination 13
Mycoplasma contamination 13
Genotypic and phenotypic drift 13
Poor success rate for establishing lines 14

References 14

2. Assessment of the immunogenicity of tumour models 17

Fred R. Miller, Bonnie E. Miller, and Gloria H. Heppner

1. Introduction 17

2. Immunogenicity and antigenicity 18

3. Statistical considerations in assessment of immunity 19

4. Tumour cell source for immunization or challenge 20

5. Host irradiation 24

6. Elimination of suppressor cells 25

7. Summary 25

Acknowledgements 25

References 25

3. Flow cytometry of lymphocytes and tumour cells 27

John Lawry

1. Introduction 27

2. Sample considerations 30
Natural sources of cell suspensions 30
Solid tumours 34
Sample storage and fixation 41

3. Standardization 45
The choice of controls 45
Alignment and calibration 46

4. Current applications of flow cytometry 47
Haematogenous and lymphoid tumours 47
Clinical applications of the analysis of solid tumours 49

Further reading 55

Acknowledgements 56

References 56

4. (Glyco-) protein antigens and peptide epitopes of tumours 59

Michael R. Price

1. Introduction 59

2. The tumour cell surface 60

3. Anti-tumour antibodies 61
Antibody storage and stability 61
Antibody purification 61

4. Immunoassays 63
Radioisotopic antiglobulin assay 64
Competitive inhibition of antibody binding 65
Sandwich or double-determinant immunoassay 66

5. Tumour homogenization and sub-cellular fractionation 68
Homogenization 68
Sub-cellular fractionation 69

6. Antigen degradation studies 69

7. Antigen solubilization 70

8. Antigen purification 70
Strategies 70
Lectin affinity chromatography of glycoproteins 71
Antibody affinity chromatography 71

9. Radiolabelling cell-surface proteins and glycoproteins 72

10. Immunoprecipitation 73

11. Immunoblotting 75

12. Epitope mapping 75

13. Conclusions 77

Acknowledgement 77

References 77

5. Isolation and characterization of human natural killer cells 81

Tuomo Timonen, Anna Maenpaa, and Panu Kovanen (with additional material by U. P. Thorgeirsson and A. R. Mackay)

1. Introduction 81

2. Characteristics of NK cells 82
Morphology and physical characteristics 82
Surface phenotype 82
Regulation of NK activity 84

3. Preparation of peripheral blood mononuclear cells (PBMC) 84

4. Purification of human natural killer cells 84
Enrichment of large granular lymphocytes from peripheral blood 84
Depletion of non-NK cells from LGL-enriched fractions 86

5. Proliferation of NK cells 86
Cultures of human NK cells 86

6. Natural killer cell cytotoxicity assays 87
Human NK cell activity 87
Murine natural killer (NK) cell assay 88

References 89

6. Isolation and characterization of mononuclear phagocytes 91

L. J. Partridge and I. Dransfield

1. Introduction 91

2. Reagents and equipment required for studying mononuclear phagocytes 91

3. Isolation of mononuclear phagocytes 92
Density-gradient techniques 92
Separation of mononuclear phagocytes by adherence 94
Counterflow centrifugal elutriation (CC) 97
Immunomagnetic isolation of monocytes 98
Isolation of mononuclear phagocytes from solid tumours 99

4. Monocyte subsets 99

5. Identification of mononuclear phagocytes 100
Histochemical staining 100
Monoclonal antibody staining 102

6. Functional characterization of mononuclear phagocytes 108
Tumour cell killing 109
Production of reactive oxygen intermediates 112
Chemotaxis 113
Phagocytosis 114
Antigen presentation 116
Cytokine production 116

References 116

7. T cells: proliferative and cytotoxic responses 119

R. Adrian Robins

1. Introduction 119

2. Media for lymphocyte preparation and assay 119
Salt base, buffer, and nutrients 119
Serum or protein supplements 120

3. Dissociation and separation of lymphocytes 120
Sources for lymphocyte isolation 121

4. Purification of lymphocytes and T cells 123
Density gradients 123
Magnetic beads 124

5. Cryopreservation of lymphocytes 124

6. Proliferation assays 125

7. Cytotoxicity assays 127
^{51}Cr release 127
Post-label cytotoxicity assays 128

References 129

8. Cloning and propagation of human T lymphocytes 131

Graham Pawelec

1. Introduction 131

2. Tissue-culture medium and growth factors 132

3. Source of T cells for cloning, and their activation 134
T-cell source 134
Activation 134

4. Cloning and propagation of human T lymphocytes 136

5. Cryopreservation 137

6. Assurance of monoclonality 138

Acknowledgements 140

References 140

9. Association of TCR expression with MHC recognition 143

Susan L. Hand, Bruce Lee Hall, and Olivera J. Finn

1. Introduction 143

2. Growth of human alloreactive T-cell cultures 145
Renal allograft-derived T-cell cultures 145
Mixed lymphocyte cultures 145

3. Preparation of total cellular RNA from T-cell cultures 146

4. Synthesis of cDNA from total cellular RNA 147

5. $V\beta$ specific, semiquantitative PCR analysis 148

6. Gel electrophoresis and quantitation of PCR products 151

7. Practical and theoretical considerations of the technique 152
Primer selection 153
Reaction conditions 154
Precision and accuracy 155

8. Representativeness of the message pool 156

Acknowledgements 157

References 157

10. Cytokines: identification and measurement of gene activation 159

F. S. di Giovine, S. Stones, D. Wojtacha, and G. W. Duff

1. Introduction 159

2. Measurement of steady-state mRNA levels 160
Northern analysis 160
Slot/dot-blot analysis 168
Nuclease protection assay 168
Reverse-transcription PCR analysis (RTPCR) 170
In situ hybridization 172

3. Transcription rate analysis (nuclear run-on assay) 174
Preparation of nuclei 174
Labelling of nascent RNA; preparation of probe 175
Membrane hybridization 176

4. mRNA transport into cytoplasm 176

5. Cytoplasmic mRNA half-life 177

Acknowledgements 177

References 178

11. Cytokine bioassay 179

F. P. Winstanley

1. Introduction 179

2. Cell proliferation bioassays 181

3. Cytotoxicity bioassays 183

4. Enzyme release bioassays 185

5. Data analysis 186
Raw data 186
Straightening the curve 187
Non-linear fitting of raw response data 188

6. Standards and quality control 189

Acknowledgements 190

References 190

12. Strategies for the production of human monoclonal antibodies 191

M. Kurpisz and G. Wilson

1. Introduction 191
2. EBV infection of human B lymphocytes: a practical approach 193
   - Source and preparation of B lymphocytes 193
   - Source of EBV 196
   - *In vitro* culture systems to improve efficiency of EBV transformation 196
   - EBV transformation of B lymphocytes 200
   - Screening for immunoglobulin production 201
   - Maintenance of EBV-transformed cell-lines 202
   - Limiting cell dilution 204
   - Fusion of EBV-transformed cell-lines 205
3. Clinical use of antibody from EBV-transformed cell-lines 205
4. Conclusions 205

References 206

13. Radiolabelling antibodies for imaging and targeting 209

M. V. Pimm and S. J. Gribben

1. Introduction 209
   - Choice of radioisotopes for antibody labelling 210
2. Handling and measurement of radioisotopes 211
   - Legal responsibilities and safety in handling radioactive materials 211
   - Detection and measurement of gamma-emitting isotopes 212
   - Specific activity of radiolabelled preparations 212
3. Labelling with radioiodine 213
   - Oxidative methods of radioiodination 213
   - Non-oxidative labelling 216
   - Causes of poor labelling 216
   - Detection of free radioiodine in labelled preparations 217
4. Labelling with radioindium 217
   - Causes of poor labelling 220
   - Detection of free radioindium in preparations 220
5. Labelling with technetium 220
   - Causes of poor labelling 222
   - Detection of free ^{99m}Tc in preparations 222
6. Materials and suppliers 222

Acknowledgement 223

References 223

14. Preparation of multispecific $F(ab)_2$ and $F(ab)_3$ antibody derivatives 225
Martin J. Glennie, Alison L. Tutt, and John Greenman

1. Introduction 225
2. Buffers used in the preparation of multispecific derivatives 226
3. Chromatography equipment 228
4. Preparation of mouse IgG and its $F(ab)_2$ fragments 230
   Preparation of mouse IgG 230
   Preparation of $F(ab)_2$ 231
5. $F(ab)_2$ and $F(ab)_3$ multispecific antibody derivatives 233
   Background 233
   Preparation of multispecific derivatives 237
   Analysis of antibody fragments on HPLC 240
   Checking and removing contaminating $Fc\gamma$ 242

References 243

15. Construction and expression of Ig fusion proteins 245
Martha S. Hayden, H. Perry Fell, and Nicholas F. Landolfi

1. Introduction 245
2. Design and construction of an immunoligand 248
3. Expression 248
   Transient mammalian expression of fusion proteins 248
   Transfection for stable expression 251
4. Detection and characterization of immunoligands 252
   ELISA 252
   Biochemical characterization by immunoprecipitation 253
   Biochemical characterization by Western immunoprecipitation 254
   Purification of immunoligands by affinity chromatography 255
   Analysis of the functional activity of the immunoligand 256
5. Antibody fusions 257
6. Conclusion 260

References 260

16. Re-shaping human monoclonal antibodies for *in vivo* diagnosis and therapy 263
M. E. Verhoeyen

1. Introduction 263

2. General strategy for re-shaping human antibodies 264

3. cDNA cloning and sequence determination of antibody variable regions 265

4. Choosing human framework regions for CDR grafting 266

5. Grafting of rodent binding sites on to human framework regions 268

CDR grafting by site-directed mutagenesis with large oligonucleotides 268

CDR grafting by *de novo* gene synthesis 272

6. Assembly of re-shaped human V-region genes in functional expression vectors 273

7. Expression of re-shaped human antibody genes in myeloma cells 273

8. Characterization of transfectomas 275

References 277

17. Single-chain Fvs 279

Marc Whitlow and David Filpula

1. Introduction 279

2. Design of the linker between the V_L and V_H domains 280

3. Genetic construction of a single-chain Fv 281

Genetic construction of a single-chain Fv from hybridoma cell-lines 281

Genetic construction of a single-chain Fv from combinatiorial libraries 284

Expression of a single-chain Fv 285

4. Fermentation and purification of a single-chain Fv 287

5. Design of single-chain Fv fusion proteins 290

References 290

18. Engineering cytokine-secreting tumour cells 293

Poulam M. Patel, Claudia L. Flemming, Suzanne A. Eccles, and Mary K. L. Collins

1. Introduction 293

2. Vectors for cytokine gene expression 294

3. Packaging cells 295

Care of packaging cells 296

Transfecting packaging cells 296

Titration of virus production 298
Assaying for helper virus 299

4. Cytokine-secreting tumours 299
Tumourigenicity assays 300
Assessing cytokine secretion of explanted tumours 301

References 303

19. *Ex vivo* activation of effector cells 305
K. E. Platts

1. Introduction 305

2. Isolation of effector populations 308
Peripheral blood mononuclear cells (PBMC) 308
Tumour-infiltrating lymphocytes (TIL) 309

3. Separation techniques to isolate enriched or purified populations of effector cells 310

4. Activation of effector populations 310
Generation of IL-2-activated human peripheral blood mononuclear cells 311
Generation of IL-2-activated human TIL 312
Modifications to the procedures for the generation of human effector cell populations 313

5. Assessment of activation 318
Cytotoxicity assays 318
Proliferation 318
Cytokine production 318
Cytokine gene expression 318

Acknowledgement 319

References 319

20. Genetic immortalization of human lymphocytes using retroviral vectors 321
Chris Darnbrough

1. Introduction 321

2. Immortalization mechanisms 322
Oncogenes 322
Autocrine loops 323
Imponderables 324
Immortalization strategies 324

3. Introducing genes 324
Retroviral vectors 325

Retroviral vector systems 325
Transfection of packaging cells 329
HIV-based vectors 335

4. Primary cells 335
Sources 335
The cell cycle 336
Stimulation of primary lymphocytes 337
Infection of primary cells 338

5. Conclusion 341

Acknowledgements 341

References 342

21. Modifying the specificity of T cells using chimeric *Ig*/*TCR* genes 345

Zelig Eshhar, Gideon Gross, and Jonathan Treisman

1. Introduction 345

2. Design and construction of the c*TCR* genes 349
Antibody selection 349
The chimeric gene construct 350
Expression vector systems 350
Cloning of c*TCR* into mammalian expression vectors 351

3. Transfection and selection of cells expressing the c*TCR* genes 355
Choosing cells for transfection 355
Sequential transfection versus co-transfection 356
Methods of DNA transfection 356
Selection of cells using antibiotic resistance 358

4. Selection of cells expressing the c*TCR* 360
Molecular analysis of transfectants 360
Functional analysis of transfectants 364

Acknowledgement 367

References 367

22. The use of pre-clinical rodent models for cancer immunotherapy 369

Robert H. Wiltrout

1. Introduction 369

2. General types of rodent tumour models 369
Transplantable primary tumours 370

Transplantable metastatic tumours 370
Primary autochthonous tumours 371
Xenografts of human tumours in athymic mice 372

3. Application and description of a transplantable murine renal cancer model 373
Intrarenal Renca as a model for treatment of a primary tumour 373
The use of Renca for the formation of experimental pulmonary metastases 376
The use of Renca for the formation of experimental hepatic metastases 377
Summary of pre-clinical immunotherapy results obtained using the Renca tumour model 378
Relationship between clinical results and pre-clinical predictions 379

4. General survey of widely used pre-clinical rodent models 380

5. Implications of biological variability that exists between rodent tumour models 380

6. Summary 382

References 382

23. Use of the tumour spheroid model in immunotherapy 385

Irma E. Garcia de Palazzo, Michele Holmes, Katherine Alpaugh, and Louis M. Weiner

1. Introduction 385

2. Methods and experimental design 386
MHTS generation and growth 386
Preparation of IL-2-activated lymphocytes 387
Antibodies 387
Co-culture of MHTS with LAK cells and antibodies 388
Histology and immunohistochemistry 388

3. Results 389
Morphology and differentiation characteristics of SW948 389
Histological and immunohistochemical characterization of LAK cell infiltration of MHTS 390

4. Concluding remarks 395

References 396

24. Characterization of metastatic tumour cells 399

U. P. Thorgeirsson and A. R. Mackay

1. Introduction 399

2. Animal models 399

3. *In vivo* metastasis assays 401
Tumour cell preparation 401
Routes of injection 401

4. *In vitro* assays to study the metastatic phenotype 404
Tumour invasion assays 404
Amnion invasion assay 405

5. Proteolytic activity 406

6. Tumour cell surface 409

References 409

Index 413

Contributors

KATHERINE ALPAUGH
Fox Chase Cancer Center, 7701 Burholme Avenue, Philadelphia PA 19111, USA.

MARY K. L. COLLINS
Chester Beatty Laboratories, Institute of Cancer Research, 237 Fulham Road, London SW3 6JB, UK.

CHRIS DARNBROUGH
Department of Immunology, University of Strathclyde, The Todd Centre, 31 Taylor Street, Glasgow G4 0NR, UK.

I. DRANSFIELD
Respiratory Medicine Unit, City Hospital, Greenbank Drive, Edinburgh EH10 5SB, UK.

G. W. DUFF
University of Sheffield, Section of Molecular Medicine, Royal Hallamshire Hospital, Sheffield S10 2JF, UK.

SUZANNE A. ECCLES
Section of Immunology, Institute of Cancer Research, 15 Cotswold Road, Sutton, Surrey SM2 5NG, UK.

ZELIG ESHHAR
Department of Chemical Immunology, The Weizmann Institute of Science, Rehovot 76100, Israel.

H. PERRY FELL
Bristol-Myers Squibb Pharmaceutical Research Institute, 3005 First Avenue, Seattle WA 98121, USA.

DAVID FILPULA
Genex Corporation (a subsidiary of Enzon Corporation), 16020 Industrial Drive, Gaithersburg, MD 20877, USA.

OLIVERA J. FINN
Department of Molecular Genetics and Biochemistry, University of Pittsburgh, School of Medicine, E1242 Biomedical Sciences Tower, Pittsburgh, PA 15261, USA.

CLAUDIA L. FLEMMING
Chester Beatty Laboratories, Institute of Cancer Research, 237 Fulham Road, London SW3 6JB, UK.

IRMA E. GARCIA DE PALAZZO
Fox Chase Cancer Center, 7701 Burholme Avenue, Philadelphia, PA 19111, USA.

F. S. DI GIOVINE
University of Sheffield, Section of Molecular Medicine, Royal Hallamshire Hospital, Sheffield S10 2JF, UK.

MARTIN J. GLENNIE
Lymphoma Research Unit, Tenovus Laboratory, General Hospital, Southampton SO9 4XY, UK.

JOHN GREENMAN
Lymphoma Research Unit, Tenovus Laboratory, General Hospital, Southampton SO9 4XY, UK.

S. J. GRIBBEN
Cancer Research Campaign Laboratories, University of Nottingham, Nottingham NG7 2RD, UK.

GIDEON GROSS
Division of Proteins and Nucleic Acids, MRC Laboratory of Molecular Biology, Cambridge CB2 2QH, UK.

BRUCE LEE HALL
Department of Microbiology and Immunology, Duke University Medical Center, Durham, NC 27710, USA.

SUSAN L. HAND
Department of Molecular Genetics and Biochemistry, University of Pittsburgh, School of Medicine, E1242 Biomedical Sciences Tower, Pittsburgh, PA 15261, USA.

MARTHA S. HAYDEN
Bristol-Myers Squibb Pharmaceutical Research Institute, 3005 First Avenue, Seattle, WA 98121, USA.

GLORIA H. HEPPNER
Breast Cancer Biology Program, Michigan Cancer Foundation, Meyer L. Prentis Cancer Center, 110 E. Warren Avenue, Detroit, MI 48201-1379, USA.

MICHELE HOLMES
Fox Chase Cancer Center, 7701 Burholme Avenue, Philadelphia, PA 19111, USA.

PANU KOVANEN
Department of Pathology, University of Helsinki, Helsinki, Finland.

M. KURPÌSZ
Institute of Human Genetics, Polish Academy of Sciences, 60-479 Pozńań, ul. Strzeszyńska 32, Poland.

NICHOLAS F. LANDOLFI
Protein Design Labs Inc., 2375 Garcia Avenue, Mountain View, CA 94043, USA.

JOHN LAWRY
Institute for Cancer Studies, Department of Experimental and Clinical Microbiology University of Sheffield Medical School, Beech Hill Road, Sheffield S10 2RX, UK.

A. R. MACKAY
Office of the Director, Division of Cancer Etiology, National Cancer Institute, National Institutes of Health, Bethesda, MD 20892, USA.

ANNA MAENPAA
Department of Pathology, University of Helsinki, Helsinki, Finland.

BONNIE E. MILLER
Department of Breast Cancer Cell and Molecular Biology, Michigan Cancer Foundation, Meyer L. Prentis Cancer Center, 110 E. Warren Avenue, Detroit, MI 48201-1379, USA.

FRED R. MILLER
Department of Breast Cancer Cell and Molecular Biology, Michigan Cancer Foundation, Meyer L. Prentis Cancer Center, 110 E. Warren Avenue, Detroit, MI 48201-1379, USA.

L. J. PARTRIDGE
Krebs Institute for Biomolecular Research, Department of Molecular Biology and Biotechnology, University of Sheffield, Western Band, Sheffield S10 2UH, UK.

POULAM M. PATEL
Chester Beatty Laboratories, Institute of Cancer Research, 237 Fulham Road, London SW3 6JB, UK.

GRAHAM PAWELEC
Section for Transplantation Biology and Immunohaematology, Second Department of Internal Medicine, University of Tübingen Medical Clinic, W-7400 Tübingen, Germany.

M. V. PIMM
Cancer Research Campaign Laboratories, University of Nottingham, Nottingham NG7 2RD, UK.

K. E. PLATTS
Institute for Cancer Studies, University of Sheffield Medical School, Beech Hill Road, Sheffield S10 2RX, UK.

MICHAEL R. PRICE
Cancer Research Campaign Laboratories, University of Nottingham, Nottingham NG7 2RD, UK.

R. ADRIAN ROBINS
Cancer Research Campaign Laboratories, The University of Nottingham, University Park, Nottingham NG7 2RD, UK.

S. STONES
University of Sheffield, Section of Molecular Medicine, Royal Hallamshire Hospital, Sheffield S10 2JF, UK.

U. P. THORGEIRSSON
Office of the Director, Division of Cancer Etiology, National Cancer Institute, National Institutes of Health, Bethesda, MD 20892, USA.

TUOMO TIMONEN
Department of Pathology, University of Helsinki, Helsinki, Finland.

JONATHAN TREISMAN
The Surgery Branch, National Cancer Institute, The National Institute of Health, Bethesda, MD 20892, USA.

ALISON L. TUTT
Lymphoma Research Unit, Tenovus Laboratory, General Hospital, Southampton SO9 4XY, UK.

M. E. VERHOEYEN
Unilever Research, Colworth Laboratories, Sharnbrook, Bedfordshire MK44 1LQ, UK.

LOUIS M. WEINER
Fox Chase Cancer Center, 7701 Burholme Avenue, Philadelphia, PA 19111, USA.

MARC WHITLOW
Genex Corporation (a subsidiary of Enzon Corporation), 16020 Industrial Drive, Gaithersburg, MD 20877, USA.

A. P. WILSON
Oncology Research Laboratory, Derby City Hospital, Uttoxeter Road, Derby DE3 3NE, UK.

G. WILSON
University Department of Surgery, Queen Elizabeth Building, Glasgow Royal Infirmary, Glasgow G32 2ER, UK.

ROBERT H. WILTROUT
Experimental Therapeutics Section, NCI-FCRDC, Building 560, Rm. 31-93, Frederick, MD 21702-1201, USA

F. P. WINSTANLEY
Department of Pathological Biochemistry, Queen Elizabeth Building, Glasgow Royal Infirmary, Glasgow G31 2ER, UK.

D. WOJTACHA
Renal Unit, The Royal Infirmary, Edinburgh, UK.

Abbreviations

Ab	antibody
ACGM	advisory committee on genetic manipulation
ADCC	antibody-dependent cellular cytotoxicity
AFP	alpha-fetoprotein
Ag	antigen
A-LAK	adherant, lymphokine-activated killer (cell)
AMV	avian myeloblastosis virus
Ap	anti-apoptosis
APAAP	alkaline phosphatase anti-alkaline phosphatase
APmA	*p*-aminophenylmercuric acetate
B-cell	lymphocyte which secretes immunoglobulin
BHK	baby hamster kidney (cells)
B-LCL	B-lymphoblastoid cell-line
BM	bone marrow
BrdU	bromodeoxyuridine
BSA	bovine serum albumin
BsAb	bispecific antibodies
CCE	counterflow centrifugal elutriation
CD	cluster of differentiation
cDNA	complementary DNA
CDR	complementarity determining regions
CEA	carcinoembryonic antigen
CFU	colony-forming units
CM	conditioned medium
CML	chronic myelogenous leukaemia
CMV	cytomegalovirus
Con-A	concanavalin-A
c.p.m.	counts per minute
CR	complement receptor
C-region	constant region
CSF	colony-stimulating factor
cTCR	chimeric T-cell receptor
CTL	cytotoxic T-lymphocytes
DCS	donor-calf serum

DEPC	diethylpyrocarbonate
DMEM	Dulbecco's modified Eagle's medium
DMF	dimethylformamide
DMSO	dimethylsulphoxide
DNA	deoxyribonucleic acid
DNase	an enzyme which digests DNA
dNTP	deoxynucleotide triphosphate
DNTP	dithio-bis(2-nitrobenzoic acid)
d.p.m.	disintegrations per minute
D-region	diversity region
DTPA	diethylenetriaminepentacetic acid
DTPAA	diethylenetriaminepentacetic acid anhydride
DTT	dithiothreitol
EBNA	Epstein–Barr virus nuclear antigen
EBV	Epstein–Barr virus
ECACC	European collection of animal cell cultures
EDTA	ethylenediaminetetraacetic acid
EIA	enzyme immunoassay
ELISA	enzyme-linked immunosorbent assay
EMA	epithelial membrane antigen
FAA	flavone acetic acid
FACS	fluorescence-activated cell-sorter
FBS	fetal bovine serum
FcR	receptor for the Fc portion of Ig molecules
FCS	fetal-calf serum
FITC	fluorescein isothiocyanate
FNA	fine-needle aspirate
FR	framework regions
G0, G1, etc.	stages of the cell-cycle
G6PDH	glucose-6-phosphate dehydrogenase
G-CSF	granulocyte colony-stimulating factor
GLU	glutamic acid
GLY	glycine
GM-CSF	granulocyte-macrophage colony-stimulating factor
HAMA	human anti-mouse antibody
HAT	hypoxanthine, aminopterin, thymidine
HBS	HEPES-buffered saline
HBSS	Hank's balanced salt solution
HCG	human chorionic gonadotrophin
HITES	hydrocortisone, insulin, transferrin, oestradiol, selenium
HIV	human immunodeficiency virus
HLA	human leucocyte antigen
HMFG	human milk-fat globulin
HPLC	high-pressure liquid chromatography

HS	human serum
HSV	herpes simplex virus
HTLV	human T-cell leukaemia virus
ICAM	intra-cellular adhesion molecule
Id	idiotype
IDMEM	Iscove's modification of DMEM
IFN	interferon
Ig	immunoglobulin
IL	interleukin
Im	immortalization
i.p.	intraperitoneal
i.r.	intrarenal
IRMA	immunoradiometric assay
i.v.	intravenous
J-region	joining region
LAK	lymphokine-activated killer (cell)
LALS	large-angle light scatter
LCA	leucocyte common antigen
LD	limiting dilution
LEU	leucine
LGL	large granular lymphocyte
LMP	low melting-point
Lp	lymphoproliferation
LPS	lipopolysaccharide
LT	lymphotoxin
LTBMC	long-term, bone-marrow cultures
LTR	long terminal repeat
LYS	lysine
MAb	monoclonal antibody
MAPPing	message amplification phenotyping
MDP (1)	muramyl dipeptide
MDP (2)	methylene diphosphonate
MDR	multi-drug resistance
2-ME	2-mercaptoethanol
MEM	minimal essential medium
MHC	major histocompatibility complex
MHTS	multicellular human tumour spheroids
MLC	mixed lymphocyte cultures
MLR	mixed lymphocyte reaction
MLTC	mixed lymphocyte tumour culture
MMLV	Moloney murine leukaemia virus
MMTV	mouse mammary tumour virus
MMP	matrix metaloproteinases
MNC	mononuclear cells

MoAb	monoclonal antibody
MoMLV	Moloney murine leukaemia virus
MOPS	3-[*N*-morpholino]propanesulphonic acid
MPA	mycophenolic acid
mRNA	messenger RNA
MTT	3-[4,5-dimethylthiazol-2-yl]-2,5-diphenyltetrazolium bromide
NCA	normal cross-reacting antigen
NCS	newborn-calf serum
NEM	*N*-ethylmaleimide
neo	neomycin
NFM	nuclear freezing medium
NK	natural killer (cell)
NTP	nucleotide triphosphate
O.D.	optical density
OPD	*o*-phenylenediamine dihydrochloride
o-PDM	*o*-phenylenedimaleimide
Osmol	osmolarity
PA	plasminogen activator
PAGE	polyacrylamide gel electrophoresis
PAI	plasminogen activator inhibitor
PBL	peripheral blood lymphocytes
PBMC	peripheral blood mononuclear cells
PBS	phosphate-buffered saline
PCNA	proliferating cell nuclear antigen
PCR	polymerase chain reaction
PD	population doublings
PDT	photodynamic therapy
PE	phycoerythrin
PHA	phytohaemagglutinin
PI	propidium iodide
PLAP	placental alkaline phosphatase
PMA	phorbol myrisic acatate
PMN	polymorphonuclear leucocytes
PMSF	phenylmethylsulphonylfluoride
PPD	purified protein derivative (of tuberculin)
PSA	prostate-specific antigen
PTFE	polytetrafluoroethene
PWM	poke-weed mitogen
QC	quality control
RB	reaction buffer
RBC	red blood cells
RCV	replication-competent helper virus
RENCA	renal-cell carcinoma
RIA	radioimmunoassay

RNA	ribonucleic acid
RNase	enzymes that can digest RNA
ROI	reactive oxygen intermediate
RPMI	Rockwell Park Memorial Institute
rRNA	ribosomal RNA
RSB	reticulocyte standard buffer
RSV	raos sarcoma virus
RT	reverse transcriptase
RTPCR	reverse-transcriptional polymerase chain reaction
SAC-1	staphylococcus aureous Cowan-1
SBTI	soyabean trypsin inhibitor
sc	subcutaneously
SCID	severe, combined immunodeficiency
SDS-PAGE	PAGE, incorporating sodium dodecylsulphate
SER	serine
SF	serum-free
SFM	serum-free medium
SIN	self inactivating (virus)
SPDP	*N*-succinimidyl-3-(2-pyridyldithio)-propionate
SRBC	sheep red blood cells
STE	sodium chloride/Tris/EDTA buffer
TBS	Tris-buffered saline
Tc	translocations
TCA	trichloroacetic acid
TCC	T-cell clone
T-cell	thymus-derived lymphocyte
TCGF	T-cell growth factor(s)
TCLL	T-cell chronic lymphocytic leukaemia
TCR	T-cell receptor
TDAC	tumour-derived activated cell
TdT	terminal deoxynucleotidyl transferase
TE	Tris–EDTA buffer
Tg	transgenics
TGF	transforming growth factor
TIL	tumour-infiltrating lymphocytes
TIMP	tissue inhibitors of metalloproteinases
TK	thymidine kinase
Tm	tumorigenesis
TNF	tumour necrosis factor
t-PA	tissue type plasminogen activator
TPA	12-*o*-tetradecanoylphorbol-13-acetate
TRIS	Tris[hydroxymethyl]aminomethane
tRNA	transfer RNA
TsAb	trispecific antibodies

UV	ultraviolet
VLA	very late antigen
V-region	variable region
WEHI	Walter and Elisa Hall Institute

1

Preparation of tumour cell-lines

A. P. WILSON

1. Introduction

The importance and relevance of tumour cell-lines as an experimental aid for biological studies on human cancer is becoming increasingly recognized. Whilst the numbers of human tumour cell-lines and the different types of tumour represented by one or more cell-lines are increasing, there may be restrictions around the availability of those lines used by others and such cells as can be obtained may not possess specifically desired properties or they may be inadequately characterized for your own purpose. It is therefore very useful to have the expertise to develop one's own cell-lines from clinical material or from animal models. The uses of cell-lines in the field of tumour immunobiology are multiple and include:

- evaluation of cellular antigenicity
- use as targets for investigation of cell-mediated immune responses
- evaluation of the cytotoxicity and fate of antibody-conjugated drugs
- studies on cytokines
- the development of pre-clinical predictive models and animal models for *in vivo/in vitro* comparisons

Whether a tumour cell-line is truly representative of the parent tumour is a matter for debate, but given the diversity of the same disease between individuals and the heterogeneity within each tumour, a cell-line's relevance stands on its own merit and the validity of any *in vitro* model is more dependent upon adequate characterization. This includes exclusion of the possibility of intraspecies and interspecies contamination and identification of base-line characteristics for assessing phenotypic and genotypic stability during the history of the cell-line's use.

In this chapter, protocols for handling cells from clinical material to frozen stock are included. Steps which should be taken to characterize the cell-line are indicated and the reader is referred to other texts for more specialized protocols where appropriate. The protocols are general and are meant to be applicable to a wide range of tumours. Emphasis is placed on adherent cell cultures, but the information is also relevant to tumours which grow in suspension. References for a range of tumour types are given in *Table 1*.

2. Materials required for the preparation of tumour cell-lines

It is assumed that the reader has access to routine tissue culture facilities and has a basic knowledge of tissue-culture techniques. Information on these basics can be obtained from several reference manuals, which also include more specialized information (1–3). You will need the following equipment and reagents to hand and they should be sterile:

Basic equipment

- conical-bottomed universal containers
- pipettes (non-graduated)
- glass petri dishes
- dissecting instruments (scissors, forceps, scalpels)
- conical flasks
- culture flasks
- nylon mesh (20–30 μm, available from Henry Simon)
- 2 ml freezing vials
- polystyrene foam boxes

Basic reagents

- Hanks balanced salt solution (HBSS)
- culture medium containing 10% foetal calf serum (FCS)

Table 1. Media and identification markers for specific tumour types

Tumour type	Medium	Markers	Reference
Colorectal adenocarcinoma (6)[a]	DMEM, 10% FCS	CEA	5
Ovarian adenocarcinoma (7)	DMEM or DMEM/F12, 10% FCS, insulin	OC125, HMFG2	21
Ovarian adenocarcinoma (9)	RPMI 1640 10% FCS, insulin	CEA, PLAP, HMFG1	22
Ovarian adenocarcinoma (4)	α-MEM, 20% FCS, vitamins	Growth in soft agar	11
Ovarian adenocarcinoma (4)	RPMI 1640, 10–20% FCS	CEA, hormone production, hormone receptors	23
Breast (1° culture)	DMEM/F12, 20% FCS, insulin	Keratin, CEA, EMA	10
Breast (1° culture)	DMEM/F12, 20% FCS, insulin	G6PDH	24

Table 1. *Contined*

Tumour type	Medium	Markers	Reference
Lung (13)	Hams F12, 20% DCS or HITES	Neural enzymes	9
Lung	Hams F12, HITES		25
Squamous carcinoma (10)	DMEM, 10% FCS	Morphology	4
Breast carcinoma (1)	RPMI 1640, 10% FCS, insulin, hydrocortisone, galactose, thioglycerol	Differentiation features	26
Myeloma (3)	RPMI 1640 or Hams F12, 20% FCS, feeder cells	EBV negative Production of monoclonal IgG	27
Lung (20)	ACL-4 chemically defined	Secretion of tumour markers	28
Chronic B-cell leukaemias (4)	RPMI 1640, 10% FCS with polyclonal B-cell activators	Karyotype IgG gene rearrangements	29
Gliomas (4)	Eagles MEM, 10% FCS		30
Pancreas (6)	RPMI 1640, 10% FCS, EGF, HC, transferrin, selenite	CEA, tumourigenicity in nude mice	31
Childhood acute leukaemia (8)	GM-CSF	Cytogenetics	32
Myelomonocytic leukaemia (4)	RPMI 1640, 10% FCS, 5% human serum and irradiated human macrophages as feeders		33
Burkitt's lymphoma (60)	RPMI 1640, 20% FCS (HI), with feeder layer of irradiated human embryo fibroblasts	BL translocation	34
Sarcoma (8)	Hams F12, 15% FCS, NEAA		35
Lung (6)	RPMI 1640, or Hams F12, 10% FCS	Neuron-specific enolase, peptide products	36
Lymphoma	Pooled HS, diploid feeder layer, L-cysteine, transferrin, bathocuproine disulphonate (copper chelator)		37

[a] Number of cell-lines established.

DMEM = Dulbecco's modification of Eagle's medium; FCS = foetal calf serum; α-MEM = α minimal essential medium; DCS = donor calf serum; HITES = hydrocortisone, insulin, transferrin, estradiol, selenium; GM-CSF = granulocyte-macrophage colony-stimulating factor; CEA = carcinoembryonic antigen; HMFG2 = human milk fat globulin; PLAP = placental alkaline phosphatase; G6PDH = glucose-6-phosphate dehydrogenase; HCG = human chorionic gonadotrophin; EMA = epithelial membrane antigen.

- phosphate-buffered saline (PBS)
- red blood cell lysing buffer (Sigma)
- Ficoll–sodium diatrizoate (e.g. Histopaque (Sigma), lymphocyte separation medium (ICN-Flow))
- enzymes—trypsin, trypsin/versene, collagenase (available from Sigma, Gibco BRL, ICN-Flow)
- DNase Type I (Sigma)
- dimethylsulphoxide (DMSO)

3. Collection of clinical material

It is important to develop a good collection system which ensures that medical or nursing staff have appropriate containers for receiving tumours, a labelling system which clearly identifies patient and registration number for follow-up, and a transport system which gets the specimen into the laboratory without too much delay. If your laboratory is within a hospital, you'll probably find it best to go to theatre yourself.

Effusions are generally drained from the patient directly into paracentesis bags, the contents of which can be transferred to large sterile bottles for ease of handling. Sterility of the fluid during transfer is easier to maintain if the bags are not first filled to capacity. It is common practice to add heparin at 10 U/ml as an anti-coagulant, but this is not essential.

Solid tumour specimens should be collected in sterile containers appropriate to the amount of tissue and containing a sterile transport medium. Suitable transport media include phosphate-buffered saline (PBS), Hanks balanced salt solution (HBSS), or culture medium (about 10 ml/cm^3 of tissue). Tumours from skin and gut are certain to be infected and inclusion of suitable antibiotics may reduce the risk of contaminated primary cultures (4, 5), but extra care is needed with such samples. If the tissue is to be stored for several hours prior to processing, it may be advantageous to use a serum-containing culture medium rather than PBS or HBSS. The viability of tumour tissue is best preserved if the tumour is cut up into small pieces of no more than 1 cm diameter; tissue stored in this way may be kept for at least 24 h (and possibly longer) at 4°C without significant loss of viability. A representative piece of tissue should always be fixed in 10% formol saline for histopathology. This allows comparison of pathologies and also provides essential information on the cellular composition of the tumour which may be enlightening if cell yield is low or viability is poor (see Section 9.4).

4. Disaggregation of solid tumours

Solid tumour tissue can be disaggregated mechanically or with enzymes. The most commonly used enzymes are trypsin or collagenase but others such as pronase, neuraminidase, hyaluronidase, and dispase may also be used (Boehringer and Sigma are good sources of enzymes). There are advantages and disadvantages associated with each method, which are outlined in the relevant section.

4.1 Mechanical disaggregation of tumours

Some tumours can be disaggregated without resorting to enzymatic digestion. This may be because the tumour is very soft or because differential recovery of cell type is required (e.g. the 'spill-out' technique for breast tumours (6)). Mechanical disaggregation has the advantage of being quick and is particularly useful for small tumours. However, cell viability may be poor due to damage and it is tedious when large amounts of tumour are to be disaggregated. This method can be used as the starting point for enzyme digestion, to obtain cells for primary culture, or for explant culture (see reference (3) for a protocol).

Protocol 1. Mechanical disaggregation of tumours

The method shown describes tissue disruption by chopping. It is also possible to disrupt the tissue by mashing it through sieves of decreasing size (see reference (3) for protocol).

1. Transfer the tumour tissue into a glass petri dish. Discard any fat, muscle, fibrous capsule, and necrotic material.
2. Add a small amount of HBSS (~2 ml) to keep the tumour moist and chop the tumour into smaller fragments of about 2–3 mm in size. For hard tumours, crossed scalpel blades in a glass petri dish are most effective. For soft tumours, curved scissors work well though damage to cells may be less using scalpel blades. The addition of more culture medium (~ 5 ml) after the initial chopping is complete, separates the fragments and it is then easy to see the larger fragments which need further disaggregation. For ease of chopping, this volume should, however, be kept as small as possible.
3. These pieces can be frozen for disaggregation at a later date, or as surplus stock. Re-suspend the fragments in culture medium containing 10% DMSO and 10% FCS (3–4 fragments/ml) and freeze (*Protocol 9*).

4.1.1 Recovery of cells for primary cultures

When the tumour has been disaggregated into very small fragments there may be a sufficiently high yield of viable cells to allow initiation of a primary culture.

Protocol 2. Recovery of cells from mechanically dissociated tissue

1. Continue chopping fragments obtained from step **2**, *Protocol 1* to reduce their size to about 1 mm^3.

Protocol 2. *Continued*

2. Add about 10 ml of medium to the petri dish and gently agitate the dish to suspend the free cells and small clumps; pipette these fragments a few times to increase the release of cells into the medium.
3. Tip the dish to allow larger fragments to settle in one corner and harvest the cell suspension into a sterile universal.
4. Repeat steps **1–3** until the harvested medium is clear and contains very few cells.
5. Centrifuge the harvested cell suspension at 400*g* for 5 min.
6. Discard the supernatant and re-suspend the cell pellets in culture medium—about 10 ml/1 ml of cell pellet; the pellets can be pooled if necessary.
7. Store at 4°C until ready to proceed.
8. Refer to Section 6 (clean-up procedure) and Section 7 (setting up primary cultures).

4.2 Disaggregation of tumours by enzyme digestion

Tumours may be disaggregated using trypsin, collagenase, or collagenase-containing cocktails. Enzyme digestion provides a more efficient release of viable cells, a higher cell yield, and is more convenient for large tumours. Trypsinization is carried out in the absence of serum and is therefore potentially damaging to the cells. Warm trypsinization is comparatively fast, but labour intensive; the disadvantages of trypsinization can be overcome using a cold trypsinization technique (see reference (3) for a protocol). Collagenase digestion is potentially less damaging because it can be done in the presence of serum, but it can take up to three days for complete disruption of tissue. Stromal cell contamination can be more of a problem with collagenase digestion, since cells are released more easily from connective tissue than from tumour. With either trypsin or collagenase it is common practice to include DNAase in the enzyme solutions because the release of DNA from damaged cells can reduce proteolytic activity and tends to cause re-aggregation of cells (seen as an increase in viscosity of the cell-containing enzyme solution), which makes cell recovery very difficult and which is prevented by the inclusion of DNAase. Other enzymes (such as dispase) have also been used in conjunction with collagenase and examples of different cocktails can be found in the literature (7–11).

Protocol 3. Warm trypsinization of solid tumours

1. Rinse the fragments (obtained at step **2** in *Protocol 1*) in HBSS to remove all traces of serum.

2. Re-suspend them in warm trypsin (0.25%, w/v) containing DNAase Type I (0.002%, w/v) and transfer to a conical flask securely capped with foil to maintain sterility. Make the mixture to a final volume of 20 ml per cm^3 of tissue.
3. Gently agitate the suspension at 37°C. Agitation methods include:
   - intermittent shaking by hand (e.g. every 5 min)
   - use of a water bath with shaking attachment
   - gentle use of magnetic stirring devices (which may also increase mechanical damage)
4. After 15–30 min incubation allow the tissue fragments to settle under gravity and aspirate the cell-containing enzyme solution into universals. The length of time required for digestion depends on the consistency of the tumour, which in turn influences the rate of release of the cells. For soft tumours 15 min will probably be sufficient, whilst 30 min or more may be needed for harder tumours. Centrifuge at 400*g* for 5 min, discard the supernatant, and re-suspend the cell pellet in 10 ml of culture medium containing 10% FCS. Store at 4°C labelled as 'trypsin 1'.
5. Add fresh trypsin to the remaining fragments in the flask and repeat steps **3** and **4**. Label cells as 'trypsin 2'.
6. Continue trypsinization until tissue disaggregation is complete. Residual connective tissue will appear as soft, white, floating fragments.
7. Check each trypsin fraction for cell yield, using trypan blue to check cell viability, and pool those which contain the highest yields of viable cells. The first fraction may have low viability, as may the washings from the various stages of mechanical dissociation; the last fraction may have a low cell yield.
8. Store the pooled fractions at 4°C until you are ready to proceed.
9. Refer to Sections 6 and 7.

Protocol 4. Collagenase digestion of solid tumours

1. Suspend the tissue fragments (from step **2** in *Protocol 1*) in a culture medium containing the selected enzyme cocktail (20 ml/cm^3 tissue).
2. Transfer the mixture to tissue-culture flasks and incubate horizontally at 37°C for 18 h–3 days. The time depends on the rate of release of cells from the fragments.
3. Gently pipette the fragments to release the cells.
4. Harvest the cell suspension into sterile universals and centrifuge at 400*g* for 5 min. Re-suspend the cell pellet in culture medium and store at 4°C until ready to proceed.
5. Refer to Sections 6 and 7.

5. Effusions

Cells can be easily recovered from effusions by centrifugation at 400–500*g*. Some fluids contain very few malignant cells and it is useful to check the cellularity of a small sample prior to processing. The final cell pellet should be re-suspended in culture medium (10 ml/ml cell pellet) and then handled as for cell suspensions obtained by any of the other methods described. Mesothelial cell overgrowth can be a problem with cultures from effusions; the characteristics of cultured mesothelial cells are well documented (12) and you should be able to identify them in order to avoid embarrasing mistakes!

6. Clean-up procedures

The cell suspension obtained by any of the above methods may need additional treatment to prepare it for primary culture. Further treatment is indicated when red blood cell contamination is heavy, cell viability is low, or preliminary separation of epithelial (tumour) cells from stromal cells is desirable.

6.1 Removal of red blood cells and dead cells

There are several methods available for removal of red blood cells. These include the use of ammonium chloride buffer and layering over a mixture of Ficoll and sodium diatrizoate. Ammonium chloride is quick but removes only red blood cells. Layering over Ficoll–diatrizoate is more time-consuming but has the advantage that dead cells are removed with the red blood cells, thereby improving the overall viability of the remaining cell suspension. This is therefore a valuable option if cell yield is low and viability poor.

Protocol 5. Use of ammonium chloride

1. Add 10 ml of ammonium chloride buffer (red blood cell lysing buffer (Sigma)) to 1 ml of cell pellet and gently re-suspend the cells.
2. Incubate for 2–5 min at 37°C, until the red blood cells are lysed.
3. Centrifuge the cell suspension at 400*g* for 5 min and re-suspend the cell pellet in culture medium.
4. Repeat step **3** once to wash cells free of buffer and re-suspend the cell pellet in culture medium.

Protocol 6. Use of Ficoll–diatrizoate

1. Add 6 ml Ficoll–diatrizoate solution (Histopaque 1077 (Sigma); lymphocyte separation medium (ICN-Flow); Ficoll–Paque (Pharmacia)) to a universal.

2. Gently layer 9 ml medium containing up to 2×10^7 cells on to the Ficoll 'cushion'.
3. Centrifuge at 600*g* for 15 min.
4. Carefully remove the medium from the top of the Ficoll–diatrizoate and collect the viable cells from the interface, using a pipette or syringe.
5. Re-suspend the cells in 20 ml of culture medium and centrifuge them at 400*g* for 5 min. Repeat once more to wash cells.
6. Re-suspend the cell pellet in culture medium.

6.2 Preliminary separation of epithelial and stromal cells

Epithelial tumours may yield a mixture of single stromal cells and epithelial clusters which can be separated from each other by sedimentation or filtration. For separation by sedimentation, re-suspend the cells in 20 ml of medium and allow the clusters to settle out over a period of 2–3 min. Remove the supernatant gently and discard it, then repeat the process using fresh medium. The sedimented pellet is enriched for epithelial cells.

The cells can also be separated by filtration.

Protocol 7. Separation of stromal cells and epithelial cells by filtration

1. Secure a sterile piece of 30 μm nylon mesh over a sterile beaker, so that there is a depression in the middle. Two aluminium plates (~1 mm thick), 8 cm square, with a hole of about 5 cm diameter can be conveniently used. A piece of mesh about 8–9 cm square is inserted between these plates, which are secured with paperclips on each edge. The unit can be sterilized by autoclaving.
2. Pre-wet the nylon mesh with medium and gently pipette the cell suspension on to the filter. Allow it to run through and wash single cells through by gently pipetting on more medium.
3. Invert the filter unit and place it over a second beaker.
4. Recover the epithelial clusters from the underside by gently pipetting culture medium through the filter.
5. Centrifuge the cell suspension and re-suspend the cells in culture medium.

---

7. Setting up primary cultures

The cell suspension is now ready for use and primary cultures can be initiated. The concentration of cells should be adjusted to about 5×10^5 viable cells/ml in the appropriate culture medium (see *Table 1* for examples) and seeded into culture flasks. A high concentration is desirable, since the plating efficiency of primary cells may be low. It is important at this stage to gain familiarity with the expected morphological appearance of the cell types which may grow. Illustrations of growth patterns can be obtained from the relevant research literature and some text-books also provide a comprehensive catalogue of examples (3.13). Possible outcomes which will be apparent after about 7 days in culture are:

- non-adherent cell populations
- heterogeneous adherent population of mixed tumour cells and stromal cells
- homogeneous confluent populations of cells

Obviously, some tumour types will be non-adherent and the main problem lies with providing a medium which permits cell proliferation; some tumours which are expected to be adherent can also be induced to proliferate in suspension. The likelihood of adherence can be increased in several ways (see references (2) and (3) for more details):

- use of attachment factors such as collagen Types I and IV, fibronectin, laminin, or gelatin (all available from Sigma), or as ready-coated plastics (e.g. Bibby Tissue Culture Plastics)
- increase in the positive charge of plastic by poly-L- or poly-D-lysine (Sigma), or modified plastics (e.g. Primaria—Falcon Plastics)

Overgrowth of tumour cells by stromal cells is a common problem, even if initial attempts have been made to separate cell types. The growth of fibroblasts can be reduced by the use of metabolic inhibitors (14–16), media modification (17), variations in surface characteristics of the plastic (3), provision of a feeder cell layer (3), or by the use of monoclonal antibodies directed against fibroblasts (18). Mesothelial cell growth can be inhibited by the use of 5% serum and the absence of hydrocortisone. Further attempts can also be made to separate cells using differential enzyme treatments, which depend on differences in the sensitivity of epithelial cells and stromal cells to trypsin, and on differences in their rates of adherence to plastic.

Optimum conditions for cell separation need to be established for the culture system in use. Variations to try include trypsin concentration (0.1%–0.25%), presence or absence of versene (which may detach epithelial cells), and incubation times for detachment and re-attachment of stromal cells.

Protocol 8. Differential enzyme treatment

1. Gently rinse the cell monolayer three times in HBSS without Ca^{2+}/Mg^{2+}. Retain any loosely adherent tumour cell clumps from areas of three-dimensional growth which detach during this washing.

2. Add about 2 ml of enzyme solution (e.g. 0.1% trypsin) at 37°C and tip the flask so that the solution is evenly distributed over the whole surface.
3. Place the flask on to the stage of an inverted microscope and find an area of adjacent stromal cells and tumour cells.
4. When the stromal cells have rounded up and are beginning to detach, add about 5 ml of warmed HBSS and gently tap the side of the flask against the palm of the hand three to four times to detach them.
5. Remove the cell-containing medium and wash the monolayer with more HBSS to remove non-adherent cells. Discard these, unless the stromal cells are specifically needed.
6. Add 2 ml of enzyme solution (e.g. 0.25% trypsin +0.004% versene) to the residual monolayer and incubate at 37°C for 5–10 min to detach any remaining cells.
7. When all the cells have detached, neutralize the trypsin by adding 5 ml of serum-containing culture medium and centrifuge the cells for 5 min at 400*g*.
8. Add 10 ml of fresh medium to the cell pellet, re-suspend the cells, and re-inoculate them to a new culture flask. Return any detached clumps from the initial washings (step **1**) at this point.
9. Incubate at 37°C for 1–2 h and check for attachment of the residual single-cell stromal component. When these have attached, decant off the floating tumour cell suspension and transfer it to a new culture flask for incubation at 37°C.

The length of time spent trying to obtain pure confluent cultures of tumour cells will depend on the resources available, as well as availability of tumour material, specific points of interest about an individual tumour, and knowledge of the success rate for establishing lines from a particular tumour type. A confluent primary culture should initially be subcultured using a low split ratio (1:2) and better results may be obtained by using enzyme-free dissociation medium (Sigma). Careful records of the cell-line's history must be kept and freezing of material for back-up should also be considered (Section 8), though detailed characterization can wait until the growth potential of the culture is obvious.

8. Characterization

When it is clear that a cell-line has been developed with sufficient growth potential for amplification of stocks and repeated use, it is appropriate to consider its characterization.

This should include defining:

(a) species of origin
(b) tissue of origin
(c) karyotype
(d) absence of mycoplasmal, viral, or bacterial contamination
(e) biological characteristics

It is important to freeze material throughout the life history of the cell-line, and this should ideally include:

(a) uncultured material (reserve stock, verification of origin of cell-line)
(b) primary culture cells (seed stock, determination of cell type, identification of base-line characteristics)
(c) sub-cultures 3–10 (seed stock for use in obtaining working stocks)
(d) sub-cultures 10–100, e.g. every 10 sub-cultures (seed stocks in case of changes in genotype/phenotype, working stocks to allow experiments to be done on similar passage levels without depleting seed stocks, comparison of working stock, and seed stock to check for later introduction of cell contaminants)

Information on characterization procedures can be found elsewhere (2, 3, 19). The nomenclature of the cell-line needs to be considered and it is also important to record the number of generations through which cells have passed (e.g. one subculture using a split ratio of 1:4 = two generations).

Protocol 9. Freezing and thawing cells

1. Re-suspend cells at 10^6/ml in culture medium containing 10% FCS and 10% DMSO.
2. Dispense 1 ml aliquots of the cell suspension into an appropriate number of vials.
3. The optimum recovery of cells is obtained when cells are cooled at a rate of −1°C/min, down to −60°C to −80°C. A programmable cell freezer is an asset, but good results can be obtained without, by placing the vials in a polystyrene box and storing at −70°C for a minimum of 2–3 h before transferring to liquid nitrogen. The rate of cooling approximates to −1°C/min and a viable inoculum of cells can be obtained to initiate new cultures.
4. To thaw cells, remove the vial from the cell-bank and immediately warm it rapidly to 37°C in a water bath, taking appropriate safety measures in case the vial explodes. Transfer the contents to a 75 cm^2 culture flask.
5. The cell recovery is improved by slow dilution of cells to avoid osmotic shock. Dilute the 1 ml of cell suspension to 10 ml by slowly adding culture

medium warmed to 37°C. Initially, add a drop at a time with gentle shaking of the flask and slowly increase the volume added, so that the addition is spread over about 5 min.

6. Incubate the flask at 37°C and change the medium the following day when the cells have adhered.

9. Pitfalls and trouble-shooting

9.1 Cross-line contamination

Contamination of established cell-lines by other cells has been detected; HeLa cells are particularly common as contaminants in many older cell-lines. This can be avoided by careful attention to characterization in the early stages of establishment and comparison with other lines in use. It can be prevented by:

(a) handling each cell-line separately
(b) keeping media for each cell-line separate
(c) adding media to flasks before adding the cell suspension
(d) never using a pipette twice. This is particularly important when a cell-line has a rapid growth rate and grows well from a low inoculum.

9.2 Mycoplasma contamination

Mycoplasma contamination is common in cell-lines and may affect specific characteristics of the line, e.g. antigenicity. It is not always grossly visible, though the appearance of a culture may indicate its presence. Common signs include extracellular graininess, increased acidity of the medium and a slowed growth rate. Mycoplasma can be eliminated by use of mycoplasma removal agent (ICN-Flow) or B. M. Cyclin (Boehringer Mannheim), though it is questionable whether it can be completely eradicated once present. Lines should be screened regularly (e.g. once a month) and, ideally, lines which are known to be mycoplasma-contaminated should be handled and incubated in completely separate facilities. Bacterial/viral contamination should also be checked for regularly. The routine use of antibiotic-free medium ensures that low levels of infection are always obvious.

9.3 Genotypic and phenotypic drift

It is a common finding that the ploidy of a cell-line gradually increases with the length of time it is maintained in culture, although this is not always accompanied by a change in phenotype. Regular checks on karyotype will detect this and adequate freezing of seed stocks will ensure that cells are available which approximate more closely to the original genotype. Note that the proportion of sub-populations recovered from freezing may be different from that laid down (20).

9.4 Poor success rate for establishing lines

The success rate for establishing cell-lines from human tumours is notoriously low, though some tumour types are easier than others. It has been a common finding that tumours from advanced disease are more likely to give rise to cell-lines, though this is not a solution if you are interested in early disease. Other problems include bacterial contamination, stromal cell overgrowth, and non-adherence of cells. Bacterial contamination can be more of a problem with gut and skin tumours (see Section 3), though it may also indicate poor aseptic technique in the collection system. If stromal cell overgrowth is a continuing problem, then attention to cell selection methods may be appropriate or it may be partly due to the nature of the sample being taken, in which case more careful selection of the material to be disaggregated would help. A check on the histology of the tumour received for culture will reveal this problem. Non-adherence of cells which will not proliferate in suspension can be improved by modifications to the surface (Section 7).

References

1. Paul, J. (1975). *Cell and Tissue Culture*. Livingstone, Edinburgh.
2. Freshney, R. I. (ed.) (1986). *Animal Cell Culture: A Practical Approach*. IRL Press, Oxford.
3. Freshney, R. I. (1987). *Culture of Animal Cells. A Manual of Basic Technique.* Wiley Liss, New York.
4. Easty, D. M., Easty, G. C., Carter, R. L., Monaghan, P., and Butler, L. J. (1981). *Br. J. Cancer,* **48,** 772.
5. Kirkland, S. C. and Bailey, I. G. (1986). *Br. J. Cancer,* **53,** 779.
6. Lasfargues, E. Y. and Ozzello, L. (1958). *J. Natl Cancer Inst.,* **21,** 1131.
7. Rong, G. H., Grimm, E. A., and Sindelar, W. F. (1985). *J. Surg. Oncol.,* **28,** 131.
8. Slocum, H. K., Pavelic, Z. P., and Rustum, Y. M. (1980). In *Cloning of Human Tumor Stem Cells (Prog. Clin. Biol.* **48**), (ed. S. Salmon), p. 339. Liss, New York.
9. Duchesne, G. M., Eady, J. J., Peacock, J. H., and Pera, M. F. (1987). *Br. J. Cancer,* **56,** 287.
10. Muller, D., Fricker, J-P., Millon-Collard, R., Abecassis, J., Pusel, J., Eber, M., *et al.* (1987). *Biol. of the Cell,* **61,** 91.
11. Bertoncello, I., Bradley, T. R., Webber, L. M., Hodgson, G. S., and Campbell, J. J. (1985). *Aust. J. Exp. Biol. Med. Sci.,* **63,** 241.
12. Connell, N. D. and Rheinwald, J. G. (1983). *Cell,* **34,** 245.
13. Fogh, J. (1975). *Human Tumour Cells in Vitro.* Plenum, New York.
14. Gilbert, S. F. and Migeon, B. R. (1975). *Cell,* **5,** 11.
15. Whei-Yang, K. W. and Prockop, D. J. (1977). *Nature,* **266,** 63.
16. Fry, J. and Bridges, J. W. (1979). *Toxicol. Lett.,* **4,** 295.
17. Peehl, D. M. and Ham, R. G. (1980). *In Vitro,* **16,** 526.

18. Edwards, P. A. W., Easty, D. M., and Foster, C. S. (1980). *Cell Biol. Intl Rep.,* **4,** 917.
19. Rooney, D. E. and Czepulkowski, B. H. (ed.) (1986). *Human Cytogenetics: A Practical Approach*. IRL Press, Oxford.
20. Yaseen, N. Y., Watmore, A. E., Potter, A. M., Potter, C. W., Jacob, G., and Rees, R. C. (1991). *In Vitro Cell Dev. Biol.,* **27,** 185.
21. Wilson, A. P., Lee, H., Dent, M., Hubbold, L., Scott, I. V., and Golding, P. G. (1992). In preparation.
22. Langdon, S. P., Lawrie, S. S., Hay, F. G., Hawkes, M. M., McDonald, A., Hayward, I. P., *et al.* (1988). *Cancer Res.,* **48,** 6166.
23. Woods, L. K., Morgan, R. T., Quinn, L. A., Moore, G. E., Semple, T. U., and Stedman, K. E. (1979). *Cancer Res.,* **39,** 4449.
24. Petersen, O. W., Briand, P., and van Dews, B. (1984). *Acta Path. Microbiol. Immunol. Scand.,* **92,** 103.
25. Carney, D. N., Bunn, P. A., Gazdar, A. F., Pagan, J. A., and Minna, J. D. (1981). *Proc. Natl Acad. Sci. USA,* **78,** 3185.
26. Whitehead, R. H., Bertoncello, I., Webber, L. M., and Pedersen, J. S. (1983). *J. Natl. Cancer Inst.*, **70,** 649.
27. Jernberg, H., Nilsson, K., Zech, L., Lutz, D., Nowotny, H., and Scheirer, W. (1987). *Blood,* **69,** 1605.
28. Masuda, N., Fukuoka, M., Takada, M., Kudoh, S., and Kusonoki, Y. (1991). *Chest,* **100,** 429.
29. Melo, J. V., Foroni, L., Brito-Babapulle, V., Luzzatto, L., and Catovsky, D. (1988). *Clin. Exp. Immunol.,* **73,** 23.
30. Jacobsen, P. F., Jenkyn, D. J., and Papadimitriou, J. M. (1987). *J. Neuropathol. Exp. Neurol.,* **46,** 431.
31. Kobari, M., Hisano, H., Matsuro, S., Sato, T., Kan, M., and Tachibana, T. (1986). *Tohoku J. Exp. Med.,* **150,** 231.
32. Lange, B., Valtieri, M., Santoli, D., Caracciolo, D., Maviolo, F., Gemperlein, I., *et al.* (1987). *Blood,* **70,** 192.
33. Treves, A. J., Barak, V., Halperin, M., Biran, S., Leizerowitz, R., and Polliack, A. (1986). *Immunol. Lett.,* **12,** 225.
34. Lenoir, G. M., Vuillame, M., and Bonnardel, C. (1985). *IARC Sci. Publ.,* **60,** 309.
35. Bruland, O., Fodstad, O., and Pihl, A. (1985). *Intl J. Cancer,* **35,** 793.
36. Bergh, J., Nilsson, K., Ekman, R., and Giovanella, B. (1985). *Acta Pathol. Microbiol. Immunol. Scand.,* **93,** 133.
37. Epstein, A. L., Variakojis, D., Berger, C., and Hecht, B. K. (1985). *Intl J. Cancer,* **35,** 619.

2

Assessment of the immunogenicity of tumour models

FRED R. MILLER, BONNIE E. MILLER, and
GLORIA H. HEPPNER

1. Introduction

The 'science' of tumour immunology began in the 1950s, with the work of Foley (1) and Prehn and Main (2) and, later in the 1960s, with that of the Klein's laboratory (3), of Sjogren (4), of Habel (5), of Weiss (6), and many others. Prior to this time, there had been numerous published reports claiming the experimental demonstration of tumour-induced immune reactions (7, 8), as well as a considerable body of theoretical and anecdotal literature arguing for the existence of tumour-associated antigens and for host reactivity against them. In hindsight, however, it is clear that the earlier experimental work contained a major flaw, namely, the failure to recognize the difference between immune reactivity to tumours versus reactivity to normal immunogens, including histocompatibility and organ-specific antigens. The development of inbred strains of animals and the recognition of the laws of transplantation and histocompatibility were necessary prerequisites for approaching the question of the existence of 'tumour-specific' antigens. Only then were cancer biologists and immunologists able to return to the problem of tumour immunogenicity. At first, great care was taken to assure that histocompatibility problems were minimized: only autochthonous tumours, or very early transplant generations were utilized, grafts of normal skin from tumour donors were done to test for syngenicity, and much attention was given to the origin and inbreeding methods of the inbred strains. Over time, however, there was a relaxation of these stringent standards. In part, this was due to logistical and practical considerations. Autochthonous tumours are extremely difficult to work with; given the great behavioural heterogeneity among tumours of even common origin, the experimentalist is forced to choose experimental variables before knowing the necessary base-line information upon which these variables can be chosen rationally. Furthermore, no matter how clever the experimental design, an autochthonous tumour (and host) is only a group of 'one', a statistical shortcoming at best. Tumour transplants have their own problems. Since the dynamics of tumour progression are also heterogeneous, there is no firm theoretical reason to believe that a first-generation tumour is necessarily any more representative of a natural cancer than is a tumour of a later passage generation.

In addition to these practical forces, encouraging results from tumour immunology research also deflected attention from the initial zeal to maintain experimental purity. It came to seem likely that there are no truly tumour-specific antigens, a conclusion which might have been expected from thoughtful considerations of the principles of basic cancer biology. An effect of this insight was to diminish emphasis on the importance of maintaining rigid standards for the biological tools necessary to demonstrate specific reactivity. A second counteractive influence has been the heavy reliance on *in vitro* techniques for assessing tumour immunogenicity. Quite often it has been found that *in vitro* observations do not correlate well with *in vivo* results. Rather than questioning the *in vitro* methods, many investigators responded to this unwanted outcome by downplaying the *in vivo* results as being 'too' complex (which they may be) but, in so doing, ignored the methodological lessons of the *in vivo* experience.

The authors of this chapter are certainly not immune to the practical and theoretical forces that have reduced reliance on *in vivo* methodology or, once again, driven *in vivo* systems toward long-term transplantable tumours. Furthermore, advances in our understanding of clonal tumour heterogeneity and of the interlocking complexity of the many arms of the immune system have revealed many of the earlier concepts about host 'defence' reactions to cancer to be too simplistic. We believe, however, that there still is much value in well-designed *in vivo* experimentation because, ultimately, the whole organism must be the validator of all our ideas. What follows are our protocols, with some caveats and complications, for assessment of tumour immunogenicity. They come from our experience with a particular model system, and so can only serve as a starting point for work in other systems.

2. Immunogenicity and antigenicity

Antigens are molecular structures which elicit an immune response in an animal. Tumour cells can exhibit a variety of antigens including common viral antigens (9, 10), oncofetal, often tissue-specific, antigens (11), as well as putatively tumour-specific transplantation antigens (12, 13). These cell-surface determinants can be differentially able to induce an immune response (defined here as immunogenicity) and to be susceptible targets to efferent immune mechanisms (defined here as antigenicity). We have described the immunogenic and antigenic activity and cross-reactivity of five tumour sub-populations of a single mouse mammary tumour (14). Two determinants were variably expressed by these sub-populations, one a murine mammary tumour virus antigen and one an apparently unique antigen. Three sub-populations possessed both antigens, one expressed only the viral antigen, and one expressed only the unique antigen. A determinant could be both antigenic and immunogenic on cells of one sub-population but only antigenic for cells of another sub-population. One of the sub-populations, 410, immunizes syngeneic mice against other sub-populations (including sub-population 168) in transplantation resistance tests, but sub-population 168 does not render mice resistant to either 168 or 410 (15). Thus, 168 and 410 share a determinant which is both immunogenic and antigenic as expressed on 410 cells but is antigenic, not immunogenic, as expressd on 168 cells. Such patterns of 'one-way cross reactivity' are a complication in establishing tumour specificity.

3. Statistical considerations in assessment of immunity

If a tumour is highly immunogenic and antigenic, immunization may completely protect from challenge transplants and a simple chi-squared analysis of differences in incidence between control and experimental groups is sufficient. However, with weakly immunogenic/antigenic models, only a few of the sensitized animals may be completely protected. Rather, the latency may be extended in a few animals or the growth rate of palpable tumours may be slowed. In these cases statistical analysis of any single parameter may reveal no differences between the sensitized and control groups. Because weakly immunogenic models are deemed more relevant to human cancer than strongly immunogenic models, it becomes necessary to assess host reactivity in a composite way, which deals with all these endpoints of tumour growth control. We use a method of analysis which is affected by changes in incidence, latency, and growth during lag and exponential growth phases.

Following inoculation of a known number of tumour cells (subcutaneously) animals are examined periodically (at least twice a week but more frequently for very fast growing tumours) for palpable tumours. Tumour diameters are measured in two perpendicular directions with Vernier calipers and the volume estimated according to the formula $ab^2/2$, where b is the smaller of the two diameters. *Figure 1A* depicts a typical growth curve of a transplanted tumour in a normal, non-immunized host. After a latent period during which tumours are not detectable, small palpable tumours often grow slowly at first (lag phase) but then enter a faster, exponential phase of growth before slowing again into a plateau. The day at which each tumour reaches a size of 500 mm^3 (size parameter selection depends on tumour model but should be reached during the middle or latter part of the exponential phase) is calculated by regression analysis, using only the measurements made during the exponential phase of growth. This value is sensitive to alterations in latency period, length of the lag phase, and growth rate during the exponential phase. In *Figure 1*, B depicts an extended latency, C depicts a decreased growth rate

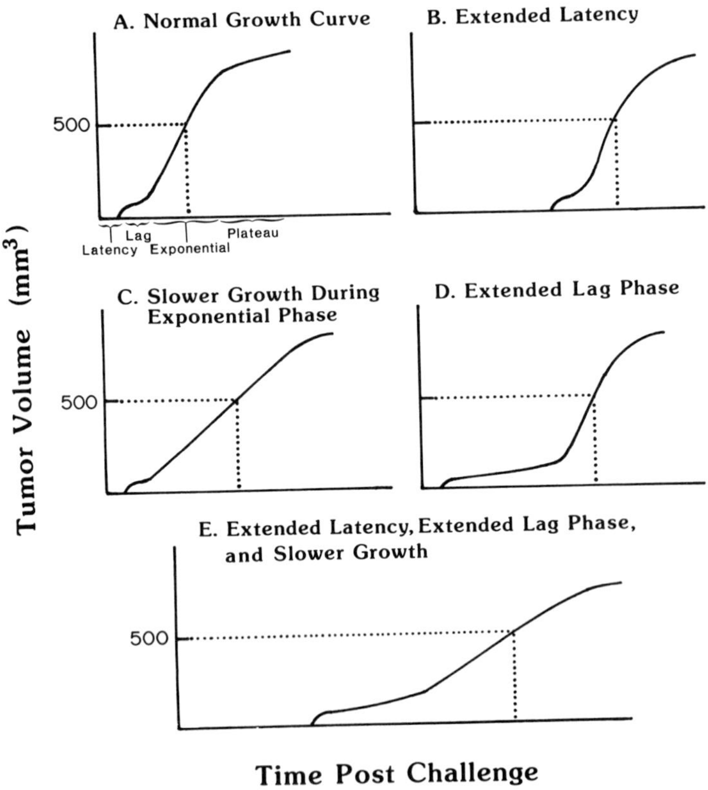

Figure 1. Possible effects of immunity on tumour growth. These idealized curves represent the time taken to reach a predetermined tumour volume.

during the exponential phase, D depicts an extended lag phase, and E depicts alterations in all three. Each of the three alterations shifts the growth curve to the right resulting in an increase in number of days necessary for the tumour to reach the designated size. If immunization completely protects some animals from the challenge tumour, these tumours are treated statistically as having reached the designated size on the last day of measurement. A non-parametric rank test is then used to determine the significance of differences between groups.

4. Tumour cell source for immunization or challenge

For immunization we use cells (or tumour pieces) from tumours growing in animals rather than cells growing in tissue culture to avoid complications of immune responses to the serum proteins typically used for maintaining cell-lines *in vitro*. For challenging animals, we use cells from tissue culture to avoid the problems presented by infiltrating host cells contained within suspensions or pieces of tumours. Not only is it difficult to determine accurately the number of neoplastic cells versus normal host cells in suspensions prepared from tumours, the growth of the challenge tumour inoculum is influenced by the adoptively transferred, sensitized host cells as well as by the immune response of the new host. Although one can separate malignant cells and infiltrating cells by various means, including isokinetic gradients (16, 17) and centrifugal elutriation (18), some contamination with infiltrating host cells is inevitable. We find it both more convenient and more reliable to use tissue culture cells for the challenge.

Protocol 1. Concomitant immunity (immunity directed against a challenge inoculum or implant of tumour in an animal already bearing that tumour)

1. Remove tumours from animals, dissect away any surrounding tissue, and finely dice healthy looking material with scalpels. Generally, the healthy tissue is located in the peripheral shell of tumours, rather than necrotic centres, but one must avoid selecting only the fibrotic capsule which surrounds tumours in some experimental models.

2. (a) If tumour pieces are to be used directly, make an incision through the skin of the animals to be immunized and place a 1 mm^3 piece of tumour under the skin, then close the incision with a wound clip.

(b) If a suspension of tumour cells is desired, digest the tumour pieces enzymatically (19, 20) and inject 1×10^3 to 1×10^6 cells (depending on the tumourigenicity of the model) in 0.1 ml of a physiological buffer *s.c.*, with a 23-gauge needle.

(c) Alternatively, cell suspensions, prepared as in step **2**(b), may be injected into an *orthotopic* site. For example, mammary tumour cells in a 20 μl volume are injected into a #4 mammary gland (21). For this procedure, animals are anaesthetized (for BALB/c mice we use 65 mg/kg body weight of sodium pentobarbitol) and an incision made through the skin so that the mammary gland can be observed. The incision is then closed with a wound clip.

3. Establish the dose of tumour cells at which 50% of animals develop tumours (TD50) separately for each tumour. Inoculate each animal with a standard multiple of this, e.g. 10 × TD50.

4. Ten to fifteen days after injecting tumour cells or implanting tumour pieces, inject challenge tumour cell suspensions prepared from tissue cultures into the contralateral side of the animal. A challenge dose range is recommended, e.g. 1×10^3–1×10^5 cells per mouse, but the range

Protocol 1. *Continued*

selected depends upon the tumour model used. We typically use 5–10 mice per group but highly immunogenic tumours require fewer mice than poorly immunogenic tumours.

5. Growth of the challenge tumours is monitored as described above (Section 3).

Protocol 2. Pre-immunization by temporary growth and surgery ('transplantation test')[a]

1. Initiate tumours at the site of choice. This site is sometimes chosen for ease of surgical removal of the resulting tumour. Because we work with a mammary model, we immunize by injecting cells into a #4 mammary gland.
2. Once the tumours reach the size of approximately 120 mm^3, anaesthetize the animals and remove the tumours. Make an incision through the skin and pull the skin flap away from the abdominal wall. Use a pencil cautery to cut through the blood vessels and connective tissue, taking great care not to touch the abdominal wall. If the tumour has invaded and become firmly attached to the abdominal wall such that removal without cutting through the wall is not possible, the animal should be humanely euthanased. Use scissors to cut the skin around the tumour so that the tumour and overlying skin are removed intact. Remaining skin is then juxtaposed and the wound closed with stainless steel clips. Surgery should be carried out on all the animals in an experiment on the same day post-tumour-initiation. Animals will display a range of tumour sizes and must be randomized if more than one experimental immune group is to be challenged.
3. Seven to ten days following surgery, inject challenge tumour suspensions into the contralateral side. We inject a range of 1×10^3–1×10^5 tumour cells, into different groups of mice, from tissue culture into the contralateral #4 mammary gland.
4. Growth of the challenge tumours is monitored as described (Section 3).

[a] Tumours which spontaneously metastasize cannot be removed efficiently and are therefore not suitable for pre-immunization experiments by this method.

Protocol 3. Lung colonization assay ('experimental metastasis')

Metastasis is a process consisting of several sequential steps culminating in replication of malignant cells at a metastatic site. We have found that replication of malignant cells in the lung is inhibited by pre-immunization or by concomitant immunity, using *Protocols 1* and *2* (22). Recently, we have found that replication of malignant cells in the lung is a more sensitive indication of immune resistance than is growth of a primary tumour in a subcutaneous or mammary gland site. For studies on immunity to metastatic cells, we use tumour cells that contain selectable 'markers' (i.e. resistance to specific drugs) that allow quantitation of clonogenic tumour cells in the secondary organs.

1. Groups of control and immunized (see *Protocols 1* and *2*) mice are gently and carefully warmed by placing cages on a heating pad, until tail veins are prominent.
2. Inject tumour cells with drug-resistance markers (such as thioguanine, ouabain, diaminopurine, or neomycin) into lateral tail veins as single cell suspensions in 0.2 ml of a physiological buffered salt solution.
3. Humanely euthanase groups of control and immunized mice (minimum of three mice per group) at days 1, 3, 7, 10, . . . (at least three time points are desirable) and remove the lungs.
4. Prepare single-cell suspensions from each individual lung by mincing each into 1–3 mm^3 pieces, that are then placed in plastic blender bags and pre-soaked for 60 min in 5 ml of an enzyme cocktail containing 1 mg/ml collagenase type-IV and 36 units of elastase, at 4°C (see also Chapter 1).
5. Mechanically disperse the samples with four sequential 30 sec and three sequential 1 min periods in a Stomacher blender. Remove cell fractions after each dispersion period and add 2.5 ml of serum-containing tissue-culture medium to the undigested portion each time.
6. Pool all fractions containing cells, pellet by centrifugation, rinse, and resuspend. Determine the total number of cells recovered by haemocytometer or Coulter counter.
7. Pipette cell suspensions repeatedly to break up any remaining cell clumps and then plate out at multiple concentrations in tissue-culture medium containing the appropriate selective drug. The drug kills all wild-type (host) cells but allows tumour cells to form colonies.
8. Incubate for 10–14 days at 37°C in 10% CO_2–air, fix the colonies with methanol/acetic acid, stain with crystal violet, and count. The total number of clonogenic tumour cells present in each lung is then calculated.
9. The doubling time for the clonogenic cells in the lung is calculated by regression analysis. If immunization is effective, a reduction in the number of colonies visible in the lungs at necropsy should also be seen. However, a reduction in the number of visible lung colonies which develop does not necessarily reflect increased specific immune resistance (22).
10. This protocol is adaptable for colonization of other organs, such as liver or spleen.

Protocol 4. Local adoptive transfer

This procedure, commonly known as the Winn assay (23), mixes immune effector cells with tumour cells *in vitro* prior to injection into normal, non-immune animals. The source of effector cells can be peripheral blood leukocytes, lymph node cells, splenocytes, or tumour-infiltrating inflammatory cells. Effector function of the tumour-bearer or immunized host cells is very dependent upon the cell source (24).

1. Remove and pool inguinal, cervical, axillary, and mesenteric lymph nodes from immunized animals 7 to 14 days after surgical removal of immunizing tumour or from tumour-bearing animals, remove excess fat, and tease the nodes apart in tissue-culture medium.
2. Re-suspend tumour cells from tissue culture together with lymph node cells (or lymphocytes from other sources) in saline, at a ratio of 100 lymph node cells to one tumour cell. The ratio required may vary depending upon the antigenicity of the tumour model. Inject the mixtures into the subcutis or a mammary fatpad (0.1 ml or 0.02 ml volumes, respectively). With our mouse mammary tumour lines, 1×10^4 tumour cells mixed with 1×10^6 lymph node cells are injected.
3. Control groups receive tumour cells mixed with the same proportion of lymph node cells from normal, non-immunized animals.
4. Growth of the tumours is monitored as described.

5. Host irradiation

Low-dose X-irradiation or γ-irradiation of animals can be used to temporarily suppress host immune responses. We have used 450 rads whole-body γ-irradiation to suppress immunity in BALB/c mice. Mice were shown to be immunosuppressed on day 2 after irradiation by their ten-fold decrease in splenocyte number and by the profound loss of ability of the remaining splenocytes to respond to either a T-cell or a B-cell mitogen in blastogenesis assays (19). Both functional assays and splenocyte numbers recovered gradually, but had not returned to normal values by day 10 after irradiation (19). Using a similar irradiation protocol, and injecting cells 2 days after irradiation, we showed that the incidence and growth rate of the strongly immunogenic tumour line 410 were increased, and its latency was decreased, in irradiated mice (25). In the same experiment, the less immunogenic tumour line 168 grew only slightly better in irradiated animals (25). However, since whole-body irradiation can have profound effects on the host beyond that of immunosuppression, this technique can only suggest a possible role for host immune response in limiting or slowing growth in non-irradiated animals.

6. Elimination of suppressor cells

It is possible that immunogenicity is masked in some tumour models by a suppressor T-cell response. Low-dose cyclophosphamide treatment may enable the host to express anti-tumour immunity (26, 27).

7. Summary

A number of methods have been described using irradiated cells, vaccines, and adjuvants to immunize against specific tumours. Undoubtedly, individual tumour models require somewhat unique protocols for optimal immunization. However, we find that the handful of protocols described allows us to study the interplay of tumour and host without getting mired in attempts to define an optimum protocol for each new tumour model studied.

We have not discussed *in vitro* methods to assess either immunogenicity or antigenicity. This reflects the independent and collaborative experiences of the authors in which *in vitro* and *in vivo* results have been discordant. We suggest that the study of a host response requires a host.

Acknowledgements

The authors gratefully acknowledge the continuing support of the US Public Health Service (NIH grants CA 27419, CA 54926, CA 28366) and Concern/ Concern II Foundation. We also thank Margaret Peterson for preparation of the manuscript.

References

1. Foley, E.I. (1953). *Cancer Res.*, **13**, 835.
2. Prehn, R. T. and Main, J. M. (1957). *J. Natl Cancer Inst.*, **18**, 769.
3. Klein, G., Sjogren, H. O., Klein, E., and Hellstrom, K. E. (1960). *Cancer Res.*, **20**, 1561.
4. Sjogren, H. O., Hellstrom, I., and Klein, G. (1961). *Exp. Cell Res.*, **23**, 204.
5. Habel, K. (1961). *Exp. Biol. Med.*, **106**, 772.
6. Weiss, D. W., Faulkin, L. J. jun., and DeOme, K. B. (1964). *Cancer Res.*, **24**, 732.
7. Southam, C. M. (1960). *Cancer Res.*, **20**, 271.
8. Kidd, J. O. (1961). *Cancer Res.*, **21**, 1170.
9. Klein, G. (1966). *Ann. Rev. Microbiol.*, **20**, 223.
10. Sjogren, H. O. (1966). *Prog. Exp. Tumor Res.*, **6**, 289.
11. Gold, P. and Freedman, S. O. (1965). *J. Exp. Med.*, **122**, 467.
12. Vaage, J. (1968). *Cancer Res.*, **28**, 2477.
13. Morton, D. L., Miller, G. F., and Wood, D. A. (1969). *J. Natl Cancer Inst.*, **42**, 289.
14. Miller, F. R. and Heppner, G. H. (1979). *J. Natl Cancer Inst.*, **63**, 1457.

15. Miller, B. E., Miller, F. R., Leith, J., and Heppner, G. H. (1980). *Cancer Res.,* **40,** 3977.
16. Blazar, B. A. and Heppner, G. H. (1978). *J. Immunol.,* **120,** 1876.
17. Rios, A. M., Miller, F. R., and Heppner, G. H. (1983). *Cancer Immunol. Immunotherapy,* **15,** 87.
18. Wei, W.-Z., Malone, K., Mahoney, K., and Heppner, G. H. (1986). *Cancer Res.,* **46,** 2680.
19. Miller, B. E., Miller, F. R., Wilburn, D., and Heppner, G. H. (1988). *Cancer Res.,* **48,** 5747.
20. Miller, B. E., Aslakson, C. J., and Miller, F. R. (1990). *Invasion and Metastasis,* **10,** 101.
21. Miller, F. R., Medina, D., and Heppner, G. H. (1981). *Cancer Res.,* **41,** 3863.
22. Aslakson, C. J., McEachern, D., Conaway, D. H., and Miller, F. R. (1991). *Clin. Exp. Metastasis,* **9,** 139.
23. Winn, H. J. (1961). *J. Immunol.,* **86,** 228.
24. Blazar, B. A., Laing, C. A., Miller, F. R., and Heppner, G. H. (1980). *J. Natl Cancer Inst.,* **65,** 405.
25. Miller, B. E., Miller, F. R., Leith, J., and Heppner, G. H. (1980). *Cancer Res.,* **40,** 3977.
26. Hengst, J. C. D., Mokyr, M. B., and Dray, S. (1981). *Cancer Res.,* **41,** 2163.
27. North, R. J. (1982). *J. Exp. Med.,* **55,** 1063.

3

Flow cytometry of lymphocytes and tumour cells

JOHN LAWRY

1. Introduction

Flow cytometry is a technology capable of the rapid and precise analysis of many thousands of cells in only a few seconds. The level of monoclonal antibody binding to antigen expressed on the surface of a cell, or to cytoplasmic or nuclear epitopes, can provide quantitative measurements of antigen density while fluorochromes with preferential binding abilities may be used to label the cellular DNA/RNA content, to identify organelles and to indicate intracellular pH, Ca^{2+} content, etc.

When flow cytometers were developed in the 1960s, the cell sample of choice was peripheral blood (or any other natural suspension of cells) and this resulted in the development of an extensive range of monoclonal antibodies (MoAbs) against leucocyte antigens. These now comprise the majority of the CD (cluster of differentiation) antibody series (1). Sales of flow cytometers still reflect the success of this application, with most new installations being into haematology laboratories. The reasons for this success included improved sample throughput, accuracy of measurements, and technical simplicity. Immunohistochemical and APAAP (alkaline phosphatase anti-alkaline phosphatase) techniques were highly time-consuming and the resultant staining was of variable quality. Difficulties arose in the (subjective) classification of a positive versus a negative cell, as well as an inability to quantitate staining intensity. Fluorescence microscopy was restricted by fluorescence quenching during analysis of individual slides.

Of secondary importance was the analysis of the DNA content of cells. This was of value to both pathology and haematology laboratories but initially was restricted by the availability of suitable fluorochromes. However, it was not until reliable techniques were developed for the disaggregation of solid tumours that applications in oncology became readily accepted. Evidence of this can be seen in the literature, yet few centres currently use DNA analysis in routine clinical diagnosis, with pathological staging and histological grading forming the 'gold standards' for prognosis.

One limitation of single-parameter DNA analysis is that whilst aneuploid populations of tumour cells can usually be identified, diploid tumour cells cannot be distinguished from infiltrating leucocytes, stromal cells, etc. Histochemical staining techniques for DNA or cycling cells (such as Feulgen staining, or the silver precipitation method for staining nuclear organizer regions (AgNOR) (2, 3)), do enable the identification of cell populations but are highly subjective in resolving diploidy from aneuploidy, or cycling from non-cycling cells. There are also limitations with flow cytometric techniques. For example, ploidy populations often overlap, making accurate determination of cell-cycle phases impossible; this may in turn reduce the efficiency of detection of low levels of aneuploid cells. In part, this can be overcome by dual-parameter analysis using a tumour-specific marker in combination with the DNA fluorochrome (4). Thus, tumour populations identified by antibody binding can be analysed for their DNA content and cell-cycle profile independently of non-tumour cells. This may open up important applications in the use of flow cytometry in cervical and breast screening clinics by the analysis of biopsy material, as well as in other clinical situations where fine-needle aspirates are taken, or samples obtained by other biopsy methods such as needle-core, diathermy, or scrapes.

Flow cytometric karyotyping is a highly specialized, yet important application of this technology, with clinical significance in the detection of trisomy, chromosome deletion, and (in some cases) chromosome translocations. While most reports in the literature are of karyotypes made from chromosome suspensions of peripheral blood cells, it is also possible to extract cells from samples of solid tumour and obtain chromosome suspensions (5).

With the current interest in molecular biology, it is not absurd to suggest an expansion in the application of flow cytometry to this field. Dual-parameter analysis techniques with either chromosome preparations or intact cells, stained with a DNA fluorochrome (6) and a fluorescent conjugated gene probe are possible (7). However, this technology suffers from the absolute sensitivity of fluorescent detection of the cytometer, typically in the order of 1000 molecules of FITC. Finite sensitivity is totally dependent on the level of natural autofluorescence of a cell, which may be equivalent to 1500 molecules of FITC; genes with a low copy number will not therefore be detected. This may be resolved by using fluorochromes with comparatively long fluorescence emission periods compared to that of autofluorescence (0.1 μsec), for example selenium (half-life 50 μsec) or europium (half-life, 500 μsec), so that proportionally more light may be collected from each labelled particle. This would, however, require the use of time-delayed fluorescence measurement to enable the fluorescence emission to reach a maximum. Such technology has been termed time-resolved fluorescence (8). This technique, together with *in situ* hybridization and traditional immunohistochemistry are all possible by flow cytometry, and should (in theory) provide a reliable, objective and accurate service for the clinical laboratory, and be valuable tools in cancer research. Hence, a wide range of samples may be analysed by flow cytometry using a whole spectrum of techniques.

Detailed information on the phenotype, karyotype, and cell-cycle state of a cell can be obtained, as well as other biological parameters, by using the range of antibodies or fluorochromes currently available. There are further characteristics of cells that can be analysed, without the need of a marker. Light scatter is a property that all cells exhibit when passed through an excitation light source. Light scattered in the same angle as the beam is termed forward (low-angle) scatter and is often used to indicate the relative size of a cell. Light scattered at a wide angle (usually collected through the 90° optics pathway) can be used to indicate relative granularity. Thus, in a sample of peripheral blood, neutrophils, monocytes, lymphocytes, red blood cells, and platelets can all be identified. If required, exclusion gates can be set to analyse only the cell population of interest. Similarly, if a suspension contains tumour cells and infiltrating leucocytes, light scatter can be used to distinguish these populations with a reasonable degree of accuracy. Examples which yield such mixed populations include peritoneal washings, bone marrow, or peripheral blood. Finally, wide-angle light scatter can provide important additional information when used in combination with DNA fluorochromes, or with antibodies. *Figure 1* illustrates the use of light scatter in dual-parameter (scatter/MoAb) contour plot of density-gradient-harvested peripheral blood mononuclear cells. CD3-stained lymphocytes can be clearly seen with the unstained monocyte populations above.

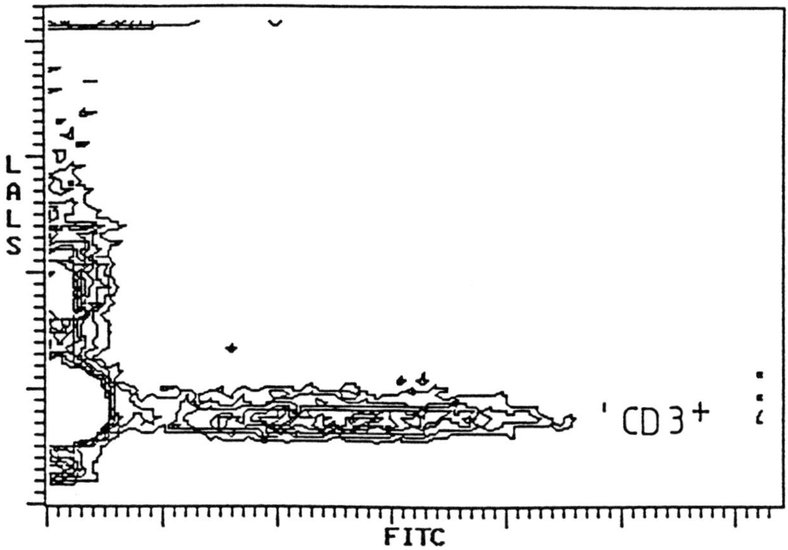

Figure 1. Two-dimensional contour plot of peripheral blood mononuclear cells stained with FITC CD3. Note: Large-angle light scatter (LALS) distinguishes monocytes from lymphocytes, the latter also being FITC CD3 positive.

This chapter will now proceeed to address the above, with emphasis on the source of cells or tissue, and of the techniques employed in obtaining cell suspensions. Staining procedures will be reviewed, together with examples of application areas.

2. Sample considerations

2.1 Natural sources of cell suspensions

2.1.1 Peripheral blood samples

Peripheral blood is a natural source of cells already in suspension. However, serum elements such as clotting factors have to be removed, and partial or total separation of cell types be undertaken to enable precise measurements to be made. Routine phenotyping in the haematology laboratory is now usually carried out on whole blood. Here, blood is taken by venipuncture with EDTA as the anti-coagulant of choice, cells stained with fluorescent-conjugated antibodies, and the red cell populations lysed to enable the detection of leucocyte populations. The flow cytometer first gates out all but the lymphocyte or monocyte populations prior to the measurement of antibody binding on the cells of interest (*Protocol 1*).

Protocol 1. Whole blood techniques: direct antibody stain. (Protocol supplied by Mrs Janet Peel, Department of Haematology, Royal Hallamshire Hospital, Sheffield, UK)

Reagents

- phosphate-buffered saline (PBS) pH 7.4
- fresh blood (EDTA) held at room temperature
- fluorescent-conjugated monoclonal antibodies
- 1% paraformaldehyde solution in PBS
- lysing solution

Method

1. Label plastic microcentrifuge tubes, or disposable polystyrene tubes appropriately.
2. Carefully add 50 μl blood (EDTA) to each tube.
3. Add the appropriate amount of antibody (according to manufacturers' recommendations) to each tube.
4. Vortex gently and incubate in the dark at 21°C or below for 15 min.
5. Add 1 ml of lysing solution[a] (FACS-lyse, Becton Dickinson Ltd, Oxford) to each tube, gently vortex, add an additional 1 ml lysing solution and vortex again.

6. Incubate the sample at room temperature in the dark for 10 min (over-incubation may result in general cell damage).
7. Centrifuge the samples at 1200 r.p.m. (approx. 400*g*) for 5 min and remove the supernatant. Add 2 ml PBS to wash and centrifuge again at 1800 r.p.m. (approx. 600*g*) for 3 min.
8. Remove the supernatant, dislodge the cell pellet and re-suspend it in 200 μl 1% (v/v) paraformaldehyde in PBS (pH 7.4). Store at 4°C until analysed.

[a] Other lysing solutions which do not require centrifugation stages are available from other manufacturers (e.g. Ortho Diagnostics Ltd); not all allow for the use of fixatives, and some require sample analysis within one hour. Also, antibodies from one company may not be compatible to lysing solutions from another.

Should a 'pure' population of cells be required, blood may be separated on a density gradient by centrifugation (in this instance, the anti-coagulant of choice would be heparin). This may be specific for lymphocytes or monocytes (see Chapters 6 and 19), or neutrophils, red blood cells, or platelets. Regardless of the technique used, antibody staining can then be undertaken with conjugated antibodies as a single step, or with two-stage techniques using the appropriate primary antibody followed by a secondary, fluorescent-conjugated antibody. Primary antibodies are generally raised in mice against human determinants and the secondary antibody in an animal species such as goat, raised against whole or fragment mouse immunoglobulin (*Protocol 2*). Flow cytometric analysis commences with the identification of lymphocytes and monocytes using light scatter, and perhaps a monocyte MoAb to aid the setting of exclusion gates. The phenotype analysis of lymphocytes alone can then be performed. *Figure 2* illustrates this approach.

Protocol 2. Indirect antibody staining

Reagents

- PBS containing 1% serum (BSA, new born or foetal calf serum)[a]
- 1% paraformaldehyde solution in PBS, pH 7.4
- primary antibody, titrated for good intensity staining whilst still being at saturating levels
- secondary antibody, titrated as above (Caltag. Ltd titre approximately 1:40 to 1:60, for example) in PBS

Method

1. Label the tubes and add (0.5–1.0) × 10^6 cells in 100 μl PBS containing 1% serum to each.

Protocol 2. *Continued*

2. Add 100 μl of the primary (test) antibody at an appropriate titre, and incubate for 30 min at 4°C, with occasional mixing.
3. Wash off the excess antibody with 1 ml PBS/serum at 4°C by centrifuging at 1800 r.p.m. (600*g*) for 5 min. Discard the supernatant and then repeat this stage.
4. Add the second-stage antibody (FITC-conjugated goat anti-mouse f(ab)^{1}2 fragment immunoglobulin) at an appropriate dilution, and incubate at 4°C, in the dark for 30 min, with occasional mixing.
5. Wash off the excess antibody with two centrifugation stages as above (step 3).
6. Re-suspend the cell pellet. Use PBS/serum for immediate analysis; 1% paraformaldehyde/PBS for subsequent use or if the samples are of a hazardous nature.

[a] Where there is a danger of 'false positive' results occurring from antibodies binding 'backwards' into Fc receptors on the target cells, care should be taken to include Ig-containing sera in the staining buffer.

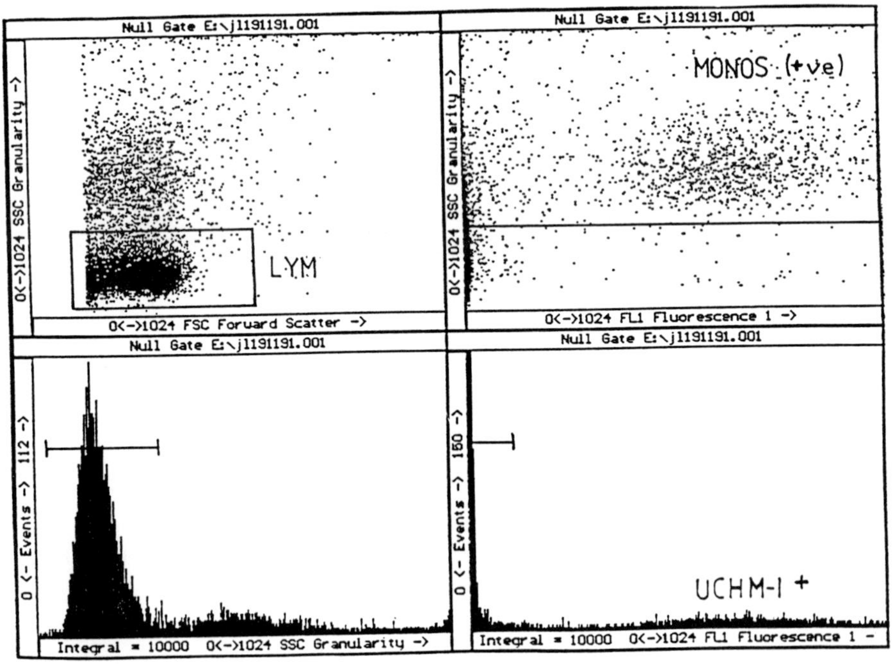

Figure 2. Combined scatter and MoAb data set for peripheral blood mononuclear cells stained with anti-monocyte UCHM1, showing gate regions to only include lymphocytes.

Peripheral blood from cancer patients may also be analysed for the presence of abnormal, possibly neoplastic cells, by light scatter, DNA fluorochrome, and MoAb analysis. The presence of aneuploidy would be conclusive evidence of tumour cells, whilst light scatter or MoAb staining may be subjective. *Figure 3* shows abnormal cells identified by scatter from a patient with prostatic cancer, which were sorted and identified as being of tumour origin.

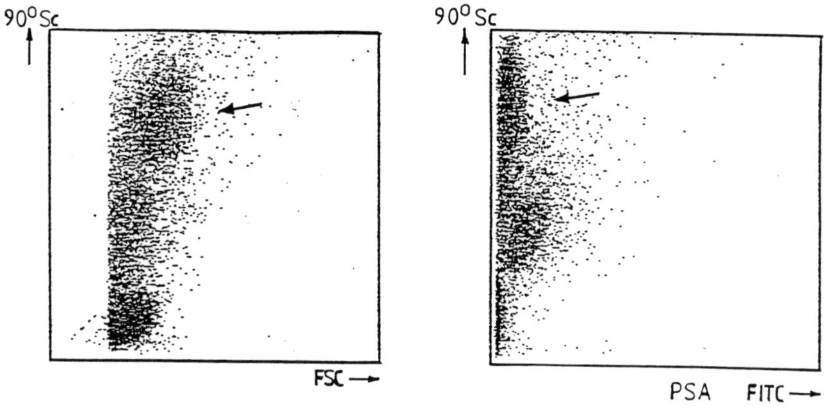

Figure 3. Density-gradient-separated blood sample from a prostate cancer patient showing abnormal cells, being of high scatter but prostate-specific antigen negative.

2.1.2 Bone marrow

Bone marrow samples may be readily made into single-cell suspensions by gentle pipetting. DNase (100 units/ml), EDTA (3 mM) and 1% serum may all be incorporated into the PBS solution to minimize cell aggregation. Whole blood or cell separation procedures may then be used if monoclonal antibody analysis is required, or if the cells are to be stained with a DNA fluorochrome alone or with an antibody. Megakaryocyte populations may be isolated by dual-parameter techniques using flow cytometry, or by the use of centrifugation over a 30% (v/v) Percoll density gradient using the methods described by Lawry *et al.* (9), even though the frequency of megakaryocytes in the normal bone marrow may be less than 0.05% of cell population.

2.1.3 Peritoneal washings

During abdominal surgery, saline washings of the peritoneal cavity may be made, and following centrifugation the harvested cells can be analysed. These cells will include macrophage and lymphocyte populations, but in cancer patients may include tumour cells which may have migrated to the peritoneal cavity and be of potential metastatic phenotype, or may have been shed during the surgical procedure. The wound-healing process taking place after surgery would result in this region being flooded with cytokines and growth factors, which of course would provide ideal stimuli for the growth and development of any neoplastic cells still remaining.

Cell samples can be stained with monoclonal antibodies as illustrated above, using direct or indirect techniques, as well as by DNA fluorochromes (10) and dual DNA/antibody techniques as described below. In contrast, light-scatter differences can also be used to identify abnormal (neoplastic) cells. *Figure 4* illustrates the forward (*x*-axis) and wide angle (*y*-axis) scatter dot-plot of a peritoneal washing taken before the removal of a colon carcinoma (PE21a) and immediately after resection (PE21b). Initially, only mononuclear and phagocytic cells were present (identified by MoAbs and histochemistry), but following surgery abnormally large, granular cells (which were found to be CEA positive, and identified as tumour cells by histopathology) were visible. They were, however, DNA diploid, as was the colon carcinoma.

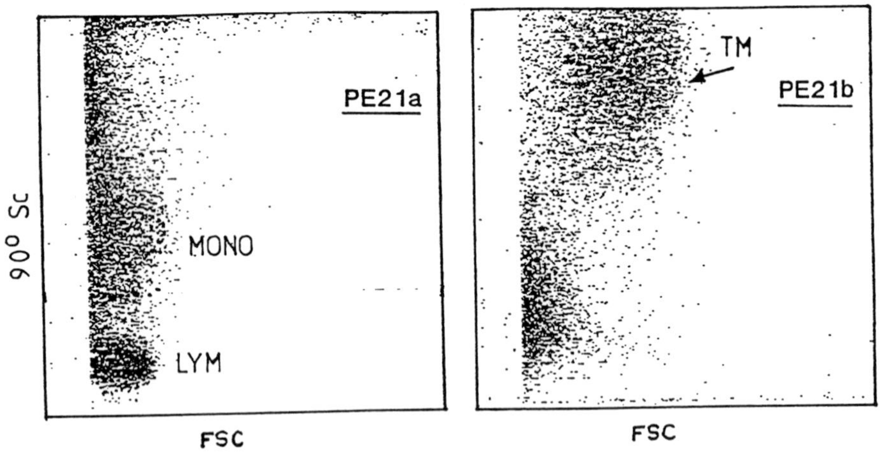

Figure 4. Scatter analysis of a colon cancer patient peritoneal washing sample. High levels of tumour cells are visible post-surgery.

2.2 Solid tumours

2.2.1 Dissociation of fresh or frozen tissue

The analysis of cell suspensions taken from samples of solid tumour can be readily achieved by using mechanical and enzymatic dissociation techniques, releasing cells bound to connective tissue, other cells, or basement membrane structures within the tumour. Any dissociation process should be a balance between being too aggressive or prolonged, causing cell damage or death, and being too mild or rapid, perhaps resulting in the selective release of peripheral or loosely associated cells only, or a low yield. Enzymes in common use are summarized in *Table 1*. All but collagenase and EDTA may be considered to be aggressive and may result in cell death, loss of surface epitopes, and functional damage. *Table 2* illustrates the effect of the three of these enzymes

Table 1. Enzymes used in tissue dissociation

Name	Type, concentration	Properties
Collagenase	(II), 0.2 mg/ml	Digests BM components
EDTA	(versine), 0.02% PBS	Calcium chelator
Hyaluronidase	(VIII), 0.25 mg/ml	Breaks down mucous
Pepsin	(porcine stomach mucosa), 0.5% in PBS pH 1.5	General enzyme
Trypsin	(pancreatic), 0.2% soln.	General enzyme [a]
DNase	(bovine pancreas), 2000 U/ml	Breaks down DNA [b]
RNase	(bovine pancreas), 1 mg/ml	Breaks down RNA

[a] Trypsin made up in Dulbecco's saline containing calcium (0.1% $CaCl_2$) and magnesium (0.1% $MgCl_2$) in PBS, pH 7.4.

[b] DNase is used to break down extracellular DNA released by lysed or dead cells, thereby minimizing cell aggregation.

Table 2. The effect of enzymatic dissociation on MoAb binding to peripheral blood lymphocytes

MoAb	Untreated		Collagenase		Trypsin	
	(%)	($\bar{x}$ ch)	(%)	($\bar{x}$ ch)	(%)	($\bar{x}$ ch)
Control	0.3	–	0.7	–	0.4	–
CD8 (Leu 2a)	19.6	368	18.1	366	4.3	26
CD4 (Leu 3a)	46.3	136	49.7	116	0.5	–
CD3 (Leu 4)	66.8	162	66.2	159	59.7	137
CD57 (Leu 7)	7.6	752	6.4	864	4.1	664
CD16 (Leu 11b)	7.9	177	8.3	157	5.6	173
CD19 (Leu 12)	12.3	85	12.9	81	12.7	58
CD15 (Leu M3)	16.2	190	16.0	155	22.3	84
CD45 (LCA)	97.7	312	98.5	334	97.6	166

MoAb	Untreated		Hyaluronidase	
	(%)	($\bar{x}$ ch)	(%)	($\bar{x}$ ch)
Control	0.3	–	1.7	–
CD8	31.1	438	27.8	448
CD4	50.6	146	46.7	112
CD3	77.7	192	76.8	86
CD2	82.8	26	84.9	22
CD57	18.9	374	16.8	362
CD16	16.8	124	15.9	161
CD19	8.2	102	7.9	63
CD15	24.6	142	27.9	149
CD45	99.3	209	98.6	200

% = per cent positive cells; $\bar{x}$ ch = median fluorescence channel

(collagenase, trypsin, and hyaluronidase) on the surface epitopes of a range of lymphocyte markers. Cells were incubated in the enzyme for a 15 min period, washed, and then stained using the indirect staining technique (*Protocol 2*). Collagenase shows no effect on either the percentage of stained cells, or the fluorescence intensity (antigen density), whilst trypsin has a detrimental effect on CD2, CD4, CD8, and CD15; hyaluronidase reduces the intensity of CD3 and CD19.

Tumour samples must be placed on ice as soon as possible and be processed as rapidly as possible, either for storage or for the generation of a single-cell suspension. Considerations such as retaining a portion for histological analysis, paraffin-wax embedding, and for molecular biology studies (such as DNA extraction) should also be made. If tissue is required for chromosome karyotype analysis, for oncoprotein analysis, or RNA extraction, or for establishing cell cultures, tissue must be handled aseptically and processed immediately. *Protocol 3* illustrates one possible routine for handling samples of solid tumour, and methods for obtaining cell suspensions from such tissue are described in detail in Chapter 1.

Protocol 3. Handling and cryopreservation of tumour samples

1. The tissue sample should be either placed in a tissue culture medium such as HBSS, or serum-free medium such as AIM-V (Gibco) if it is to be used for tissue culture or chromosome karyotype analysis, or in a plastic universal, plastic bag, or aluminium foil to prevent dehydration, and should be transported on ice.
2. As soon as possible after resection, fat should be trimmed off the tissue sample, which should then be divided so that representative portions may be frozen, processed to paraffin wax, and dissociated to produce a single-cell suspension.
3. The portion for freeze storage could be placed either in aluminium foil, covered with OCT freezing medium to prevent dehydration, and rapidly frozen; or simply be placed in a 'cryovial' and frozen directly. Liquid nitrogen in a flask may be used, and the wrapped tissue placed on to a cotton-wool plug just above the liquid level, but still in the vapour; or freezing spray may be used until the whole tissue sample is white with frost. Tissue should then be stored at −70°C, or in liquid nitrogen.
4. The portion for wax embedding must be placed in approximately 10 ml buffered formal saline for a 12 h period prior to dehydration in increasing concentrations of alcohol (50%, 70%, 95%, 100%), clearing in xylene, and embedding in paraffin wax.
5. The portion required for the generation of a single-cell suspension should be mechanically or enzymatically dissociated as described in Chapter 1.

2.2.2 Dissociation of paraffin-embedded tissue

Since the method of Hedley *et al.* (11) was first published, wax-embedded tissue has been used as a source of tumour-cell nuclei for the flow cytometric measurement of DNA ploidy and cell-cycle analysis. Not all archival samples can be used, as mercury-based fixatives were frequently used during the 1950s, and these samples do not yield reliable numbers of nuclei. The choice of section thickness must also be addressed, and a compromise reached. Too thin a section, i.e. that normally used for haematoxylin and eosin staining (4 μm), will slice through all cells, and high numbers of nuclei, resulting in large amounts of debris in the sample. Excessively thick sections (greater than 40 μm) may be hard to dissociate, but will also use large portions of what may be rare tissue blocks. Hence, an optimum section thickness is generally selected at approximately 30 μm (12).

The generally accepted method for the extraction of nuclei from paraffin blocks is summarized in *Protocol 4*, but modified protocols have been reported in the literature, including the use of alternative enzymes (13, 14) and the use of ultrasonication to enhance yields of nuclei (15). *Figure 5* shows two

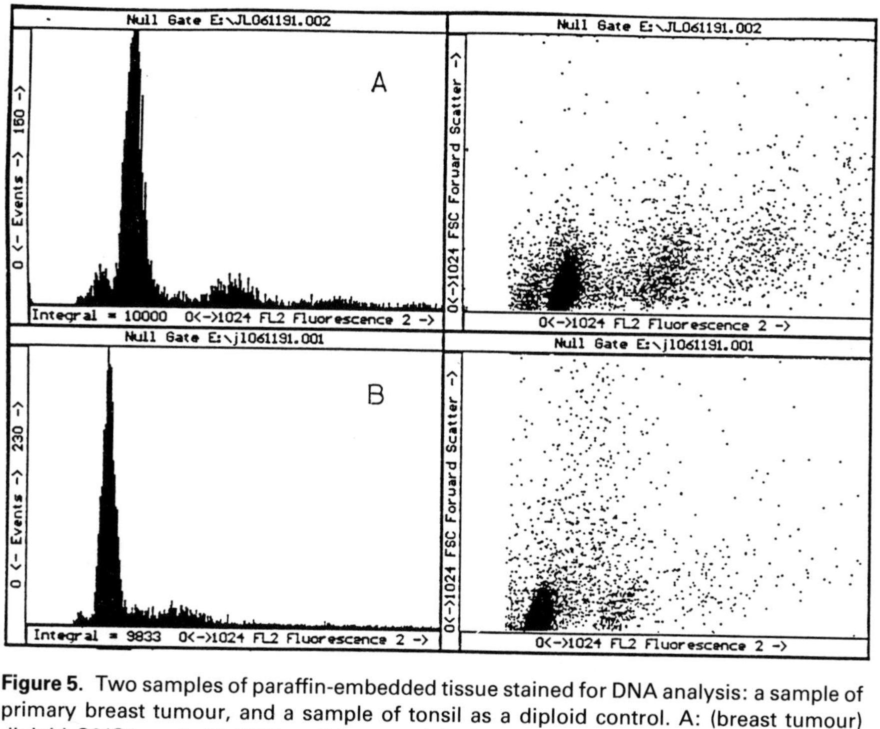

Figure 5. Two samples of paraffin-embedded tissue stained for DNA analysis: a sample of primary breast tumour, and a sample of tonsil as a diploid control. A: (breast tumour) diploid G0/G1 = ch 48, 5.7% cv 7.1; aneuploid G0/G1 = ch 65, 62.5% cv 5.8; PI = 1.35. B: (tonsil) diploid G0/G1 = ch 50, 68.1%, cv 6.9.

such preparations, a sample of breast tumour containing a diploid population of only 6%, the rest being aneuploid cells (Ploidy index 1.35). Note the use of light scatter to detect cell aggregates.

Protocol 4. The extraction of nuclei from sections of paraffin-embedded material

Reagents
- xylene
- graded concentrations of alcohol (absolute to 50%)
- distilled water
- PBS for washing nuclei
- pepsin (0.5% in PBS, pH 1.5)
- RNase (1 mg/ml in PBS)
- propidium iodide (PI; 50 μg/ml in PBS)

Method
1. Cut 30 μm sections from blocks of paraffin-embedded tissue, and de-wax them in glass tubes or bijous containing 5 ml xylene. Decant off the xylene after 15 min and replace with 5 ml fresh xylene for a further 15 min.
2. Decant off the xylene (store it until it can be disposed of correctly) and add 5 ml absolute alcohol for 15 min. Decant off and replace with decreasing concentrations of alcohol (repeating the 100% stage), followed by 95%, 70%, and 50% solutions of alcohol in water for 15 min each.
3. Remove the 50% alcohol and add distilled water. Swirl the sample gently and replace this water with a fresh 5 ml. Leave in water overnight to fully rehydrate at 4°C.
4. Remove the water from the sections and add 2–5 ml pepsin (0.5% solution in PBS, pH 1.5) depending on the amount of tissue, and incubate at 37°C for 1–3 h, or until the sections fragment and the solution becomes cloudy with extracted nuclei. Mix the sample well during this incubation period.
5. Pipette off the nuclear suspension and wash twice by centrifugation in PBS (400*g*, 5 min).
6. Add 50 μl RNase (1 mg/ml in PBS) to the pellet, re-suspend the nuclei and incubate for 30 min at room temperature.
7. Add 0.5 ml PI solution to stain the DNA, for a period of at least 30 min at room temperature. Samples may be held overnight in PI at 4°C.

One problem with the use of paraffin-embedded tissue for flow cytometric DNA measurements, is the identification of the diploid cell population (as opposed to hypo-diploid cells or total aneuploidy), due to the absence of a suitable control, other than cells within the tissue sample (see below). There are, however, reports in the literature of the successful use of antibodies with DNA stains in nuclear suspensions from paraffin sections, which may facilitate the distinction between tumour populations and normal stromal or infiltrative cells, perhaps by virtue of the presence or absence of tumour suppressor gene transcription (see for example reference (16), p. 57).

2.2.3 Dissociation of lymph-node tissue

Lymph-node tissue forms an important potential source of metastatic tumour cells in breast and other cancers. This tissue is usually highly cellular, and readily dissociated by mechanical techniques, or with very mild and rapid exposure to collagenase.

2.2.4 Needle biopsies

Other forms of tissue sample can be obtained from screening and outpatient clinics, as well as surgical procedures. For example, breast screening frequently demands the cytological analysis of fine-needle aspirates (FNAs). These may be used as a source of cell or nuclear suspensions, using mechanical and/or enzymatic dissociation procedures. Care must be taken on the choice of holding medium used, the presence or absence of fixatives and also of preservatives such as 'Carbo-wax', which may make analysis difficult. 70% methanol is usually recommended (17).

Needle-core biopsy material may be available from patients, as is the case when prostate cancer is suspected. This tissue can be readily dissociated by mechanical techniques alone.

2.2.5 Analysis of brush specimens

Cervical screening has always been plagued by the labour-intensive analysis of thousands of samples, and is perhaps an area in which most effort has been made to provide automation. To date this is far from ideal, and is therefore a potential area in which flow cytometry can be applied (18). What would be required would be a means of generating a cell suspension from the sampling brush or spatula; a suitable protocol for fixation; and one for dual-parameter analysis by flow cytometry of the DNA ploidy and cell-cycle status of cells, together with a suitable marker of neoplasia. Unfortunately, the latter has yet to be identified. Various candidates have ranged from the transferrin receptor to the C-myc oncoprotein. *Protocol 5* outlines a successful technique used for the generation of a nuclear suspension for the dual analysis of DNA and C-myc protein expression, and is illustrated in *Figure 6*, in which both aneuploid and diploid cells were present. This technique may also be suited to other mucoid samples such as the lung mucosa. Poorly bound cells are first collected by vortex mixing; and then pronase is added to digest cervical mucus to release more cells. Finally, pepsin is used to generate a nuclear suspension.

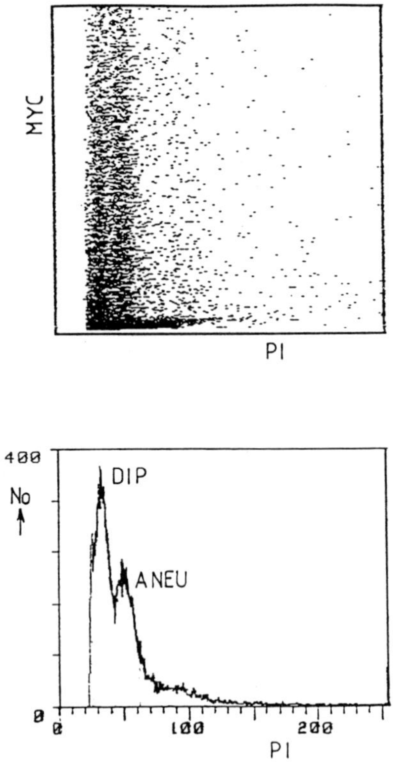

Figure 6. Dual-parameter DNA/C-myc 6E10 MoAb staining of a nuclear suspension obtained from a cervical brush specimen, showing the presence of both diploid and aneuploid cells positive for myc. Diploid G0/G1 = ch 34, 45.1%, cv 8.8; aneuploid G0/G1 = ch 51, 30.8%, cv 7.8, PI = 1.52.

Protocol 5. The preparation of cytology brush samples from the uterine endocervix. (Protocol supplied by Marina Flynn, Department of Obstetrics and Gynaecology, Clinical Sciences Centre, Northern General Hospital, Sheffield, UK)

Reagents
- PBS with and without 1% serum (0.22 μm filtered)
- 50% and 100% ethanol for fixation
- pronase E, 0.1% in PBS
- pepsin A, 50 μg/ml in 0.1 M HCl

To obtain a cell suspension:

1. Place the brush (immediately) in a 30 ml universal container containing either 5 ml PBS for immediate processing or storage at −20°C or 5 ml 50% ethanol for techniques that require fixed cells.

2. Remove the sample from the brush into the PBS by vortexing the tube gently for 10 min. Remove the brush and place it in a 10 ml conical-bottomed tube. Transfer the solution to another conical-bottomed tube and hold on ice.
3. Incubate the brush in 2 ml pronase (Type E, 0.1% in PBS) for 30 min at 37°C, with regular mixing.
4. Remove the brush and discard it.
5. Centrifuge the pre- and post-enzyme-treated solutions (10 min at 600*g*) and discard the supernatant. Wash any harvested cells in PBS.

To obtain a nuclear suspension:

6. Break up the cell pellets and add 2 ml pepsin (Type A, 50 μg/ml in 0.1 M HCl) for 45 min at 37°C. Vortex gently every 10 min; wash the nuclei in PBS and harvest by centrifugation.
7. Unfixed samples should now be fixed in 1.5 ml ice-cold ethanol with mixing, for 15 min, and can be stored at 4°C.
8. Prior to MoAb and/or DNA staining the nuclei must be washed in PBS to remove all traces of alcohol; re-suspended in PBS/1% serum to minimize cell aggregation.

2.3 Sample storage and fixation

Tissue samples for flow cytometric analysis should be stored frozen and not paraffin-wax embedded as cytoplasmic or membrane antigens cannot be detected (19). However, if part of the sample can be spared, it will provide a useful reference for histological grading, and immunohistochemistry. Freezing should be completed as soon as possible after ischaemic isolation during surgery and should be a rapid procedure (*Protocol 3*). In comparison, samples of cell suspensions should be frozen slowly to minimize large ice crystal formation (*Protocol 6*).

Protocol 6. Cryopreservation of cell suspensions

1. Re-suspend the cells in tissue-culture medium containing 10% FCS at a density of one to ten million cells per ml.
2. Add DMSO dropwise to a 10% concentration, slowly, with mixing, and on ice.
3. Aliquot the cell suspension into 1 ml amounts into sterile vials.

Protocol 6. *Continued*

4. Wrap the vial in polystyrene and freeze slowly to −70°C overnight before transfer to nitrogen storage.
5. Cells should be thawed in a 37°C water bath and washed well.

Fixation results in sample preservation, maintains the macromolecular framework and allows for processing at a convenient time. It can, however, produce artefacts which may lead to the generation of false results. The most common is the loss of antibody-binding abilities due to antigen loss, conformational changes in the protein preventing antibody binding, or for alterations in adjacent molecules causing obstruction of the epitope. Fixation may also prevent the entry of large molecules into the cell or the nucleus, and therefore prevent complete DNA staining. This should be particularly noted when using paraffin-wax-embedded tissue for flow cytometry.

Fixatives may also act as coagulants and aggregate or clot protein globules or be non-coagulant in altering protein viscosity. They may be additive and retain cell structure by the formation of cross-linkages or be non-additive and result in protein denaturation and the disorder of structure. Aldehydes (formaldehyde, gluteraldehyde, and paraformaldehyde) are examples of additive, non-coagulating fixatives; whilst alcohols (ethanol and methanol) are examples of coagulating, non-additive fixatives (20). Peripheral blood or bone marrow cell suspensions are routinely fixed in a 1% paraformaldehyde solution once antibody staining is complete, to prevent the capping or the polarized migration of surface antigen/antibody complexes. In addition, fixation reduces the biohazard risk of category 3 samples. However, samples fixed in paraformaldehyde should not be analysed for at least four hours, to ensure complete fixation. *Table 3* shows the changes in lymphocyte antibody binding seen following fixation in 1% paraformaldehyde upon completion of

Table 3. Sequential analysis of lymphocyte staining following paraformaldehyde fixation

MoAb	Unfixed		2 h fix		12 h fix		3 day fix	
	(%)	($\bar{x}$)	(%)	($\bar{x}$)	(%)	($\bar{x}$)	(%)	($\bar{x}$)
FITC	1.4	–	1.5	–	1.5	–	1.9	–
CD3	95.5	102	92.4	34	94.3	80	93.2	77
CD4	72.4	300	76.1	58	70.4	224	80.8	191
CD8	25.5	576	25.3	104	26.1	388	23.1	243
CD16	5.6	63	6.1	38	8.0	50	8.9	41
CD19	7.6	72	7.1	41	8.0	66	8.0	40
CD11c	6.9	161	5.9	41	6.4	55	7.5	43

% = per cent positive cells; $\bar{x}$ = median fluorescence channel

the staining procedure (*Protocol 1*). Whilst the percentage of stained cells remains constant over the three-day period, it can be seen that fixation initially causes a loss of fluorescence intensity that is generally restored by 12 hours. Hence, fixed samples should be stored overnight prior to analysis.

Many cell suspensions have to be stored prior to analysis. Whilst cells can be stored frozen, it is sometimes an advantage to fix them if for example, dual DNA/MoAb staining is required, or if the cells are too delicate to survive freeze/thawing. *Table 4* shows the range of fixatives commonly used on cell suspensions for flow cytometric analysis and also includes the effects fixation may have on the quality of DNA results on a sample of peripheral blood lymphocytes. It is clear that formaldehyde fixatives prevent uniform staining and result in a reduction in the level of fluorescence (lower peak channel), and wider peaks (higher coefficient of variation, cv). Acetone results in severe cell clumping as seen by an apparent reduction of cells in the G0/G1 peak.

In summary, fixation is a most convenient process, enabling the long-term storage of unique samples, or the short-term preservation of tests prior to cytometric analysis. However, all fixatives must be regarded as being potentially damaging to the cell and to molecular structures, so good controls must be established to ensure that results are as comparable as possible to the natural state. Morkve and Hostmark (21) describe the attention they took when analysing p53 expression with DNA staining, in nuclear samples from fixed-embedded tissue. Their first question was whether the binding of the p53 antibody (PAb 1801) was influenced by fixation and enzyme treatment. Their conclusion was that there were minimal differences between fresh, paraffin-embedded, or paraformaldehyde-fixed tissue, but that a loss of fluorescence intensity occurs with ethanol fixation. A similar approach was taken in the preparation of *Protocol 7*, which outlines one fixation system that has been successfully used for the analysis of membrane, cytoplasmic, and nuclear monoclonal antibody binding in combination with the DNA fluorochrome,

Table 4. The choice of fixatives, and their effect on DNA staining of lymphocytes

Fixative	G0/G1 peak	% G0/G1	Peak cv
Unfixed	50	98.5	4.2
Formal saline	20	88.2	13.8
70% Ethanol	50	87.5	8.2
Acetone	49	61.7	10.7
Ethanol/acetic acid (95%/5%)	54	79.3	7.7
Ethanol/acetone (50%/50%)	50	63.2	9.5
Paraformaldehyde (1%)	22	89.7	12.1
Para. then ethanol (1%, 70%)	38	96.4	6.8
Para. then eth/acetic acid	39	88.0	9.7

All incubations with propidium iodide were for 15 min at room temperature

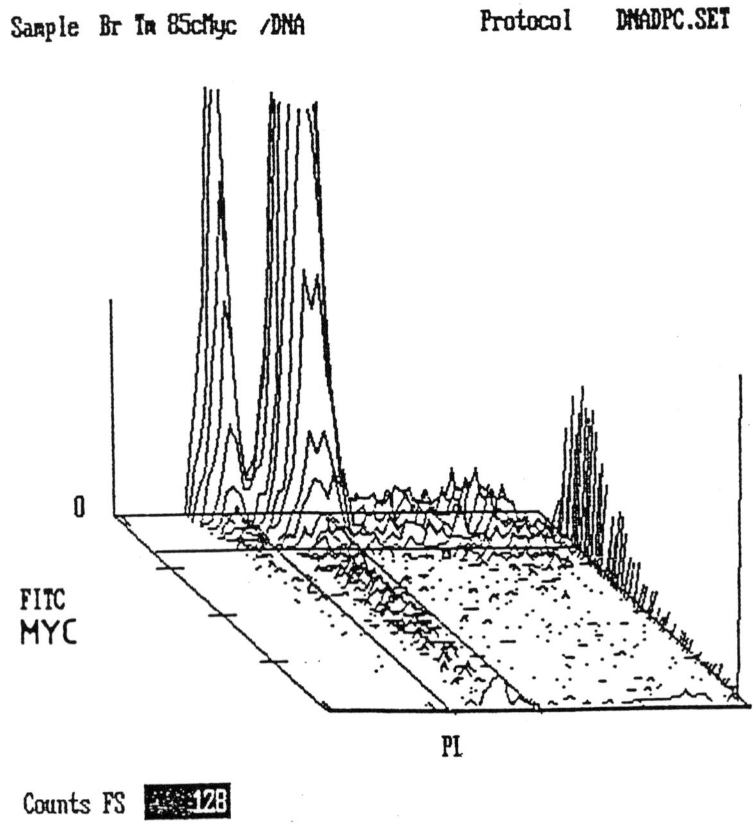

Figure 7. Dual parameter net-plot of DNA/C-myc 6E10 MoAb staining of a suspension of primary breast tumour cells showing selective positivity within the aneuploid G0/G1 peak. Diploid G0/G1 = ch 59, 9.2%, cv 5.4; aneuploid G0/G1 = ch 102, 66.6%, cv 7.2; PI = 1.73; aneuploid C-myc positive cells = 11%.

PI. Paraformaldehyde is used to maintain membrane integrity, whilst methanol is used to permeabilize the cells. An example of this type of analysis is shown in *Figure 7*, with breast carcinoma cells stained with anti-C-myc antibody (6E10, Cambridge Research Biochemicals Ltd), together with PI. Diploid and aneuploid cells can be seen together with a discrete population of myc-positive cells within the aneuploid G0/G1 peak.

Protocol 7. The preparation of breast tumour cells for dual DNA/MoAb staining of membrane, cytoplasmic, and nuclear proteins

Reagents

- 1% paraformaldehyde solution in PBS
- 70% methanol

- PBS with 1% serum added
- primary antibody (titrated)
- secondary antibody—FITC conjugate (titrated)[a]
- propidium iodide (PI; 50 μg/ml in PBS)[a]

Method

1. Dice and enzymatically/mechanically dissociate the tumour.
2. Wash the cell suspension twice in PBS to remove all traces of serum.
3. Re-suspend the pellet, and add 1–2 ml 1% paraformaldehyde[b] (in PBS), and mix well. Allow to fix for 15 min.
4. Wash the cells in PBS, re-suspend the pellet and add 1–2 ml 70% ice-cold methanol and mix well. Allow the sample to fix for 15 min.[c]
5. Wash the cells, first in PBS alone, then PBS/1% serum, and count the cells.[c]
6. Label small tubes (e.g. Falcon 2054) appropriately and add one million cells to each. Reduce the volume by centrifugation and remove the supernatant. Re-suspend the pellet.
7. Stain with either a directly conjugated (FITC) antibody, or a primary and then a secondary antibody as in *Protocols 1* and *2*.
8. Stain with the DNA fluorochrome, propidium iodide (PI) (50 μg/ml in PBS) for 15–30 min prior to analysis and hold on ice.

[a] FITC and PI staining should be protected from light.
[b] Paraformaldehyde will only dissolve when heated to 56°C.
[c] Samples may be stored long-term at −20°C in methanol or short-term at 4°C after stage **4**; and overnight at 4°C after **8**.

3. Standardization

3.1 The choice of controls

All assays must include appropriate controls. Negative controls identify background levels of reagent binding, or antigen expression, and should be subtracted from the positive test result. Positive controls are markers that are known to be expressed and are used to indicate the efficiency of the protocol. Immunoglobulin isotype control antibodies are most suited as the negative control for direct antibody assays using conjugated MoAbs; whilst the fluorescent second-stage antibody, or an irrelevant antibody, form convenient negative controls for indirect assays. Positive controls include the CD2 MoAb (E-rosette receptor), CD45RB (leucocyte common antigen) for samples of lymphocytes; the CAM 5.2 anti-cytokeratin MoAb cocktail, PHM5 (Silenus Ltd), berEP4 (Dako Ltd) antibodies may also be suitable for cells of epithelial origin (see Section 4.2). More general reagents may be of use for other tumour types, such as the epithelial membrane antigen (EMA), human milk fat globule antibody (HMFG), carcino-embryonic antigen (CEA), or prostate-specific antigen (PSA).

DNA analysis also requires the use of controls. If cultured cells are used to measure the relative frequency of cells in each phase of the cell cycle under the modulatory effect of chemicals (growth factors or cytokines for example) the control should simply be untreated cells. If a tumour sample is being analysed for ploidy and cell cycle, control diploid cells should be stained in parallel with the test cells. Frozen or fixed lymphocytes are suitable depending on the source of tumour, although fresh cells should not be used to control fixed cells and vice versa. There is not, however, a suitable control for the analysis of archival paraffin-wax-embedded tissue, as the original fixation procedure cannot be determined or reproduced. It may be possible to trace 'normal' tissue samples processed at the same time; if a new study is being established with fresh tissue, control tissue should be included (*Figure 4*). Most tumour samples do, however, contain control marker cell populations in the form of diploid stromal and infiltrative cells. In addition, other marker cells may be introduced into the cell suspension, such as chick or trout red blood cells, with DNA contents of approximately one third that of normal human cells. PI is considered to be the fluorochrome of choice for most applications, but as it can also stain single-stranded RNA that has folded back on itself it is advisable to use RNase (100 μl 1 mg/ml, 15 min, 37 °C prior to PI staining) on cell suspensions where active proliferation is suspected (e.g. cell cultures).

Quality control (QC) may be taken one step further by enrolling your laboratory for a national or international (European Community) scheme (22). These normally address issues related to the phenotype analysis of lymphocytes using MoAbs and are thus targeted to haematology or immunology laboratories. The aim of a QC scheme is to help registrants maintain their cytometers in good order, as well as ensuring that methodologies used generate results which are comparable to those of other laboratories. This is achieved by sending aliquots of a standard sample of cells to each participating laboratory for them to analyse. Their data are then correlated to data from other registrants, and errors can then be identified and, hopefully, problems traced (23). The quality control of DNA analysis is somewhat harder to address, reflected by limited reports in the literature (24, 25).

3.2 Alignment and calibration

Glutaraldehyde-fixed chick red blood cells may be used as fluorescent alignment controls; although it is more common to use fluorescent beads, both for alignment and for fluorescence calibration. In this case, fluorescent beads with known levels of a fluorescent molecule (usually fluorescein iso-thiocyanate

(FITC) or phycoerythrin (PE)) are run through the cytometer and the arbitrary channel numbers given are then converted into numbers of molecules of fluorescein. If the valency of binding of antibody to antigen, and the fluorescence conjugation ratio of the antibody, are known, accurate values of antigen density can be determined.

4. Current applications of flow cytometry

4.1 Haematogenous and lymphoid tumours

Leukaemia phenotyping is possibly the most significant application of flow cytometry in haematology. The percentage of cells stained with antibody within a cell suspension can be measured, together with an indication of the average fluorescent intensity (equivalent antigen density). Light scatter is simple to analyse, and gates can be set to select for particular populations. DNA analysis is also possible, but being more common for solid tumour analysis, is discussed later in Section 4.4. Patients' blood can now be analysed by both direct (fluorescent MoAbs) and indirect (primary MoAb, then fluorescent second stage) staining techniques for the rapid determination of the lineage of the leukaemia (T-cell, B-cell, or monocytic) and then of the particular stage of maturation of the predominant cell present, using phenotype-specific MoAbs. *Table 5* illustrates the primary reagents used in the Department of Haematology of the Royal Hallamshire Hospital, Sheffield, to diagnose acute and chronic (lympho-proliferative) leukaemias by flow cytometry;

Table 5. Monoclonal antibodies used in leukaemia diagnosis

Acute leukaemia	Chronic leukaemia
Control	Control
CD3	CD2
CD7	CD5
CD10	CD10
CD13	CD14
CD14	CD19
CD15	CD23
CD19	FMC7
CD33	4B8
CD34	IA
CD61	Kappa
HLA-DR	Lambda
RBC	SMIG A
	SMIG G
	SMIG M

SMIG = surface immunoglobulin

although light microscopy may also be used for acute patients for the measurement of cytoplasmic immunoglobulins (CD3, CD22, IgM, and the terminal deoxy-nucleotidyl-transferase (TdT) nuclear antigen); and with chronic patients for the measurement of cytoplasmic immunoglobulin light (kappa and lambda) and heavy (IgA, IgG, IgM) chains, by APAAP staining. There are reports in the literature on the significance of DNA staining in, for example, non-Hodgkin's and Hodgkin's lymphoma (26, 27), but this method is not routinely used in clinical diagnosis. There may be instances, however, when cells stained for MoAb phenotyping are also required for the measurement of cell cycle, in for example lympho-proliferative disorders. This can be readily achieved on density-gradient-purified cells, by the addition of 0.2% Triton-X 100 to permeabilize cells, followed by the addition of PI. Thus, the phenotype of cells in each phase of the cell cycle can be determined. An example is shown in *Figure 8*, with control cells (FITC isotype) and CD3 stained cells.

Lympho-proliferative disorders can be divided into categories which can be used to aid diagnosis: the intermediate B-cell disorders, such as chronic lymphocytic leukaemia (the marker of choice being CD23 expressed at high levels) and prolymphocytic leukaemia (identified by surface immunoglobulins

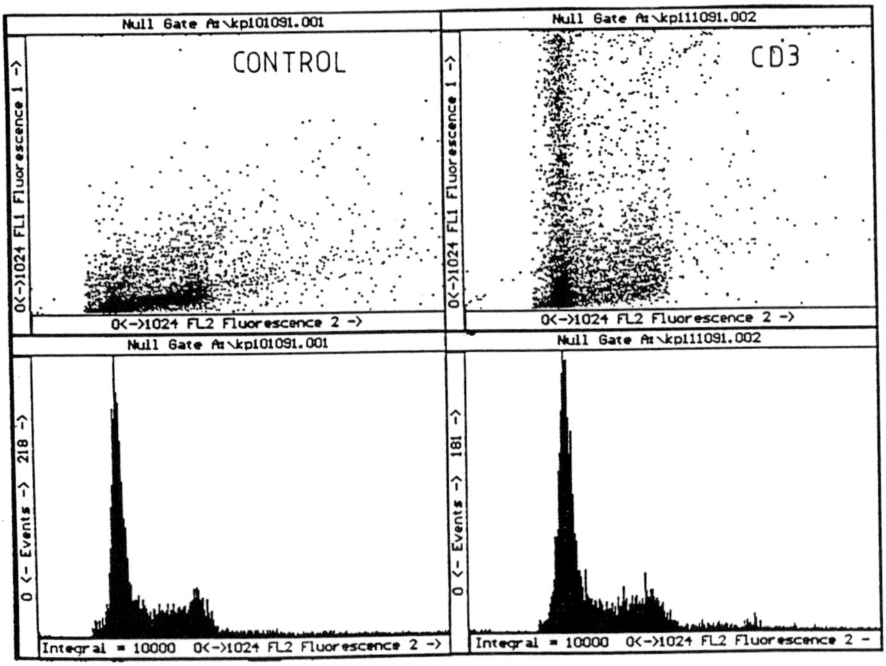

Figure 8. Application of the use of secondary DNA staining of separated lymphocytes, pre-stained with FITC isotype and CD3, to determine the phase of the cell cycle of the labelled cells.

and FMC7 expression); secondly, the mature B-cell disorders, including Hairy-cell leukaemia (expressing high level FMC7, as well as surface and cytoplasmic immunoglobulin), lymphoma, Waldenstrom's syndrome, and myeloma. Finally there are T-cell disorders, including TCLL, T-gamma, ATCL lymphoma, and Segary's syndrome, and reactive lymphocytosis disorders. Each disease state can be defined by a characteristic marker profile, although not all are easily defined as the 'simple' T- or B-cell leukaemias, which are distinguished by the presence or absence of CD2 (sheep E-rosette receptor) or CD19 positively, which is the earliest B-lineage-specific marker known to date (28, 29).

Phenotype MoAb binding can thus be used to monitor progression from the chronic phase to the acute phase, and treatment administered accordingly.

Using similar phenotype markers, bone marrow transplantation can be monitored in leukaemics, with, for example, changes in bone marrow cell types being proportional to the acceptance and regrowth of the donor marrow, as compared to the diseased/neoplastic host marrow, which should have been destroyed by radiotherapy and/or chemotherapy.

4.2 Clinical applications of the analysis of solid tumours

4.2.1 DNA analysis

For many years primary cancer diagnosis was achieved by histochemical means on tissue sections, cell smears, or cytocentrifuge preparations. Immunohistochemistry was then employed to confirm difficult diagnoses. It would seem to be a logical step for flow cytometry to assist in the diagnostic process, with DNA ploidy and cell-cycle analysis, or with the identification of cell types using MoAbs. DNA analysis is possible with fluorochromes such as PI or ethidium bromide that intercalate non-specifically in the double helix of DNA, and fluoresce red; acridine orange fluoresces green when intercalated with DNA, and also binds to single-stranded nucleic acids to fluoresce red (i.e. RNA); whereas fluorochromes such as mithramycin bind to the GC-rich regions of DNA and benzimides, such as Hoechst 33342, bind preferentially to AT-rich regions in the small groove of DNA and fluoresce blue with UV excitation. Irrespective of the dye used, the measurement of DNA content is simply considered to be proportional to the intensity of fluorescence, which is in turn proportional to the amount of dye bound in the nucleus. Thus, as cells progress through the cell cycle, their DNA content increases, causing an increase in fluorescence. Similarly, chromosomal trisomy, etc., will also result in the increased fluorescence seen in cell samples termed aneuploid.

However, although flow cytometric DNA measurements have been applied to a wide range of tumour types, and prognostic significance has been recorded, routine use has not been adopted. This may in part be due to the apparent simplicity of the data presented following flow cytometric analysis.

Data may be in the form of the percentage of cells in each phase of the cell cycle, i.e. G0/G1, S and G2/M-phases, or expressed as the overall DNA content or ploidy of cell populations. Cell-cycle calculations are based on the increase in fluorescence intensity, associated with DNA synthesis, generating normal distributions for each cell-cycle phase. Gaussian curves can be fitted into the G0/G1 and G2/M phase peaks by computer models, and the S-phase approximated, using linear regression of the area between the mid-points of the G1 and G2 peaks; S-phase overlap can thus be accounted for. However, complex aneuploid/diploid mixtures are still difficult to analyse (30, 31). *Figure 9* shows one such example using the MultiCycle package, in which diploid and aneuploid populations have been calculated from a sample of paraffin-embedded bladder tumour. In contrast, DNA ploidy is easier to determine, being the ratio of the peak channel of the abnormal (tumour) population to that of the normal diploid control (either within the same sample, or between two samples stained and run under exactly the same conditions). Thus, DNA diploid cells (2n) have a ploidy index of 1.00, and DNA tetraploid cells (4n) an index of 2.00. Controversy exists with the exact definition of 'near' diploid or tetraploid cells, but from a ploidy index range between 1.4 and 1.9, the notation 'DNA aneuploid' is generally given (32). Cells of DNA content below diploid would be termed hypo-diploid, and

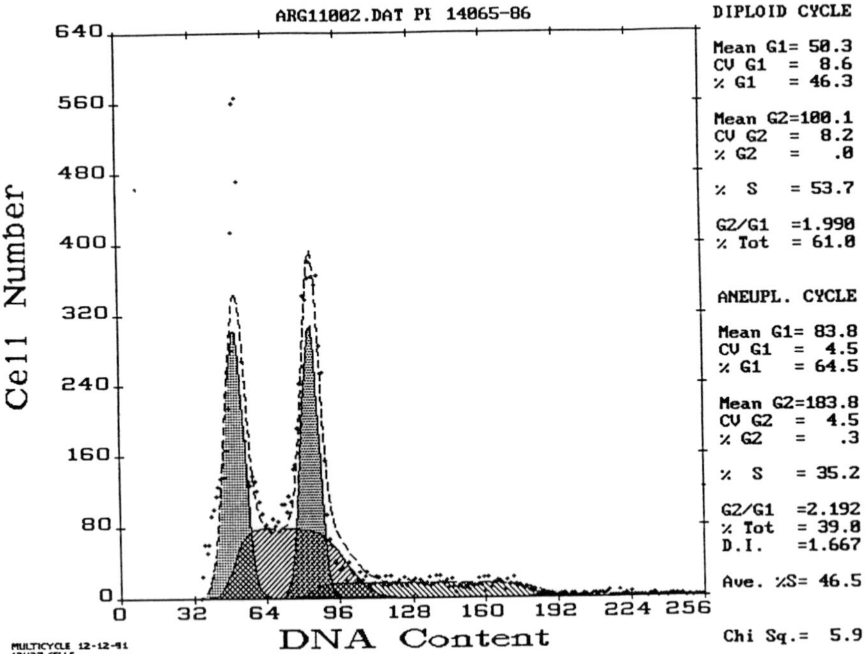

Figure 9. Example of the MultiCycle software package for the measurement of ploidy and cell cycle, on a sample of paraffin-wax-extracted nuclei of a bladder tumour.

above tetraploid, hyper-tetraploid; whilst tetraploidy can only be suspected if the peak (which is at the same location as the diploid G2/M peak) exceed 15% of the total, with a possible tetraploid G2/M peak visible further along the fluorescence axis (33).

One attempt at improving the prognostic credibility of DNA ploidy and cell cycle, has been to categorize S-phase fraction data in ranges of 2–5% (good prognosis), at 7% (intermediate prognosis), and at 12% (poorest prognosis) (34); whilst other attempts have been to combine DNA ploidy data with S-phase data as a score for prognosis and survival (35).

4.2.2 Anti-tumour antibodies

One problem with the single parameter measurement of DNA ploidy and cell cycle, is that tumour cells cannot be distinguished from infiltrative or normal host or stromal cells. By using an antibody in combination with a DNA fluorochrome, tumour cells of epithelial origin can be distinguished from stromal and infiltrative cells.

Antibodies should be selected for their specificity, and matched to the tumour type. For example, colon carcinoma cells should be identified by their positivity with CEA, whilst HMFG would identify breast tumour cells and PSA cells of prostate origin. Numerous other antibodies are of a more general nature. Ber-EP4 (Dako) reacts with two glycoproteins present on the surface and in the cytoplasm of all epithelial cells except squamous epithelia, hepatocytes, and parietal cells, and is shown in *Figure 10* staining circulating (tumour) cells in the peripheral blood of a patient with prostate cancer. PHM5 (from Silenus) can similarly be used for epithelial and endothelial cells, and is shown in *Figure 11* staining the diploid (high-intensity) and aneuploid (lower-intensity) tumour populations in a sample of ocular melanoma.

Cytokeratin antibodies, however, are those most commonly used. Cytokeratins are a group of structural proteins of the cytoskeleton, forming intermediate-sized filaments. Cytokeratins are characteristic of epithelial cells and have been catalogued numerically, from 1 to 19 (36). Cytokeratins 7, 8, and 18 are specific for simple and transitional epithelia, and cocktails of 8, 18, and 19 are frequently used for the detection of breast tumour cells as the reagent CAM 5.2. CK 19 is the earliest (embryonic) form and has been postulated to be a useful marker of stem cell or undifferentiated cell tumours (37). An alternative cocktail is presented in the Dako reagent CK-MNF116, reactive for CKs 10, 17, and 18. CK 7 distinguishes ovarian (+) from gastro-intestinal tract (−) carcinomas, and CK 10 and 14 are markers for keratinizing squamous and stratified epithelia. CK 10 has been demonstrated in squamous cell carcinomas but not adenocarcinomas or transitional cell carcinomas of the cervix, while CK 14 has been used to identify neoplasms of myoepithelial origin, and to distinguish squamous cell (+) from adenocarcinoma (−) of the cervix. CK 14 may also be an indicator of benign breast disease (38). CK 16 is expressed in normal and abnormal human breast

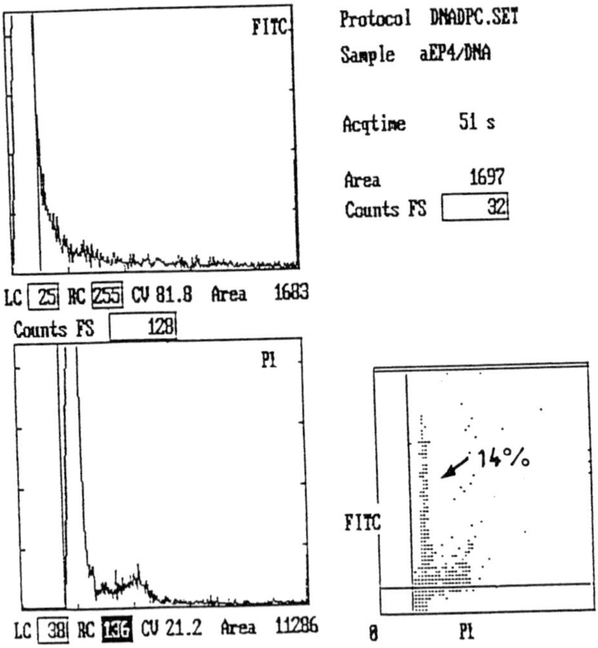

Figure 10. Example of the use of Dako Ber-EP4 anti-epithelial cell MoAb in detecting circulating tumour cells from a patient with prostate cancer.

epithelium, together with CK 13, which is also present in some ductal carcinomas and benign lesions. Together, these markers may be capable of classifying subsets of ductal carcinomas (39).

4.2.3 Proliferation antibodies

i. Ki67

An alternative form of measuring proliferation is by the use of MoAbs against epitopes whose expression is restricted to particular phases of the cell cycle. Examples of Ki67 (Dako Ltd), which is an antibody raised against an epitope in the nucleus thought to be revealed when histone and non-histone proteins cleave during DNA transcription (40). The antigen can be identified on chromosomes in all phases of mitosis, as well as interphase nuclei, but not cells in G0.

ii. PCNA

A second, comparable antibody is the proliferating cell nuclear antigen (PCNA)/cyclin and is an intranuclear polypeptide antigen found in both normal and transformed proliferating cells (41). It may be an auxiliary protein of DNA polymerase delta and several antibodies have been raised against the

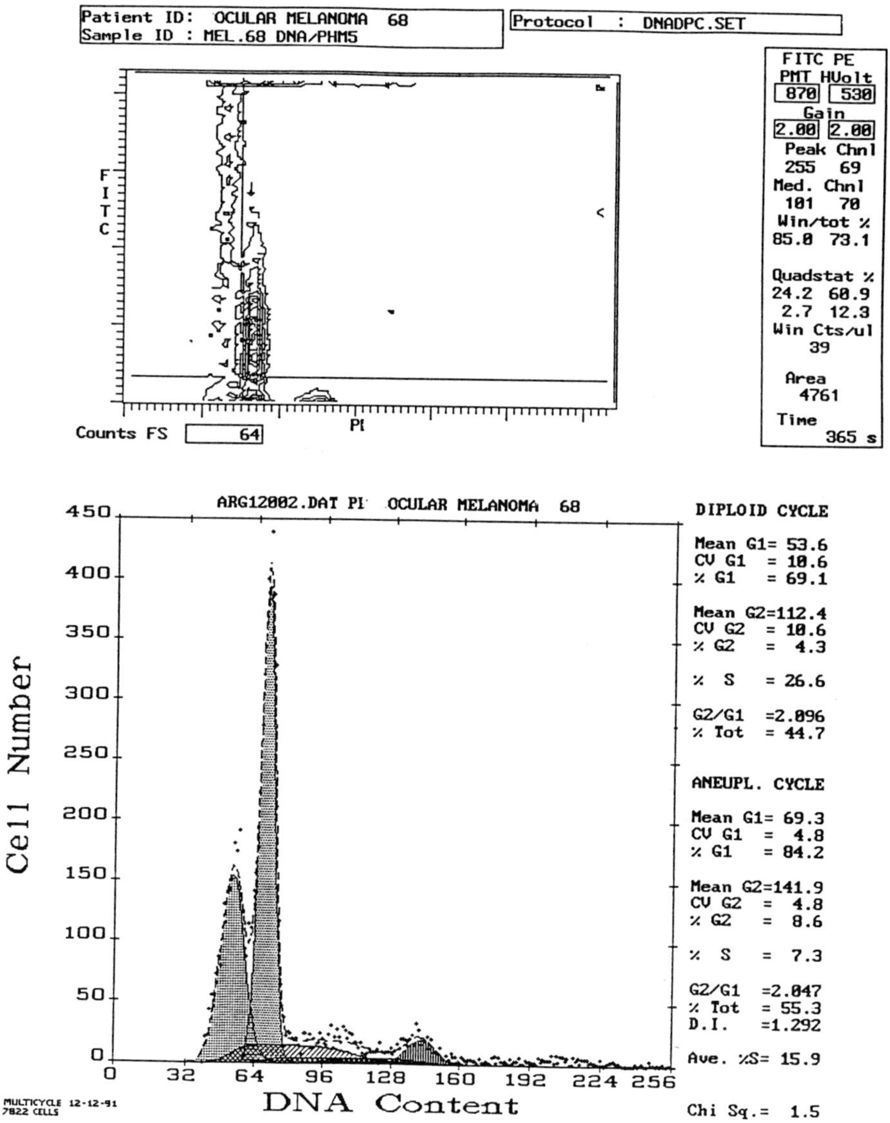

Figure 11. Differential staining of the epithelial/endothelial cell Silenus MoAb PHM5 between diploid and aneuploid cells of an ocular melanoma.

molecule. PC10 (Dako Ltd) is one such antibody, but its use must be carefully controlled, as the antibody binds to different epitopes depending upon the fixation procedure used. PCNA should only be detected during S-phase, yet when fixed cells are analysed, cells in G1, S, and G2/M-phase are all detected. This is because part of the epitope is detergent soluble and part is insoluble. Only the detergent-insoluble form is exposed during S-phase and hence can be used as a marker for these cells. Thus, tissue sections or cell suspensions must be detergent treated prior to analysis, using triton, tween, or NP40. If detergent is not used, the generalized staining pattern is seen (42) with antibody binding to cells in G1, G2, and M-phase, as well as all cells in S-phase.

iii. BrdU

The third technique that can be used to measure cell proliferation, is to incubate cells in the presence of bromodeoxyuridine (BrdU), a thymidine analogue, which is incorporated into the DNA of S-phase cells (43). *In vivo* or *in vitro* incubation can be used and the time period carefully controlled before either resection or harvesting the cells. By using an anti-BrdU antibody (either in a direct FITC conjugate, or indirect staining technique), BrdU-labelled cells can be detected. PI is added to enable the determination of cell cycle phase and total DNA content and S-phase cells are easily distinguished from G1 and G2/M-phase cells by their FITC stain. By controlling the time period between BrdU incubation and the final analysis with MoAb, potential doubling times of the cells can be calculated (44). *Figure 12* shows a schematic diagram of the nature of BrdU staining in combination with DNA fluorescence analysis.

4.2.4 Radiobiology

Flow cytometry has been used to monitor the efficacy of radiotherapy particularly in patients with bladder cancer, leukaemics, and bone marrow

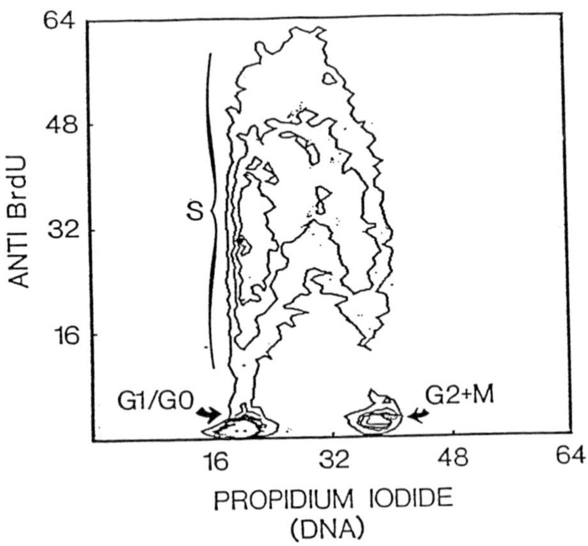

Figure 12. Schematic representation of BrdU MoAb staining in combination with propidium iodide DNA staining, to identify S-phase cells.

transplantation. This has been achieved by the use of tumour-specific MoAbs, including those identifying the nature and stage of the leukaemia, when minimal residual disease presence can be monitored, and therefore the success or failure of radiotherapy in killing the tumour cells. Alternatively, the application of MoAbs capable of detecting cells with abnormal levels of proliferation (PCNA/Ki67/BrDu), or by the use of simple DNA fluorochromes, can be considered. If radiotherapy is successful, tumour proliferation should cease.

4.2.5 Chemotherapy

The measurement of the level of multi-drug-resistance (MDR) protein expression on the cell membrane of tumour cells can provide important information on the potential efficacy of chemotherapy. Multi-drug resistance is conferred on a cell by a specific membrane pump, the P-glycoprotein (p-170), capable of removing all toxic molecules from the cytoplasm, and as a result of this normal function, can also remove chemotherapeutic agents. Resistance can be broad, covering the anti-mitotics (vincristine, vinblastine, colchicine), anthracyclines (doxorubicin, daunorubicin, dihydroxy-anthracenedione, mitoxantrone), antibiotics (mithramycin, actinomycin-D, puromycin), epipodophyllo-toxins (etoposide, tenopside), and others including emetine, mitomycin, gramicidin-D, ethidiun bromide, taxol, and cytochalasin-B. MDR expression will thus result in widespread therapy failure following drug administration (45).

A further effect that can be utilized by flow cytometry is that some chemotherapy agents (adriomycin, dornomycin, etc.) are naturally fluorescent when excited by a suitable energy source. Thus, cells taking up the drug can be identified from those either failing to take up the molecule, or those capable of its active removal. This area also has applications in research into photodynamic therapy (PDT), in which a non-fluorescent drug is administered (typically into the bladder in cases of bladder carcinoma, or topically for skin lesions), and once bound within the tumour cells is irradiated by laser, with the resultant energy emission causing the death of the stained cell.

Further reading

Cytometry (the journal of the International Society for Analytical Cytometry). Published eight times per year by Wiley-Liss, New York.

Flow Cytometry: a Practical Approach (1990). Edited by M. G. Ormerod, published by Oxford University Press.

Flow Cytogenetics (1989). Edited by J. W. Gray, published by Academic Press.

Flow Cytometry (1991). Edited by Z. Darzynkiewicz, published by Academic Press.

Flow Cytometry in Haematology (1991). Edited by O. D. Laerum and R. Bjerknes, published by Academic Press.

Flow Cytometry, First Principles (1992). Edited by A. L. Givan, published by Wiley-Liss, New York.

Acknowledgements

I am most grateful for methods supplied by Janet Peel (Department of Haematology, Royal Hallamshire Hospital, Sheffield, UK) and Marina Flynn (Department of Obstetrics and Gynaecology, Northern General Hospital, Sheffield, UK), for practical examples from Freddie Hamdy (Department of Urology, Royal Hallamshire Hospital, Sheffield, UK) and David Cottam (Institute of Cancer Studies, University of Sheffield Medical School, UK), for technical information from Becton-Dickinson, Ortho, Dako, and Silenus, and to the Yorkshire Cancer Research Campaign for their support. The flow cytometry unit of the Institute for Cancer Studies, University of Sheffield Medical School is funded by the Yorkshire Cancer Research Campaign.

References

1. McMichael, A. J. (1987). *Leucocyte Typing III. White Cell Differentiation Antigens*. Oxford University Press.
2. Ploton, D., Menager, M., Jeanasson, P., Himber, G., Pigeon, F., and Adnet, J. J. (1986). *Histochem. J.*, **18,** 5–14.
3. Giri, D. D., Nottingham, J. F., Lawry, J., Dundas, S. A. C., and Underwood, J. C. E. (1989). *J. Pathol.*, **157,** 307–13.
4. Lawry, J., Rogers, K., and Duncan, J. L. (1988). *Surg. Res. Commun.*, **3,** 61–70.
5. Gray, J. W. (1989). *Flow Cytogenetics*, Analytical cytology series. Academic, London.
6. Gray, J. W., Carrano, A. V., Steinmetz, L. L., Van Dilla, M. A., Moore, D. H., Mayall, B. H., *et al.* (1975). *Proc. Natl Acad. Sci. USA,* **72,** 1231–4.
7. Pinkel, D., Landegent, J., Collins, C., Fuscoe, J., Seagraves, R., Lucas, J., *et al.* (1989). *Proc. Natl Acad. Sci. USA,* **85,** 9138–42.
8. Condrau, M. A., Schwendener, R., Zimmermann, M., Rol, P., Fierz, W., Niederer, P., *et al.* (1991). *Cytometry,* **12** (Supplement 5), 101.
9. Lawry, J., Kristensen, S. D., and Martin, J. F. (1989). *Clin. Lab. Haematol.*, **11,** 361–8.
10. Stonesifer, K. J., Xiang, J., Wilkinson, E. J., Benson, N. A., and Braylan, R. C. (1987). *Acta Cytol.*, **31** (2), 125–30.
11. Hedley, D. W., Friedlander, M. L., Taylor, M. L., Rugg, C. A., and Musgrove, E. A. (1983). *J. Histochem. Cytochem.*, **31,** 1333–55.
12. Stephenson, R. A., Gay, H., Fair, W. R., and Melamed, M. R. (1986). *Cytometry,* **7,** 41–4.
13. Schutte, B., Reynders, M. M. J., Bosman, F. T., and Bijham, G. H. (1985). *Cytometry,* **6,** 26–30.

14. Lawry, J., Rogers, K., Percival, R. C., Day, C., and Potter, C. W. (1987). *Surg. Res. Commun.*, **2,** 27–37.
15. Gonchoroff, N. J., Ryan, J. J., Kimlinger, T. K., Witzig, T. E., Greipp, P. R., Meyer, J. S., *et al.* (1990). *Cytometry,* **11,** 642–6.
16. Morkve, O. and Laerum, O. D. (1991). *Cytometry,* **12,** 438–44.
17. Levack, P. A., Mullen, P., Anderson, T. J., Miller, W. R., and Forrest, A. P. M. (1987). *Br. J. Cancer,* **56,** 643–6.
18. Ellias-Jones, J., Hendy-Ibbs, P., Cox, H., Evan, G. I., and Watson, J. V. (1986). *J. Clin. Path.,* **39,** 577–81.
19. Lanier, L. L. and Warner, N. L. (1981). *J. Immunol. Methods,* **47,** 25–30.
20. Fox, C. H., Johnson, F. B., Whiting, J., and Roller, P. P. (1985). *J. Histochem. Cytochem.,* **33,** 845–53.
21. Morkve, O. and Hostmark, J. (1991). *Cytometry,* **12,** 622–7.
22. Martini, E., D'Hautcourt, J. L., Brando, B., Lawry, J., O'Connor, J. E., and Sansonetty, F. (1990). *First European Quality Control of Cellular Phenotyping by Flow Cytometry*. Frison-Roche, Paris.
23. McCarthy, R. C. and Fetterhoff, T. J. (1989). *Arch. Pathol. Lab. Med.,* **113,** 658–66.
24. Homburger, H. A., McCarthy, R. C., and Deodhr, S. (1989). *Arch. Pathol. Lab. Med.,* **113,** 667–72.
25. Lawry, J. (1992). *Proc. Royal Microscopical Society*, **27,** 16.
26. Morgan, D. R., Williamson, J. M. S., Quirke, P., Clayden, A. D., Smith, M. E. F., O'Brien, C. J., *et al.* (1986). *Br. J. Cancer,* **54,** 643–9.
27. Joensuu, H., Klemi, P. J., and Korkeila, E. (1988). *Am. J. Clin. Pathol.*, **90,** 670–3.
28. Deegan, M. J. (1989). *Arch. Pathol. Lab. Med.,* **113,** 606–18.
29. Braylan, R. C. and Benson, N. A. (1989). *Arch. Pathol. Lab. Med.,* **113,** 627–33.
30. Dean, P. N. (1980). *Cell Tissue Kinet.,* **13,** 299–308.
31. Ormerod, M. G., Payne, A. W. R., and Watson, J. V. (1987). *Cytometry,* **8,** 637–41.
32. Beerman, H., Kluin, M., Hermans, J., Van De Velde, C. J. H., and Cornelisse, C. J. (1990). *Int. J. Cancer,* **45,** 34–9.
33. Hiddemann, W., Schumann, J., Andreef, M., Barlogie, B., Murphy, R. F., and Sandberg, A. A. (1984). *Cancer Genet. Cytogenet.,* **13,** 181–3.
34. Sigurdsson, H., Baldetorp, B., Borg, A., Dalberg, M., Ferno, M., Killander, D., *et al.* (1990). *Br. J. Cancer,* **62,** 786–90.
35. Kallioniemi, O-P., Blanko, G., Alavaikko, M., Heitanen, T., Mattila, J., Lauslahti, K., *et al.* (1988). *Cancer,* **62,** 2183–90.
36. Moll, R., Franke, W. W., and Schiller, D. L. (1982). *Cell,* **31,** 11–24.
37. Lindberg, K. and Rheinwald, J. G. (1989). *Am. J. Pathol.,* **134,** 89–98.
38. Jarasch, E-D., Nagle, R. B., Kaufmann, M., Maurer, C., and Bocker, W. J. (1988). *Human Pathol.,* **19,** 276–89.
39. Pellegrino, M. B., Asch, B. B., Connolly, J. L., and Asch, H. L. (1988). *Cancer Res.,* **48,** 5831–6.
40. Gerdes, J., Schwab, U., Lemke, H., and Stein, H. (1983). *Int. J. Cancer,* **31,** 13–20.
41. Kurki, P., Ogata, K., and Tan, E. M. (1988). *J. Immunol. Methods,* **109,** 49–59.
42. Landberg, G. and Roos, G. (1991). *Cancer Res.,* **51,** 4570–4.

43. Morstyn, G., Hsu, S. M., Kinsella, H., Gratzner, H., Russo, A., and Mitchell, J. B. (1983). *J. Clin. Invest.*, **72,** 1844–50.
44. Carlton, J. C., Terry, N. H. A., and White, R. A. (1991). *Cytometry,* **12,** 645–50.
45. Morrow, C. S. and Cowan, K. H. (1988). *Oncology,* **2,** 55–66.

4

(Glyco-) protein antigens and peptide epitopes of tumours

MICHAEL R. PRICE

1. Introduction

The concept that malignant tumours possess antigens capable of eliciting immune responses which may limit tumour growth is both appealing and supported by considerable experimental evidence. It is also one of the fundamental concepts upon which the foundations of tumour immunology rest. From extensive animal studies on the induction of immunity to carcinogen-induced tumours, it was shown that most, if not all, chemical carcinogens tested are capable of inducing tumours which carry individually distinct tumour-specific rejection antigens (see Chapter 2). Classically, tumour rejection antigens have been identified on transplanted animal tumours by showing that immunization with tumour cells rendered incapable of continuous growth confers protection against subsequent challenge with viable cells of the same tumour (1–3). The expression of these antigens by malignant cells is an hereditable characteristic, the immune responses they induce are exquisitely specific but the underlying molecular basis for the recognition of tumours by the immune system has yet to be resolved—the phenomenology has been extensively researched but, as yet, the structural basis for antigen expression defies persistent enquiry (4). The lack of reproducible and consistent humoral responses of the host against its tumour has further precluded comprehensive serological investigation.

While the demonstration of tumour-specific rejection antigens has been a major influence in establishing interest in the study of tumour immunology, attention is currently focused upon other macromolecular antigens of clinical relevance to malignant disease. The use of anti-tumour antibodies raised in other species, as probes of cell-surface architecture offers an alternative route for characterizing molecules preferentially found on malignant cells. The development of murine monoclonal antibodies (5) for exploring human tumours has been particularly rewarding and has facilitated the introduction of novel strategies for diagnosis and therapy. It should be emphasized here that such molecules, while being elevated on malignant cells, may have no relevance whatsoever to host immunity to tumours. Even so, the application of these reagents in tumour immunobiology may lead to the identification of other cellular features and their associated macromolecules which may be manipulated to affect the growth of tumours. Therefore, while these approaches with monoclonal antibodies may not necessarily lead to an understanding of the structural basis of tumour immunity, they may focus attention upon other functionally relevant targets for therapeutic manipulation (e.g. growth factor receptors, adhesion molecules, specific transport systems, etc.).

The purpose of this chapter is to offer the immunobiologist a number of basic strategies leading towards a molecular definition of their antigens of interest. Attention will be somewhat directed towards protein (or glycoprotein) antigens defined by monoclonal antibodies since these represent a major class of tumour-associated products currently under investigation. The methodologies and general approaches outlined are intended to be of relevance to developing a more precise appreciation at the molecular level of antigens associated with malignant disease, whether they be defined by interaction with antibody, or indeed other elements of an ongoing immune response. Indeed, analysis of factors involved in the molecular recognition of tumours may ultimately provide a structural basis for the antigens which so often have stimulated research in tumour immunology, the tumour-specific rejection antigens.

2. The tumour cell surface

The tumour cell surface is the primary site for immune recognition of the malignant cell. The association of protein and glycoprotein tumour antigens with the lipid bilayer of the plasma membrane may be categorized into:

(a) integral (intrinsic) membrane proteins which span or are anchored within the lipid bilayer

(b) peripheral (extrinsic) proteins which are more loosely associated with the surface, interacting with the bilayer by means of weak electrostatic forces

Thus, while integral membrane proteins are bound by hydrophobic interactions and require detergents for extraction, peripheral membrane proteins may be released by treatments which leave the integrity of the membrane intact. Exogenous components (such as proteins from tissue-culture media) which support the growth of cells *in vitro* may also become incorporated into the cell plasma membrane so that care must be taken, when raising antisera for example, not to be misled by artefactually generated antigenic determinants.

There appear to be no major prominent features of the tumour cell surface which markedly distinguish it from the normal cell counterpart. In tumours, the increase (or decrease) of any particular surface component, may merely be a biochemical description of a morphological change (e.g. the loss or reduction of expression of junctional complexes in tumours will produce a different profile of plasma membrane-associated macromolecules which is unrelated to the induction or expression of neoantigens). There is evidence for elevated levels of sialic acid, a terminal sugar of membrane glycoproteins and glycolipids, so that tumour cells may exhibit an increased electronegative charge. Aberrant glycosylation of membrane glycoproteins and glycolipids, or the action of tumour glycosidases, may favour the accumulation of precursor carbohydrate structures and truncated oligosaccharide side chains (6). These are not necessarily profound changes and it could be argued that the outstanding feature of tumour and normal cell surfaces is their similarity.

3. Anti-tumour antibodies

A variety of antigens which, if not specific for tumours, are at least considerably elevated on them, have been identified using murine monoclonal antibodies (7, 8). However, even before the availability of such reagents, antisera raised in animals were successfully employed to identify clinically significant markers of human tumours including carcinoembryonic antigen (CEA) (9) and alpha foetoprotein (AFP) (10).

Having developed a monoclonal antibody using hybridoma technology, or indeed an antiserum with which antigen expression may be explored, the problems of storage and purification will be considered.

3.1 Antibody storage and stability

Antibodies in serum or ascitic fluids are relatively stable to long term storage at −20°C or below. However, since repeated freezing and thawing causes aggregation and a loss in activity, storage in appropriate aliquots is recommended. Aggregates should be removed before use by centrifugation (10 000*g* for 5 min using a bench microcentrifuge is usually sufficient) or by ultrafiltration.

Monoclonal antibodies in tissue-culture supernatants are usually stable to storage at 5°C for periods of several months and longer, provided that microbial contamination is minimized by the addition of NaN_3 to 0.05%, and the pH is adjusted to neutrality, if necessary.

Purified antibodies should be stored in isotonic solution at neutral pH (e.g. PBS, pH 7.3) in aliquots at −20°C or below, or with 0.05% NaN_3 at 5°C. Concentrations of 1 mg/ml or greater are recommended.

3.2 Antibody purification

Murine IgG monoclonal antibodies in tissue-culture supernatants and ascitic fluids may be most conveniently purified by their binding to, and elution from

Sepharose-linked Protein A or G (Pharmacia). Simple affinity chromatography (performed according to the manufacturer's instructions) frequently yields antibody preparations of greater than 95% purity. Particulate material (hybridoma cell debris) is first eliminated from the sample by centrifugation (typically, in our laboratory, 40 000*g* for 1 h) and ascitic fluids are diluted 1/10 with PBS before application to the column.

Protein A has varying affinity for the different mouse IgG subclasses and with the lowest affinity for IgG1. Adjusting the pH of the sample to 8.0 promotes IgG1 binding. After washing non-bound material from the column, bound antibody may be eluted with 0.1 M glycine–HCl, pH 2.8 or 3 M NaSCN. When fractionating mouse serum or ascitic fluid, individual sub-classes of mouse immunoglobulin may be selectively desorbed from the Protein A–agarose matrix by sequential elution with 0.1 M citrate buffers of increasing acidity (11) as follows:

- pH 6.0 for IgG1
- pH 4.5 for IgG2a (and the minor sub-class, IgG3)
- pH 3.5 for IgG2b

Clearly, the volume of each wash solution will depend upon the scale of the fractionation, but as a general rule each wash cycle with buffer should be at least five times the volume of the column.

Protein A linked to agarose matrices can be used for repeated fractionations. However, it is an expensive reagent and it is worth placing a guard column containing unsubstituted agarose beads in series immediately before the affinity column. During elution of an antibody from the column, the antibody may be rapidly separated from the potentially denaturing environment of the eluate by connecting a desalting column containing Sephadex G25 immediately following the affinity column.

For the purification of murine IgM antibodies. Sepharose-linked lentil-lectin (12) and Sepharose-linked protamine sulphate (11) have been employed.

Other methods for antibody purification include a broad range of conventional methods involving precipitation and column chromatography (13) although none produce the degree of purity achieved with relative ease using affinity techniques.

Antibody concentrations are determined by UV absorbance at 280 nm assuming that 1 mg/ml solutions of IgG and IgM give measurements of 1.43 and 1.19, respectively. Antibody purity is checked by analysis of a sample by SDS-PAGE (14, 15). A sample of the antibody solution is prepared under reducing and non-reducing conditions so that intact immunoglobulin and immunoglobulin subunits (heavy and light chains) respectively, can be identified. Sample overloading permits low-level contaminants to be located (e.g. albumin at 68 kd).

4. Immunoassays

The activity of purified monoclonal antibody is checked most conveniently by titration using an appropriate immunoassay. Comparisons with the starting material can be made and activity can be related to protein concentration. Methodologies for the quantitation of protein are described in detail by Harlow and Lane (16).

Immunoassays also provide the means to characterize the activity of purified and crude preparations of tumour antigens, as well as to probe other properties, such as relative antibody binding affinities, repeated expression of epitopes on individual antigenic molecules, and topographical relationships of different determinants on antigens. Selection of the assay procedure will obviously depend upon the nature of the information sought, but the three types of immunoassay are illustrative of commonly employed techniques. In the examples described a radioisotope, commonly ^{125}I, has been used as the trace agent, although there are a large number of methods available from the immunochemical literature (e.g. 11, 16).

Figure 1 illustrates the basic principles of the assays described. In each case, either antigen or antibody is adsorbed to a surface, most commonly the surface of wells of a standard 8 × 12 well microtitre plate. Only a small proportion of the added antigen is actually bound, but this is sufficient to work with. The preparations of antigen used for these assays include purified antigens (dispensed from solutions at concentrations in the region of 1 μg/ml), tumour membrane preparations (dispensed from suspensions containing in the region of 100 μg membrane protein/ml), and intact tumour cells which can be fixed to the surface with glutaraldehyde or cultured as adherent monolayers in the wells. Adsorption of protein or glycoprotein antigens to the surfaces of microtitre plate wells may be achieved by incubation for a few hours at room temperature or, with more stable antigens (e.g. carcinoembryonic antigen, tumour mucins), the antigen can be dried on to the plate. Antigen solutions may be prepared in a simple buffered saline solution (e.g. PBS at pH 7.3) or using carbonate buffers at pH 9.0. Once adsorbed to the plate, the antigen remains firmly associated with the surface and is not removed by repeated and vigorous washing. However, whether antigen (*Figure 1a* and *1b*) or antibody (*Figure 1c*) is immobilized at the surface, it is absolutely necessary to block any remaining unoccupied non-specific adsorption sites with an excess of an unrelated protein. Bovine serum albumin (0.1 to 1.0%), casein solutions (0.1%), or solutions containing an irrelevant serum (1 to 5%) are usually employed for this purpose, and non-specific binding may be reduced by the inclusion of a non-ionic detergent (e.g. 0.1% Tween 20) in the washing buffers (usually simple buffered saline solutions).

In our laboratories, in order to economize on the consumption of antigen, we have utilized Terasaki HLA plates with well capacities of 10 μl for various solid-phase immunoassays. The following procedures relate to the use of

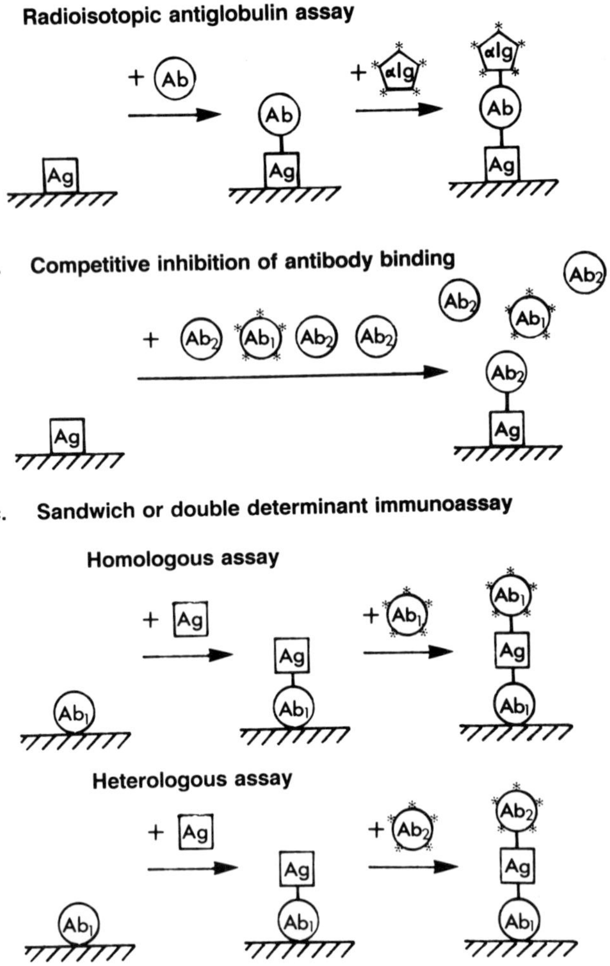

Figure 1. Solid-phase immunoassays for the analysis of monoclonal antibody reactivity with tumour-associated antigens.

these plates although the general comments are relevant to all solid-phase immunoassays.

4.1 Radioisotopic antiglobulin assay

Figure 1a illustrates the principle of this procedure and the following protocol describes the assay using CEA as an example.

Protocol 1. Measurement of antibody binding to CEA using a radioisotopic antiglobulin assay

1. Dispense CEA (at between 1 to 5 μg/ml) in PBS into the wells of Terasaki HLA plates (Nunc) at 10 μl/well.

2. Incubate the plates overnight at room temperature or for 2 h at 37°C.
3. Wash the plates four times with a washing buffer (0.1% casein in PBS) using a standard wash bottle to direct the solution into each well. During the final wash cycle, incubate the wells for at least 30 min in buffer to block any remaining non-specific adsorption sites.
4. Remove the wash buffer by plate inversion and vigorous shaking. Dispense purified monoclonal antibodies (10, 1, and 0.1 μg/ml) or tissue-culture supernatants (1/1 to $1/10^3$) or ascitic fluids ($1/10^3$ to $1/10^6$) diluted in washing buffer (or for negative controls, washing buffer alone) into the wells of the plate at 10 μl/well.
5. Incubate the assay for 60 min at room temperature, with the plate lids in place.
6. Remove the antibody solutions by aspiration and wash four times with washing buffer.
7. To each well, add 10 μl of $[^{125}I]F(ab')_2$ fragments of an affinity-purified anti-mouse Ig reagent (this can be prepared in-house or obtained commercially). The labelled antiglobulin is added at 10^5 c.p.m. per well at a concentration of about 10 ng protein per well. Radiolabelling is performed using the chloramine-T procedure using 18.5 mBq and 25 μg protein (at 1 mg/ml) (17). Specific activities of greater than 0.37 mBq/μg are achieved and the labelled antiglobulin is stored at −20°C in small aliquots.
8. Incubate the assay for 1 h, then remove excess reagent by aspiration and wash the wells with washing buffer.
9. Finally, carefully cut the plates into strips of wells with a band saw and separate the individual wells using wire cutters.
10. Determine the radioactivity remaining in each well using a gamma counter.

Table 1 illustrates the binding of several anti-CEA monoclonal antibodies to CEA and the normal cross-reacting antigen, NCA. Clearly antibodies 11.285.14, C365, and C337 are specifically reactive with CEA while antibodies C161 and C198 are not, and identify epitopes common to CEA and NCA (18).

4.2 Competitive inhibition of antibody binding

With this assay, antigen is again adsorbed to the wells of the microtest plates and remaining non-specific adsorption sites are blocked with excess protein. Radiolabelled antibody (Ab_1 in *Figure 1b*) is then added to each well in admixture with control wash buffer solution or in admixture with varying amounts of unlabelled antibody (Ab_2 in *Figure 1b*). In practice, this is most simply performed by adding 5 μl aliquots of the competing antibody or control solution to the wells followed by 5 μl of the radiolabelled antibody.

Table 1. Binding of anti-CEA monoclonal antibodies as assessed using a solid phase micro-radioisotopic antiglobulin assay

Monoclonal antibody	Mean c.p.m. ± SD bound to:	
	CEA	NCA
11.285.14	6132 ± 202	65 ± 87
C337	7341 ± 494	16 ± 21
C365	8220 ± 646	33 ± 3
C161	8532 ± 588	7174 ± 323
C198	7140 ± 356	5081 ± 135

Labelling of the antibody may be achieved as described in *Protocol 1* or using the less denaturing Iodogen procedure (19, 20). Again, the reagent is added to give 10^5 c.p.m. per well. Incubation is continued for 1 to 2 h before aspiration of unbound reagent, plate washing, and determination of radioactivity in each well. With this procedure, if the unlabelled and labelled antibodies are reactive with the same or closely related epitopes, then the binding of excess unlabelled antibody will prevent the binding of the labelled component. For a detailed discussion of how to radiolabel antibodies, see Chapter 13.

In *Figure 2*, the specific anti-CEA antibodies 11.285.14, C365, and C337, when radiolabelled with ^{125}I, are only inhibited in their binding to CEA by their unlabelled counterparts so that it can be concluded that the three antibodies define separate (CEA-specific, *Table 1*) epitopes on the antigen. Competitive inhibition experiments such as these have been carried out in extensive collaborative studies to define the major immunodominant domains (i.e. clusters of epitopes) associated with CEA (21). Similar tests have been performed upon monoclonal-antibody-defined epitopes upon breast and ovarian carcinoma-associated mucins (22).

4.3 Sandwich or double-determinant immunoassay

Using the sandwich immunoassay (*Figure 1c*), antibody is first adsorbed to the wells of the microtest plates. After washing and blocking, this is followed by antigen which is captured by the immobilized antibody. The presence of bound antigen can then be measured by the binding of a second radiolabelled antibody to complete the 'sandwich'.

The binding of antibody to the solid phase is accomplished by incubation of antibody (purified, at 1 to 10 μg/ml, or as diluted ascitic fluid or hyperimmune serum, at a dilution in the region of $1/10^3$) in the wells of the microtest plates (antibody, unlike many antigens, will not survive drying to the wells without substantial loss in activity). Antigen can be added in a purified form or, more

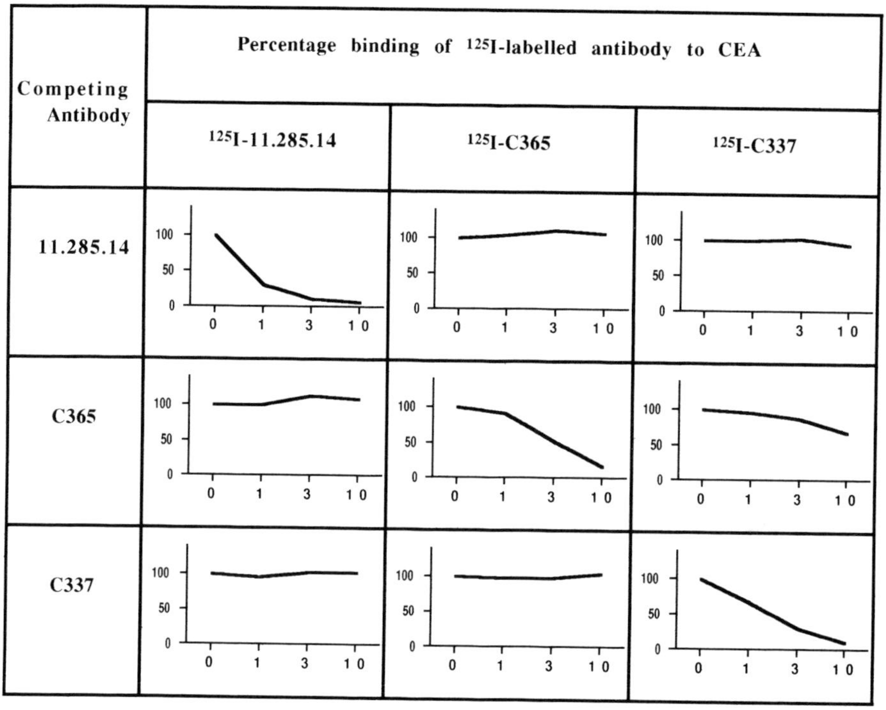

Figure 2. Competitive inhibition of binding of ^{125}I-labelled anti-CEA antibody to CEA. Unlabelled antibodies, 11.285.14, C365, and C337 were tested as 'cold' antibody inhibitors at concentrations of 1, 3, and 10 μg/ml.

commonly, in a complex solution. (This immunoassay procedure is the basis of many techniques for the quantitation of antigens in complex solutions, such as patient serum or cell membranes.) The second antibody, added as tracer, is radiolabelled as described in the previous section and the blocking and washing is performed as with the other assays (Sections 4.1 and 4.2).

If the capture and tracer antibodies are the same, then the binding of the labelled tracer antibody only occurs if the epitope is a repeated structure on the antigen (i.e. the homologous double-determinant immunoassay, *Figure 1c*). Alternatively, if the two antibodies are different, then it is only possible for the tracer antibody to bind if the epitopes defined by the two antibodies are co-expressed upon the same antigen molecule (i.e. the heterologous double-determinant immunoassay, *Figure 1c*).

Table 2 shows that the CEA-specific antibody C365, when adsorbed to the plate is able to capture CEA, and that this CEA may further bind the CEA-specific antibody 11.285.14 added as the radiolabelled tracer. The two determinants defined by C365 and 11.285.14 are therefore separate and distinct. However, CEA bound to immobilized antibody C365 is unable to

Table 2. Sandwich or double-determinant immunoassay

Monoclonal antibody used as 'capture' antibody	Binding of radiolabelled 'tracer' antibody (mean c.p.m. ± SD) to CEA bound to the plate by the adsorbed 'capture' antibody	
	[^{125}I]11.285.14	[^{125}I]C365
11.285.14	123 ± 221	23584 ± 514
C365	14687 ± 157	242 ± 44

bind radiolabelled antibody C365 suggesting that the epitope defined by this antibody is not a repeated determinant. Conversely, when 11.285.14 was employed as the capture antibody, a 'sandwich' could only be formed with radiolabelled C365 and not with radiolabelled 11.285.14, indicating again that their respective epitopes were co-expressed upon the CEA molecule and also that the 11.285.14-defined epitope is not a repeated structure of the antigen.

5. Tumour homogenization and sub-cellular fractionation

5.1 Homogenization

For the isolation of antigen from tumours, it is frequently considered useful to enrich antigenic activity within a particular sub-cellular fraction. Since most antigens of interest are expressed at the cell surface where they may interact with antibody or sensitized lymphoid cells, then homogenization and elimination of cell nuclei and the soluble intracytoplasmic protein may provide a crude membrane fraction which is considerably enriched in antigenic activity.

Several factors initially influence decisions relating to the selection of the homogenization procedure. Firstly, the amount of material to be disrupted has to be considered. For small-scale homogenizations, it is feasible to use simple hand-operated or motor-driven tight-fitting pestle-type homogenizers with which disruption is effected through shearing forces within the homogenization medium. Care has to be taken to minimize local heating effects which are potentially denaturing. Other methods applicable to small amount of tissue (of the order of a few grams) or suspensions of cells from tissue culture include sonication and nitrogen cavitation, although again care has to be taken to avoid denaturation (e.g. through heating in the case of sonication). When larger quantities of tissue are required to be processed, then it is advisable to select more powerful homogenizers of the rotating-blade type, with which it is possible to process suspensions containing several hundred grams of tissue. In this case, before starting homogenization, it is advisable to reduce the tissue essentially to a mince using simple kitchen equipment.

Homogenization may be most simply monitored by phase contrast microscopy and the increasing release of free cell nuclei is a good measure of cell disruption. The choice of homogenization medium will also influence the ease with which disruption is achieved. A hypotonic buffer (e.g. 1 mM sodium bicarbonate) assists the ease of homogenization by osmotically swelling the cells and rendering them more sensitive to mechanical trauma. However, it may be necessary here to add low concentrations of Ca^{2+} and Mg^{2+} (2 mM) which help to prevent cell nuclei from swelling and leaking their contents into the medium. Leakage of DNA into the homogenate gives rise to problems of contamination by adsorption to subcellular membranes. For tissues or cells which are particularly sensitive to homogenization, then the medium should be isotonic to preserve the integrity of intracellular organelles. Phenyl methyl sulphonyl fluoride (PMSF, 20–100 μg/ml) may be added to the homogenization medium as an inhibitor of proteolysis; other enzyme inhibitors are available for specific proteases (11).

5.2 Sub-cellular fractionation

Since plasma membranes represent only about 1% of the total cellular protein, then sub-cellular fractionation leading to membrane purification will produce a considerable enrichment of cell-surface antigens. While there are numerous procedures for this purpose, some common features can be identified. Nuclei, whole cell, tissue fragments, and connective tissue debris can all be eliminated by low-speed centrifugation (600*g* for 10 min). All particulate material remaining in the supernatant after removal of these materials, can be sedimented by ultracentrifugation (100 000*g* for 1 h). This provides a pellet of crude sub-cellular membranes which can be fractionated further by differential centrifugation or subjected to antigen extraction.

Pelleted membrane materials are re-suspended in isotonic media using syringe and needle (21 gauge) to obtain a homogeneous dispersion. Storage at −20°C or below is recommended.

6. Antigen degradation studies

Limited information concerning the characteristics of tumour antigens and their epitopes may be obtained by undertaking investigation of the susceptibility of the antigen to various denaturants. For this approach, experiments can be performed utilizing impure preparations of antigen and, it is feasible to obtain molecular information on the characteristics of an antigen using whole cells or membrane fractions. Essentially, antigenic material is subjected to treatment (physical treatments, enzymic, or chemical) and the retention of antigenic activity is assessed by appropriate immunoassay (e.g. Section 4).

Physical treatments such as susceptibility to heat may provide an indication of the overall stability of the antigenic molecule and the dependence upon protein conformation for the full expression of antigenic activity. If treatment of cells or membranes expressing the antigen of interest with proteolytic enzymes releases antigenic activity this offers a method for the solubilization of an antigenic membrane-associated protein or glycoprotein fragment, but if activity is destroyed, this implicates peptide involvement in the expression of the epitope.

The use of glycolytic enzymes may provide information concerning the nature of carbohydrates associated with the antigen or included within an epitope. Further information concerning the requirement for carbohydrates for the full expression of antigenic activity may be obtained by examining the susceptibility of antigen to agents such as sodium periodate, which cleaves vicinal hydroxyl groups. These treatments may also expose cryptic determinants previously 'masked' in the mature glycoprotein (23). Other chemical treatments that may be informative include reduction and alkylation for the examination of antigen expression upon an individual peptide chain of a complex antigen in which separate polypeptide chains are linked by disulphide bonds. Furthermore, the sequential fragmentation of a protein antigen using specific proteases and/or chemicals such as CNBr (which cleaves peptides at methionine residues), may yield antigenic fragments of a size which can be subjected to comprehensive compositional analysis and amino acid sequencing. The chemical and enzymic treatments developed for peptide mapping (24) can be particularly useful in antigen degradation studies.

7. Antigen solubilization

The prime consideration in the selection of a procedure for solubilization of antigen is that antigenic activity is preserved. Given this pre-condition, the complete range of procedures for extracting an antigenic membrane protein from its cellular environment is available. Procedures which, though effective in releasing antigenic material, are poorly understood in their mode of action, should be avoided since an interpretation of the results obtained with respect to the characteristics of the antigen will be difficult. Thus, while in the past the use of 3 M KCl was widely adopted for antigen solubilization from cells and tissues, the mode by which antigen was solubilized was generally unknown. It was not possible, therefore, to relate the findings to the overall molecular characteristics of the antigen since there was no assurance that the material isolated was not an artefact (e.g. an antigenic fragment produced by proteolysis) of the extraction process.

8. Antigen purification

8.1 Strategies

Before deciding to proceed with antigen purification it is worth considering the logistics of the exercise. In particular, the scale of the experiment needs to be defined. If, for example, a membrane protein of say, 60 kd is to be isolated and there are 10^5 copies per cell, then to obtain a few micrograms of purified antigen (e.g. 10 μg), a total of at least 10^9 cells would be required as well as 100% recovery of product at each stage of the fractionation! While it is feasible to generate such cell numbers from tissue culture, efficiencies at this level cannot be achieved. Alternatively, with an antigen such as CEA, which is produced in large amounts by liver metastases of colonic carcinomas, it is possible to begin an extraction with 1 kg of tissue and expect a recovery of 50 to 100 mg of pure product (25).

In the ideal case, with each stage in the purification, the recovery of antigenic activity should be assessed in order to maximize the efficiency of the fractionation procedure (26).

At the outset, the complete range of biochemical chromatographic and precipitation procedures are available for the purification of antigen from complex mixtures. For initial fractionation steps, it is advisable to select techniques which are able to handle large sample volumes and, indeed, concentrate the antigenic material. For example, antigen may be selectively removed from large sample volumes using affinity chromatography and eluted in concentrated form. Alternatively, ion-exchange chromatographic techniques which may also lead to product concentration, can be designed around the purification of a particular macromolecule.

It is useful to reserve techniques that require small sample volumes (e.g. molecular sieve chromatography, CsCl density gradient centrifugation, gel electrophoresis, etc.) for the latter stages of a purification when the bulk of the contaminants have been eliminated.

8.2 Lectin affinity chromatography of glycoproteins

A range of lectins immobilized on agarose beads is available commercially from companies such as Pharmacia and these are accompanied by appropriate methodological protocols for their use. Separations usually involve binding glycoproteins from a soluble extract, followed by washing to eliminate non-bound and non-specifically bound materials. The glycoproteins can then be eluted from the matrix by application of the appropriate sugar solution.

Several of the immobilized lectins function perfectly well in the presence of a detergent so that detergent-solubilized extracts of cell membrane-derived materials can be fractionated in this way (12).

8.3 Antibody affinity chromatography

The purification of antigens by affinity chromatography using immobilized antibodies represents one of the most powerful and effective separative procedures available. There are numerous protocols for this technique but one which has found application for several tumour antigens (including membrane-associated antigens) (22, 23, 27) defined by anti-tumour monoclonal antibodies is as follows:

Protocol 2. Purification of tumour membrane-associated antigens by antibody affinity chromatography

1. Substitute CNBr-activated Sepharose with antibody according to the manufacturer's instructions. Routinely, a coupling efficiency of greater than 95% should be expected. (Activation of Sepharose with CNBr can be performed in the laboratory (11) although CNBr is volatile and extremely toxic and must be handled in a fume cupboard.)
2. Pack the immunoadsorbent into a chromatography column and pre-wash the column with the agent (100 mM diethylamine, pH 11.5) to be used for antigen elution.
3. Sediment a crude tumour sub-cellular membrane preparation (Section 5.2) and extract with 0.5% NP-40 in 0.1 M Tris–HCl, pH 7.0 (added at 5 ml per g of original tissue) for 30 min at 5°C.
4. Clarify the extract by centrifugation at 100 000*g* for 60 min and pump the supernatant on to the column. For convenience, the extract may be recycled continuously through the column.
5. Wash the column[a] successively with:
   - 0.5% NP-40 in 0.1 M Tris–HCl (pH 7.6)
   - 0.2% NP-40 in 0.1 M Tris–HCl containing 1 M NaCl (pH 7.6)
   - 0.1% NP-40 in 0.1 M Tris–HCl (pH 7.6)
6. Apply 100 mM diethylamine (pH 11.5) to the column to elute the antigen. Fractions are collected into tubes containing sufficient 1 M Tris–HCl (pH 7.6) to adjust the pH of the fraction to less than 8.0.
7. Identify antigen-containing fractions using an appropriate immunoassay (e.g. Section 4). Those fractions containing antigen are pooled, dialysed against PBS (and concentrated if necessary), and stored in small aliquots at −20°C. If any aggregation has occurred during this latter processing, then insoluble material should be removed by centrifugation before storage.
8. Analyse the antigen preparation for homogeneity (e.g. SDS-PAGE) (15) and antigenic activity (e.g. Section 4).

[a] The volume of each wash solution will depend upon the scale of the fractionation, but as a general rule each wash cycle with buffer should be at least five times the volume of the column.

9. Radiolabelling cell-surface proteins and glycoproteins

Since many cell-surface proteins and glycoproteins may only be present in minute quantities, it can be an advantage to radiolabel these components so that they may be traced throughout purification and/or biochemical characterization.

Cell-surface proteins and glycoproteins may be conveniently radioiodinated by lactoperoxidase catalysed iodination (16, 28, 29). Since the high molecular weight of the enzyme precludes its passage through the plasma membrane and denies access to the cytoplasm, then only cell-surface-expressed components are radiolabelled. An example of a protocol for the radiolabelling of cells in suspension using this approach is as follows:

Protocol 3. Radioiodination of cell-surface proteins

1. Re-suspend a pellet of tumour cells (10^7, previously washed with ice-cold PBS) in 1 ml PBS.
2. To this suspension, add;
   - 10 µl 0.5 M glucose
   - 100 µg glucose oxidase
   - 20 µg lactoperoxidase
   - 10 µl ^{125}I (37 mBq carrier-free $Na^{125}I$)
3. Incubate the cell suspension at room temperature for 15 min, with frequent re-suspension of the cells.
4. Wash the cells four times by centrifugation (200*g* for 5 min) with 20 ml aliquots of ice-cold PBS.
5. The final cell pellet contains surface-membrane-iodinated proteins and glycoproteins. Using the radiolabel as a tracer, selective investigation of cell-surface-associated proteins may be achieved.

It is feasible to use other methods of labelling (reviewed in (16)) which preferentially act upon cell-surface-associated macromolecules—low concentrations of sodium metaperiodate induce specific oxidate cleavage of sialic acids which can then be reduced with sodium boro-[^3H]hydride to incorporate tritium.

Alternative procedures for radiolabelling, such as the biosynthetic incorporation of radioactive amino acids into cell protein, are less specific in labelling surface moieties compared with the methods described. However, by biosynthetic labelling with radioactive sugars, it is possible to selectively label glycosylated materials (16).

10. Immunoprecipitation

Analysis of radiolabelled antigen in immunoprecipitates provides a means to characterize the antigen by following the radioactive tracer. Determination of the (apparent) molecular weight of an antigen by SDS-PAGE (15) is a major application of this approach. A practical example of the procedure is as follows:

Protocol 4. Radioimmunoprecipitation of radiolabelled membrane-associated antigens

1. Re-suspend a cell pellet of approximately 10^7 surface-iodinated cells (*Protocol 3*) in 1.0 ml of an immunoprecipitation (IP) buffer containing TNEN (10 mM Tris, 100 mM NaCl, 1 mM EDTA, 0.5% NP-40) and 0.5% Na deoxycholate, 10 mM NaI, pH 7.5. Specific protease inhibitors may also be included in this extraction medium (11).
2. Incubate the cell suspension on ice for 60 min, centrifuge the suspension (100 000*g* for 60 min) and then collect the supernatant, which contains the soluble radiolabelled surface proteins.
3. Dispense aliquots (50 or 100 μl) of the extract into glass ignition tubes (approximately 1 × 7 cm, capacity about 5 ml) followed by equal volumes of IP buffer containing 2% BSA and 0.2% SDS.
4. Form radioactive immune complexes by adding an appropriate antibody (e.g. 5 μl aliquots of hybridoma ascitic fluid or purified antibody in the region of 0.1 to 1 mg/ml). Incubate the reaction for 60 min at 0°C.
5. Collect radioactive immune complexes upon Sepharose-linked Protein A (added at 50 μg Protein A per tube—equivalent to 100 μl of a 1/4 dilution in IP buffer). The Sepharose–Protein A is kept in suspension by gentle rocking (with care being taken to avoid the Sepharose beads collecting on the walls of the tubes) and incubated for 20 min at 0°C.
6. Wash the radioactive Sepharose–Protein A beads by low-speed centrifugation (200*g* for 5 min) with 5 ml aliquots per tube of:
   - IP buffer containing 2% BSA and 0.1% SDS (three washes)
   - 1/10 dilution of TNEN buffer (three washes)
7. Count the final pellets for radioactivity in a gamma counter. Then dissociate the radioactive antigen from the complex by adding 50 μl of SDS-PAGE sample buffer to each tube and boiling for 2 to 3 min. The sample buffer may be prepared with a reducing agent (1% mercaptoethanol) in order to analyse antigen subunits.
8. Apply the samples released from the Sepharose–Protein A complexes to an SDS-PAGE gel and perform electrophoresis (15).
9. Fix and stain the gel with Coomassie blue to reveal the position of the chosen molecular weight marker proteins.
10. Dry the gel and subject it to autoradiography (16) to trace the positions

of the radiolabelled antigen. Comparison of the mobility of the antigen revealed upon the X-ray film with that of the marker proteins on the stained gel permits an apparent molecular weight to be assigned to the antigen and/or its subunits.

11. Immunoblotting

Western blotting techniques originally described by Towbin *et al.* (30) have been extensively applied to the identification and apparent molecular weight determination of monoclonal-antibody-defined antigens, which are present in complex extracts of tumour cells or tissues (usually rendered soluble by detergent treatment). With this procedure, an SDS-PAGE gel in which antigenic proteins have been separated is placed on a sheet of nitrocellulose. The two are held in close contact in an appropriate blotting apparatus and the proteins are transferred from the gel to the nitrocellulose by application of an electric current at right angles to the face of the gel. Non-specific protein binding sites on the nitrocellulose are then blocked with an irrelevant protein and the sheet can then be probed for the presence of an antigen by incubation with antibody. Bound antibody is then revealed using an antiglobulin linked to a tracer reagent (e.g. radioactive iodine for autoradiographic detection, or an enzyme to be used in conjunction with a substrate which produces a coloured insoluble product). From the mobility of the stained antigen, an apparent molecular weight is determined by comparison with molecular weight marker proteins (which can be obtained as pre-stained markers which are visible on the nitrocellulose). The procedure of Western blotting and subsequent detection of antigens with monoclonal antibodies is the subject of several excellent articles (16, 30, 31).

12. Epitope mapping

The possibility of identifying the actual amino acids involved in the expression of a monoclonal-antibody-defined epitope expressed upon human tumours presents itself as an exciting prospect. Knowledge of an epitope sequence implies that the determinant may be synthesized, secondary structural features may be characterized using aproaches such as high field NMR (32, 33), and the problem becomes accessible to computational chemistry and molecular modelling (33, 34). With parallel developments in sequencing the variable regions of antibodies and identifying sequences of the complementarity-determining regions of antibodies (35), study of the interaction of an antibody with its epitope becomes a classic investigation upon the molecular recognition of a ligand with its receptor.

If amino acid sequence data are available for the antigenic protein, then a first approach to identify the epitope is to use the Pepscan procedure developed by Geysen *et al.* (36) and commercially available from Cambridge Research Biochemicals Ltd. Essentially, the strategy involves the detection of the binding of antibody to synthetic peptide synthesized upon the heads of polypropylene pins. The synthetic chemistry has been developed to a stage where it is feasible to produce hundreds of different peptides immobilized upon the pins within the period of a few days. Thus, for a given protein antigen of known sequence, it is then possible to produce a series of short peptides of between 6 to 12 amino acids which overlap by a constant number of residues, and these may span the complete protein sequence. With a short sequence of 20 amino acids, for example, a series of 14 heptapeptides, each of which overlaps its neighbour in six residues, would cover the complete sequence. These synthetic peptides can then be examined for antibody binding activity using standard ELISA techniques and the residues which are common to the positive antibody-binding pins represent the minimum binding structure or epitope for that antibody (e.g. reference (34)). Conversely, for a larger protein of, say 200 amino acids, it is less practical to produce a series of peptides which overlap their neighbour in all but one residue, and it becomes more realistic to produce a series of sequential 10-mers each of which overlaps its neighbour in five residues (thus spanning the complete 200-amino-acid protein) and these can be tested for antibody binding.

A major advantage of these technologies is that after finishing an analysis of binding for one particular antibody, all pins can be stripped completely of bound antibody and tracer antiglobulin reagents, leaving the immobilized peptide available for testing against a second antibody. Solid phase-linked peptides prepared in this way can be used many times for the screening of panels of related monoclonal antibodies (34, 37).

These epitope mapping procedures work exquisitely well for selected protein antigens with epitopes in which the amino acids are in a linear sequence ('continuous' epitopes). If an epitope involves secondary structural features, such as the bringing together of two or more portions of a polypeptide chain or indeed two adjacent chains to form 'discontinuous' epitopes, then the Pepscan procedure will fail to identify this type of binding site.

The strategy for production of multiple peptides for testing against an antibody has recently been considerably extended by developing procedures for synthesizing millions of different peptides to form a peptide library against which any antibody can be screened (38, 39). In the study by Lam *et al.* (38) peptides are synthesized upon bead resins, and by dividing and repooling the beads at each round of synthesis using all natural amino acids a collection of resin beads can be produced with each carrying a different peptide. The beads are tested for antibody binding using an enzyme or fluorescein-linked antibody to trace the few beads which bind antibody. A single positive bead is then separated from the rest and bound antibody is released with an appropriate dissociating agent. The peptide on the resin bead is then sequenced directly to determine the nature of the peptide recognized by that particular antibody (38).

This procedure is probably applicable to the study of any receptor ligand interaction, thereby offering the possibility of rapidly identifying particular motifs involved in the recognition of one molecule by another (38, 39).

13. Conclusions

The study of tumour-associated protein and glycoprotein antigens and peptide epitopes is reaching an exciting stage of development. Many solutions for present problems in the investigation and characterization of tumour antigens are available through application of standard methodologies of the protein chemist (40). However, novel strategies for producing peptide libraries (38, 39) for example, offer highly innovative approaches to explore the nature of molecules which can occupy the binding site of antibodies. In some instances, the fine specificity of antibody binding to its epitope appears to be controlled by immune recognition of determinants composed of as few as three, four, or five amino acids (34, 37). How such apparently minor determinants are recognized as tumour markers of real clinical utility is a puzzle yet to be resolved.

Acknowledgement

These studies were supported by the Cancer Research Campaign.

References

1. Foley, E. J. *Cancer Res.,* **13,** 835.
2. Prehn, R. T. and Main, J. M. (1955). *J. Natl Cancer Inst.,* **18,** 769.
3. Basombrió, M. (1970). *Cancer Res.,* **30,** 2458.
4. Srivastava, P. K. and Old, L. J. (1988). *Immunology Today,* **9,** 78.
5. Köhler, G. and Milstein, C. (1975). *Nature,* **256,** 495.
6. Hakomori, S. (1989). *Adv. Cancer Res.,* **52,** 257.
7. Kupchik, H. Z. (ed.) (1988). *Cancer Diagnosis In Vitro Using Monoclonal Antibodies.* Marcel Dekker, New York.
8. Boyer, C. M., Lidor, Y., Lottich, C., and Bast, R. C. (1988). *Antibody Immunoconjugates and Radiopharmaceuticals,* **1,** 105.
9. Gold, P. and Freedman, S. O. (1965). *J. Exp. Med.,* **122,** 467.
10. Abelev, G. I., Assecritova, I. V., Kraevsky, N. A., Perova, S. D., and Perevodchikova, N. I. (1967). *Int. J. Cancer,* **2,** 551.
11. Hudson, L. and Hay, F. C. (1989). *Practical Immunology,* 3rd edn. Blackwell Scientific, Oxford.
12. Takacs, B. and Staehelin, T. (1981). In *Immunological Methods*, (ed. I. Lefkovits and B. Pernis), Vol. 2, pp. 27–56. Academic, New York.

13. Stanworth, D. and Turner, M. W. (1986). In *Handbook of Experimental Immunology. Part 1. Immunochemistry,* (ed. D. M. Weir), 4th edn, pp. 12.1–12.46. Blackwell Scientific, Oxford.
14. Laemmli, U. K. (1970). *Nature,* **227,** 680.
15. See, Y. P. and Jackowski, G. (1990). In *Protein Structure: A Practical Approach*, (ed. T. E. Creighton), pp. 1–21. IRL Press, Oxford.
16. Harlow, E. and Lane, D. (1988). *Antibodies: A Laboratory Manual.* Cold Spring Harbor Press, Cold Spring Harbor, New York.
17. Jensenius, J. C. and Williams, A. F. (1974). *Eur. J. Immunol.,* **4,** 91.
18. Price, M. R. (1988). *Br. J. Cancer,* **57,** 165.
19. Fraker, P. J. and Speck, J. C. (1978). *Biochem. Biophys. Res. Commun.,* **80,** 849.
20. Pimm, M. V. and Gribben, S. J. (1993). In *Tumour Immunobiology: A Practical Approach,* (ed. Gallagher *et al.*), pp. 209–23. IRL Press, Oxford. (This volume.)
21. Hammarström, S., Shively, J. E., Paxton, R. J., Larsson, A., Ghosh, R., Bormer, O., *et al.* (1989). *Cancer Res.,* **49,** 4852.
22. Price, M. R., Edwards, S., Powell, M., and Baldwin, R. W. (1986). *Br. J. Cancer,* **54,** 393.
23. O'Sullivan, C., Price, M. R., and Baldwin, R. W. (1990). *Br. J. Cancer,* **61,** 801.
24. Carrey, E. A. (1990). In *Protein Structure: A Practical Approach*, (ed. T. E. Creighton), pp. 117–44. IRL Press, Oxford.
25. Krupey, J., Wilson, T., Freedman, S. O., and Gold, P. (1972). *Immunochemistry,* **9,** 617.
26. Williams, A. F. and Barclay, A. N. (1986). In *Handbook of Experimental Immunology. Part 1. Immunochemistry,* (ed. D. M. Weir), 4th edn, pp. 22.1–22.17. Blackwell Scientific, Oxford.
27. Blaszczyk, M., Pak, K. Y., Herlyn, M., Lindgren, J., Pesano, S., and Koprowski, H. (1984). *Cancer Res.,* **44,** 245.
28. Brown, J. P., Nishiyama, K., Hellström, I., and Hellström, K.-E. (1981). *J. Immunol.,* **127,** 539.
29. Campbell, D. G., Price, M. R., and Baldwin, R. W. (1984). *Int. J. Cancer,* **34,** 31.
30. Towbin, H., Staehlin, T., and Gorden, J. (1979). *Proc. Natl Acad. Sci. USA,* **76,** 4350.
31. Scheidtmann, K. H. (1990). In *Protein Structure: A Practical Approach*, (ed. T. E. Creighton), pp. 93–116. IRL Press, Oxford.
32. Tendler, S. J. B. (1990). *Biochem. J.,* **267,** 733.
33. Scanlon, M., Morley, D., Jackson, D. E., Price, M. R., and Tendler, S. J. B. (1992). *Biochem. J.*, **284,** 137.
34. Price, M. R., Hudecz, F., O'Sullivan, C., Baldwin, R. W., Edwards, P. M., and Tendler, S. J. B. (1990). *Mol. Immunol.,* **27,** 795.
35. Owen, M. J. and Lamb, J. (1988). *Immune Recognition.* IRL Press, Oxford.
36. Geysen, M., Rodda, S. I., Mason, T. J., Tribbick, G., and Schoofs, P. G. (1987). *J. Immunol. Meth.,* **102,** 259.
37. Burchell, J., Taylor-Papadimitriou, J., Boshell, M., Gendler, S., and Duhig, T. (1989). *Int. J. Cancer,* **44,** 691.

38. Lam, K. S., Salmon, S. E., Hersh, E. M., Hruby, V. J., and Kazmierski, W. M. (1991). *Nature,* **354,** 82.
39. Houghten, R. A., Pinilla, C., Blondelle, S., Appel, J. R., Dooley, C., and Cuervo, J. H. (1991). *Nature,* **354,** 84.
40. Creighton, T. E. (ed.) (1990). *Protein Structure: A Practical Approach.* IRL Press, Oxford.

5

Isolation and characterization of human natural killer cells

TUOMO TIMONEN, ANNA MAENPAA, and PANU KOVANEN
(with additional material by U. P. THORGEIRSSON and A. R. MACKAY)

1. Introduction

Natural killer (NK) cell activity is defined as spontaneous cell-mediated cytotoxicity against certain, mostly cultured, tumour target cells (1). The cytotoxicity is not dependent on target cell expression of MHC antigens, it is mediated by lymphocytes, and, according to several animal and *in vitro* models, appears to be involved in resistance against malignant diseases, certain viral infections, and in control of hematopoiesis (1). Also, specific alloreactivity against lymphoid cells by NK cells has been described (2–4). The early studies on NK activity revealed that the effector cells responsible for the cytotoxicity are heterogeneous and that both T cells and non-T, non-B cells are involved, these latter cells being most effective. This phenomenological background of NK cells caused an era of confusion in their exact definition and to a certain degree the confusion still prevails. However, in 1988 at the fifth NK Workshop, a definition was agreed upon: NK cells are T-cell receptor-negative, CD56-positive, mostly CD16-positive, large granular lymphocytes that kill various, mostly virus-infected and tumour target cells in a non-MHC-restricted manner (5).

Thus, the NK-like activity mediated by T lymphocytes was considered a separate entity in the field of natural immunity. The major drawback in this definition is the limited knowledge about triggering receptors and target structures of the system. Furthermore, none of the listed characteristics is specific for NK cells only. None the less, the surface marker profile and the morphology of NK cells are the basis of the current methods of their enrichment and purification and provide the means for the future development of the field.

2. Characteristics of NK cells

2.1 Morphology and physical characteristics

The large granular lymphocyte morphology of effector cells active in non-MHC-restricted cytotoxicity was initially observed from the cytological analysis of effector:target cell conjugates (6). Large granular lymphocytes (LGL) are 10–14 μm in diameter; they have a typical, often kidney-shaped nucleus, pale abundant cytoplasm with azurophilic granules, and an often polygonal shape. They represent approximately 10–15% of lymphocytes and 2–3% of leukocytes. There are very few (less than 10%) LGL in lymph nodes and thymus, whereas they are readily isolated from blood and spleen. The majority of LGLs are non-T cells and therefore represent the cells currently defined as NK cells. However, about 20–30% of LGL are T cells including those cells capable of non-MHC-restricted cytotoxicity. These LGL appear somewhat smaller, with a more basophilic cytoplasm than in NK cells.

A large body of evidence indicates that LGL are responsible for most, if not all, NK activity. However, a recent report suggests that there is a minor population of small agranular lymphocytes capable of mediating NK activity (7). Whether these represent a separate entity of killer cells, or precursors of LGL, remains to be seen. Some *in vitro* and also *in vivo* data suggest that LGL morphology is a characteristic of both T and NK cells and that the fact that most freshly isolated LGL are NK cells is due to rapid elimination of activated T cells from the circulation.

2.2 Surface phenotype

Endogenous circulating NK cells have a distinct profile of surface molecules that distinguishes them from T and B lymphocytes, as well as monocyte-macrophages (*Table 1*). NK cells are negative for T-cell receptors and CD3, the T-cell receptor-associated signal transduction structure. As mentioned above, NK cells express the low-affinity Fc receptor CD16 (on 90% of NK cells and rarely on some T cells) and the neural cell adhesion molecule CD56 (on practically all NK cells and a subpopulation of cytotoxic T cells). Monoclonal antibodies against CD16 and CD56 are potential tools for positive enrichment and purification of NK cells by flow cytometry or by using immunomagnetic beads. Expression of adhesion molecules also distinguishes NK cells from T cells to a certain degree (*Table 1*).

Receptors that mediate the triggering of NK cell cytolytic machinery against tumour cells are currently under intensive investigation. CD16 and CD2 are triggering receptors, but probably not the ones that operate in endogenous NK activity. CD16, being an Fc receptor, triggers cytolysis in antibody-dependent cellular cytotoxicity (ADCC). Perhaps the strongest candidate for the triggering receptor of endogenous NK cells is a cyclophilin homologue, expressed selectively on NK cells (8). This 150 kd molecule is

Table 1. Surface phenotype of human NK cells and T cells

Surface marker	**NK cells**[a]	**T cells**
(a) Recognition and signal transduction molecules		
T-cell receptor	−	++++
CD2	+++>++++[b]	++++
CD3	−	++++
CD4	−	+++
CD8	+	++
CD16	++++	(+)
CD56	++++	+>++
Cyclophilin homologue p150	++++	−
(b) β1 integrins		
α1	−>++++	−>++++
α2	−>++++	−>++++
α3	+>+++	+>+++
α4	++++	+++
α5	++++	+++
α6	++>−	+++>−
β1	++++	++++
(c) β2 integrins		
αL (LFA-1)	++++	++++
αM (Mac-1, OKM-1)	++++	+>++++
αX (Leu-M5)	+++	−>+++
β2	++++	++++
(d) β3 integrins		
αIIb and αV	−	−
β3	+>++++	−>++++
(e) Other adhesion molecules		
CD44	++++	++++
CD54 (ICAM-1)	+++>++++	+>++++
CD58 (LFA-3)	++>++++	++>++++
Leu-8	++>−	+++>+

[a] Expressed as per cent positive from the total subpopulation of lymphocytes: −, negative; (+), < 5%; +, 5–25%; ++, 25–50%; +++, 50–75%; ++++, > 75% positive.

[b] Effect of long-term treatment with rIL-2 on surface phenotype is expressed as > and symbols.

associated with less well-characterized 110 kd and 80 kd polypeptides. This molecular complex appears to be involved in both binding and triggering phases of the cytolytic cascade. Whether this structure is the actual NK cell receptor is yet uncertain. Future work, perhaps with transfection technology, will probably establish the function of these interesting surface molecules.

In NK cell alloreactivity, the candidate receptors are CD56 (9) and heterodimeric structures GL183 and EB6 (10). Alloreactivity against lymphoid cells is detectable in NK cell clones and also in animal *in vivo* models (2–4). According to the present evidence, separate triggering receptors are involved in NK alloreactivity and cytotoxicity against tumour cells. It has been hypothesized that alloreactive NK cells would be involved in the control of trophoblastic invasion during pregnancy (11).

2.3 Regulation of NK activity

NK activity is strictly regulated by cytokines. The major stimulators of NK cells are interferons and interleukin-2 (IL-2; ref (1)). Also IL-7 (12) and IL-12 (19) activate NK cells to a certain degree. α and β interferons boost the activity strongly, whereas γ interferon (IFN-γ) is a weak stimulator. Anti-viral and NK stimulatory effects of interferons are separate, as exemplified by the strong anti-viral but weak NK-boosting activity of IFN-γ (13). The strongest activator of NK cytotoxicity is IL-2, which also stimulates a sub-population of T-cells to non-MHC-restricted cytotoxicity. IL-2-stimulated killer lymphocytes are also called lymphokine-activated killer (LAK) cells. LAK cells are in many instances cytotoxic to uncultured, freshly isolated cancer cells that are usually resistant to endogenous NK cells. *In-vitro*-stimulated LAK cells have therefore been used in the adoptive immunotherapy of patients with widely disseminted cancers. Response rates of 10–30% have been reported in melanoma and renal cell carcinoma patients (14). Systemic IL-2 also induces responses. It is not clear, however, whether the clinical effects of IL-2 and LAK cells are due to direct killing of tumour tissue by lymphocytes, or some indirect phenomenon, such as cytokine production by IL-2-activated lymphocytes.

NK activity is down-regulated by cortisol, cyclic-AMP inducers, transforming growth factor β, platelet-derived growth factor, and prostaglandins, particularly the E series (1).

3. Preparation of peripheral blood mononuclear cells (PBMC)

PBMC can be prepared by the methods given in Chapter 7 and Chapter 19.

4. Purification of human natural killer cells

4.1 Enrichment of large granular lymphocytes from peripheral blood

The relatively high cytoplasmic:nuclear ratio of LGL enables their separation from denser small and medium-sized lymphocytes by density-gradient centrifugation. Although this method does not produce sufficient purities for all purposes, it is an efficient primary step for more stringent enrichment of LGL and depletion of the rest of the other contaminating lymphocytes. Different variants of the technique have been published, but the most commonly used is the disontinuous density-gradient centrifugation on Percoll (15).

Protocol 1. Discontinuous density gradient centrifugation of peripheral blood lymphocytes

1. Purify peripheral blood lymphocytes by Ficoll–Isopaque gradient centrifugation and subsequent nylon wool filtration (for details, see (16) and (17)). Note that the nylon wool treatment has to be very careful and extensive, since contaminating monocytes aggregate cells and disturb the sedimentation of lymphocytes in the gradient. At least 80×10^6 cells in 1 ml of medium are required for sufficient yields of LGL. The cells should be kept at 4°C for at least 4 h to inhibit spontaneous aggregation. The medium is of choice RPMI 1640 supplemented with 10% human or bovine heat-inactivated serum.
2. Adjust the Percoll (Pharmacia) to 280 mOsm/ml with 10× PBS.
3. Prepare the discontinuous density gradient in 15 ml centrifuge tubes according to the following scheme:

(a) Fraction	(b) Percoll (μl)	(b) Medium (μl)	(c) Volume	Density (g/ml)
1	2550	3450	2.5	1.053
2	2700	3300	2.5	1.060
3	2850	3150	2.5	1.063
4	3000	3000	1.5	1.068
5	3150	2850	1.5	1.073
6	3300	2700	1.5	1.077
7	4000	2000	1.5	1.080

(a) Fractions are prepared in the volumes indicated into Falcon 2089 tubes, fraction 1 on the top.

(b) Amount of Percoll (in μl) mixed with growth medium (e.g. RPMI 1640 plus 10% FCS) to the final volume of 6.0 ml.

(c) Volume added to centrifuge tube; fraction 1, top of sample–fraction 7, bottom sample.

If high-density cells (mostly dormant T cells) are needed, a gradient with the first three fractions only can be prepared. In this case, the volume of the third fraction should be 8.5 ml.

4. Layer 80–100 $\times 10^6$ peripheral blood mononuclear cells on the top of the gradient. Centrifuge the tubes at 550*g* for 30 min. LGL are enriched in fractions 2 and 3, depending on the donor. Usually, fractions 2 and 3 can be pooled.

   Check the purity of the fractions from cytocentrifuged Giemsa-stained

Protocol 1. *Continued*

slides, or preferably by flow cytometry with anti-CD16 and anti-CD56 monoclonal antibodies. The fractions should contain 60–90% LGL, 50–60% CD-16 positive cells, more than 60% CD56-positive lymphocytes, and 20–40% CD3-positive T lymphocytes. Some (1–10%) B lymphocytes and monocytes may also contaminate the population, depending on the efficiency of the nylon wool filtration.

4.2 Depletion of non-NK cells from LGL-enriched fractions

The LGL-enriched Percoll fractions can be depleted of non-NK cells in several ways. An efficient method is to label the fractions with a cocktail of anti-CD3 (anti-T lymphocyte), anti-CD14 (anti-monocyte), and anti-CD22 (anti-B cell) monoclonal antibodies and deplete the stained cells with anti-mouse IgG-coated immunomagnetic beads (e.g. Dynabeads, Oslo, Norway). With some modifications from the manufacturer's instructions, we use 800 μl of beads for 20×10^6 labelled lymphocytes in 2 ml of medium and expose the cells to the beads on ice for two hours, with intermittent shaking every fifteen minutes. After the removal of beads and cells attached to them with a magnet, the resulting purity of CD56-positive CD3-negative NK cells exceeds 90%. It is important to wash the non-adherent cells carefully, at least twice, after the exposure to the immunomagnetic beads. Equal purities of NK cells can also be reached by cell sorting of lymphocytes labelled with FITC- or phycoerythrin-conjugated anti-CD16 or anti-CD56 monoclonal antibodies.

5. Proliferation of NK cells

Although high purities of NK cells can be obtained by both of the techniques described above, they are relatively expensive and tedious and yield only limited amounts ($(1–20) \times 10^6$) of cells. This has led to difficulties in biochemical and molecular studies of NK cells. For obtaining larger quantities of NK cells, expansion of cells in *in vitro* culture is required. The essential growth factor of NK cells is IL-2. However, accessory factors are also required (*Figure 1*). It is well established that NK cells proliferate most efficiently in the presence of IL-2, feeder lymphocytes (probably CD4-positive helper cells) and certain EBV-transformed B cell-lines, such as RPMI 8866 (18).

5.1 Cultures of human NK cells

Ficoll–Isopaque-purified peripheral blood mononuclear cells at 2.5×10^6 cells/ml are combined with irradiated RPMI 8866 cells at 4×10^4 cells/ml. The growth medium is RPMI 1640 supplemented with either 10% FCS or human serum, 0.29 mg/ml of L-glutamine, and antibiotics. After ten days of

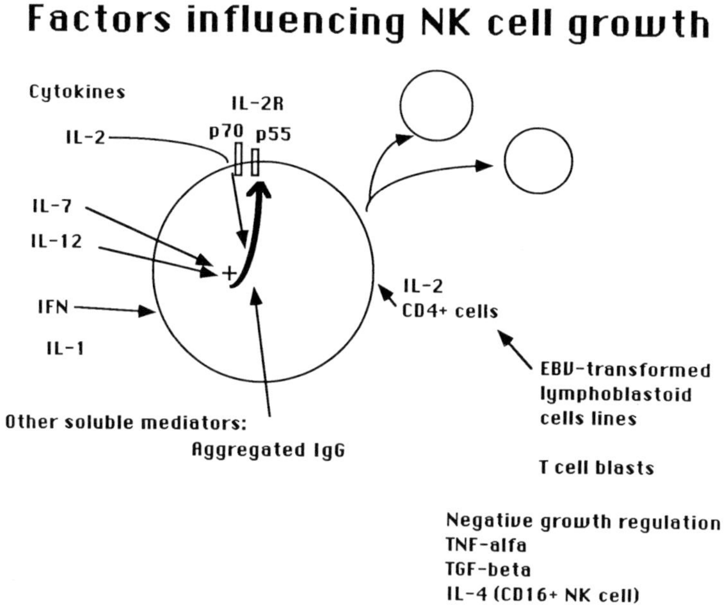

Figure 1. Regulation of NK cell proliferation. IL-2 stimulates NK cells by binding to the constitutively expressed intermediate affinity IL-2 receptor p70. This leads to the up-regulation of the p55 chain of the IL-2 receptor complex and the formation of the high-affinity IL-2 receptor p55/p70 dimers. IL-7 boosts NK cell proliferation in suboptimal IL-2 concentrations. IL-12 (also called natural killer stimulatory factor (19)) probably also up-regulates p55 when endogenous TNF production is blocked. There are also data suggesting that aggregated IgG and IL-1 up-regulate p55 expression. Interferons stimulate NK cell proliferation only *in vivo*, suggesting an indirect and IL-2-independent mechanism. EBV-transformed lymphoblastoid cell-lines efficiently induce NK cell growth, but only in the presence of IL-2 and CD4-positive T cells. Inhibition of proliferation is mediated by TNF, IL-4, and TGF-β.

culturing in standard conditions, the frequency of CD16-positive NK cells usually exceeds 50%, and the expansion of the cells is more than threefold. At this stage, rIL-2 (100 U/ml) and fresh feeder cells are added and the cells can further be expanded to the required amounts. Either after the ten days' culturing or the continued culture, the contaminating T cells are depleted as described in Section 4.2.

6. Natural killer cell cytotoxicity assays

The lytic activity of murine splenocytes or human peripheral blood lymphocytes can be detected using one of the following protocols.

6.1 Human NK cell activity

Human NK cell activity can be demonstrated using K562 target cells according to the methodology given in Chapter 7.

6.2 Murine NK cell assay

The effector cells must first be prepared and activated using the following method. NK cells are activated either *in vitro* or *in vivo*. For *in vitro* activation spleen cells should be prepared as described above. Then the following steps should be performed:

(a) Adjust the cell numbers to 5×10^6/ml in RPMI 1640 medium and plate in a 24-well tissue culture dish, 1 ml/well.

(b) Add the activator in 1 ml of medium to the cells and incubate in a humidified CO_2 incubator at 30°C for 24 h. For *in vivo* activation, inject 21-day-old mice intravenously with 0.2 ml of an activator, such as poly I:C mixed in HBSS. Repeat the injection two days later. On the third day humanely euthanase the mice, isolate the spleen cells and adjust them to 5×10^6 cells/ml. Store the effector cells on ice until used. (See also Chapter 19.)

Protocol 2. ^{51}Cr-release assay

1. Seed 100 μl of the effector cell suspension (prepared as in (b) above) into 96-well flat-bottom plates. The following numbers of NK effector cells are routinely used per well, in a volume of 0.1 ml: 5×10^5, 2.5×10^5, 1.25×10^5, and 6×10^4.
2. Add 100 μl containing 10^4 ^{51}Cr-labelled target cells (see Chapters 5 and 7 for details) to each well. Controls include radiolabelled target cells incubated alone or with unlabelled target cells at the same cell numbers as the effector cells shown above.
3. Add Triton X-100 to 10^4 target cells in 0.1 ml to determine release of total radioactivity. Plate cells in triplicate.
4. Centrifuge plates at 50*g* for 5 min and incubate in a humidified CO_2 incubator at 37°C for 4 h.
5. Centrifuge plates at 50*g* for 5 min and collect supernatants (for example 100 μl from each well) and count in a gamma counter.
6. Use the following formula to calculate per cent cytotoxicity:

$$\frac{\text{c.p.m. released from test group} - \text{c.p.m. released from control group}}{\text{total c.p.m. Triton X-100 released}}$$

Protocol 3. [^{3}H]-proline release assay

This method can be used to detect cytotoxicity against adherent target tumour cells.

1. Plate target cells in a T-75 tissue-culture flask and culture to 50% confluency. Wash the monolayer with DMEM without non-essential amino

acids, then add 0.15 ml of [^{3}H]proline in 10 ml DMEM without non-essential amino acids + 5% FCS and incubate at 37°C for 24 h.

2. Harvest the radiolabelled target cells by brief trypsinization, wash cells, and adjust the density to 5×10^4 cells/ml in DMEM + 5% FCS. Determine the total radioactive uptake into 10^4 cells by Triton X-100 lysis; this should be more than 5000 c.p.m./10^4 cells.
3. Add 200 µl containing 10^4 radiolabelled target cells to each well of a 96-well flat-bottom microtiter plate and incubate in a humidified CO_2 incubator at 37°C overnight.
4. Remove the medium and add 200 µl of effector cells (see isolation of spleen cells, *Protocol 2*) at effector/target cell ratios of 100:1, 50:1, 25:1, and 12:1. The effector cells are routinely prepared at 5×10^6/ml, 2.5×10^6/ml, 1.25×10^6/ml, and 6×10^5/ml. Each test point should be plated in triplicate. Control wells include target cells incubated in medium alone.
5. Incubate plates in a humidified CO_2 incubator at 37°C for up to 24 h.
6. Wash the wells twice with HBSS. Aspirate all the fluid from the wells. Add 0.2 ml of Triton X-100 to each well to lyse any remaining cells. Incubate at 37°C for 15–20 min. Remove 100–150 µl aliquots of lysate and count radioactivity of each well.
7. Calculate per cent cytotoxicity from the following formula:

$$\frac{\text{c.p.m./well with effector cells} - \text{c.p.m./control well}}{\text{total radioactive input per well}}$$

References

1. Trinchieri, G. (1989). *Adv. Immunol.,* **47,** 187.
2. Ciccone, E., Viale, O., Pende, D., Malnati, M., Biassoni, R., Melioli, G., *et al.* (1988). *J. Exp. Med.,* **168,** 2403.
3. Cudkowics, G. and Bennet, M. (1971). *J. Exp. Med.,* **134,** 1513.
4. Rolstadt, B. and Benestad, H. B. (1984). *Eur. J. Immunol.,* **14,** 793.
5. Hercend, T. and Schmidt, R. E. (1988). *Immunol. Today,* **9,** 291.
6. Timonen, T., Saksela, E., Ranki, A., and Hayry, P. (1979). *Cell Immunol.,* **48,** 133.
7. Inverardi, L., Witson, J. C., Fuad, S. A., Winkler-Pickett, R. T., Ortaldo, J. R., and Bach, F. H. (1991). *J. Immunol.,* **146,** 4048.
8. Frey, J. L., Bino, T., Kantor, R. R. S., Segal, D. M., Giardina, S. L., Roder, J., *et al.* (1991). *J. Exp. Med.,* **174,** 1527.
9. Suzuki, N., Suzuki, T., and Engleman, E. G. (1991). *Nat. Immun. Cell Growth Regul.,* **10,** 131.
10. Moretta, A., Tambussi, G., Bottino, C., Tripodi, G., Merli, A., Ciccone, E., *et al.* (1990). *J. Exp. Med.,* **171,** 695.

11. King, A. and Loke, Y. W. (1991). *Immunol. Today,* **12,** 432.
12. Naume, B. and Espevik, T. (1991). *J. Immunol.,* **147,** 2208.
13. Ortaldo, J. R., Herberman, R. B., Harvey, C., Osheroff, P., Pan, Y. C., Kelder, B., *et al.* (1984). *Proc. Natl Acad. Sci. USA,* **81,** 4926.
14. Rosenberg, S. A. (1991). In *Biologic Therapy of Cancer* (ed. V. T. De Vita, S. Hellman, and S. A. Rosenberg), p. 214. Lippincott, Philadelphia.
15. Timonen, T., Reynolds, C. W., Ortaldo, J., and Herberman, R. B. (1982). *J. Immunol. Methods,* **51,** 269.
16. Boyum, A. (1968). *Scand. J. Clin. Lab. Invest.,* **21** (Suppl. 97), 1.
17. Julius, M. H., Simpson, E., and Herzenberg, L. A. (1973). *Eur. J. Immunol.,* **3,** 645.
18. Perussia, B., Ramoni, C., Anegon, I., Cuturi, M. C., Faust, J., and Trinchieri, G. (1987). *Nat. Immun. Cell Growth Regul.,* **6,** 171.
19. Wolf, S. F., Temple, P. A., Kobayashi, M., Young, D., Dicig, M., Lowe, L., *et al.* (1991). *J. Immunol.,* **146,** 3074.

6

Isolation and characterization of mononuclear phagocytes

L. J. PARTRIDGE and I. DRANSFIELD

1. Introduction

It has long been suggested that mononuclear phagocytes are important in surveillance and defence against cancer. Whilst the capacity of monocytes and macrophages to kill tumour cells *in vitro* is well documented, their role in the development and growth of tumours *in vivo* has not yet been defined. Mononuclear phagocytes are, however, central to the immune response and have profound influences on the activities of leukocytes and other cells. Their status is likely to be important in determining the outcome of any anti-tumour response and therefore worthy of study. The cytotoxicity exhibited by mononuclear phagocytes towards neoplastic cells *in vitro* also suggests therapeutic potential.

This chapter will concentrate mainly on the isolation and characterization of monocytes from peripheral blood. Purification of macrophages from solid tumours is much more difficult and may be selective. Using monoclonal antibody (MAb) markers, however, it is now possible to assess the status of mononuclear phagocytes in intact tumours (Section 5).

2. Reagents and equipment required for studying mononuclear phagocytes

- Culture medium. Mononuclear phagocytes are cultured in RPMI 1640 supplemented with 2 mM glutamine (Gibco) and 10% foetal calf serum (FCS). Antibiotics can be added to reduce the incidence of bacterial contamination. A combination of penicillin (100 U/ml) and streptomycin (100 μg/ml) is usually used.
- Autologous serum. This is sometimes used instead of FCS. Whole blood anti-coagulated with citrate (1 ml of 3.8% sodium citrate per 10 ml of blood) is centrifuged for 15 minutes at 370*g* to give platelet-rich plasma (upper layer). Platelets are removed by addition of 0.2 ml of 1 M $CaCl_2$

(final concentration 20 mM) to 10 ml of platelet-rich plasma in a glass tube. After 30–60 min at 37 °C, the serum can be pipetted away from the platelet 'plug'.

- Wash buffer. HBSS (without divalent cations) is routinely used for washing cells (Gibco).
- Monoclonal antibodies (MAbs). MAbs used in characterizing mononuclear phagocytes (Section 5.2) are commercially available (e.g. from Serotec or Sigma) or in some cases from the laboratories that produced them (1).
- Second antibodies. Polyclonal antibodies labelled with fluorescein (FITC) are used to detect primary MAbs in immunofluorescence assays. We use FITC-labelled goat anti-mouse immunoglobulin from Dako, UK (see Section 5).
- Tissue-culture ware. Sterile pipettes, tissue-culture dishes (15 cm), centrifuge tubes (50 ml and 10 ml) and plugged Pasteur pipettes are used routinely. Tissue-culture plastics can be obtained from Sterilin or Nunc (Gibco).
- Refrigerated centrifuge. This is used during the isolation of mononuclear phagocytes and in some of the characterization assays. Carriers which take 96-well microtitre plates are useful for some assays.
- CO_2 incubator. Cells are cultured at 37°C in a 5% CO_2 humidified atmosphere.
- Fluorescence microscope or access to a fluorescence-activated cell sorter (FACS). These are used for examining mononuclear phagocyte antigen expression.

3. Isolation of mononuclear phagocytes

Characterization of mononuclear phagocytes *in vitro* requires a relatively pure, homogeneous population of cells. For studies of human mononuclear phagocytes, peripheral blood monocytes are a convenient source of such cells. Since approximately only 5% of circulating leukocytes are monocytes, isolation can seldom be achieved in a single step.

Isolation of minimally activated leukocytes suitable for functional analyses requires that all reagents are free of trace amounts of bacterial endotoxin. Some commonly used preparative media may also have unwanted effects upon cell function, e.g. polymers of dextran or Percoll may be internalized, possibly affecting cell surface molecule expression and function (2). Such effects must be considered when choosing isolation protocols.

3.1 Density-gradient techniques

Monocytes and lymphocytes are less dense than erythrocytes and polymorphonuclear cells (PMN) and can be separated from these relatively easily.

Typically, monocytes represent 10–30% of the enriched monocyte/lymphocyte, or mononuclear cell (MNC) fraction. Two density-gradient methods are commonly used for fractionation of blood cells as an initial enrichment step for subsequent preparation of monocytes.

3.1.1 Ficoll–Hypaque discontinuous gradient centrifugation

This involves fractionation of MNC from PMN/erythrocytes using whole blood (3).

Protocol 1. Isolation of MNC using Ficoll–Hypaque [a]

All procedures are performed at room temperature unless otherwise stated.

1. Add 10 units of heparin (1000 U/ml) for each ml of freshly drawn blood. Dilute the blood 1:1 with HBSS.
2. Carefully layer 30 ml of diluted blood on to 12.5 ml of Ficoll–Hypaque (e.g. Lymphoprep, density 1.077 g/ml, Nycomed) in a 50 ml tube.
3. Centrifuge for 20 minutes at 800*g*.
4. Collect the MNC from the interface of the dilute plasma layer (top) and the Lymphoprep layer (bottom).

[a] We have used commercial preparations from Flow (Lymphocyte separation medium), Sigma (Histo-paque), and Nycomed (Lymphoprep) with similar results.

3.1.2 Percoll discontinuous-gradient centrifugation

This is usually used in conjunction with Dextran sedimentation of leukocytes and erythrocytes (see *Protocol 3*). Further fractionation of the leukocyte-rich preparation is then achieved using Percoll of differing densities (4).

3.1.3 Escalated density-gradient media

Density-gradient media have been developed that permit further fractionation of monocytes and lymphocytes (Sepracell MN) and isolation of monocytes in a single step from whole blood (Nycoprep 1.068).

i. Sepracell MN

This density-gradient medium is, like Percoll, based upon colloidal silica. In this method, however, the gradient medium is mixed with the cells prior to separation. Since separation of large numbers of monocytes from whole blood requires large amounts of Sepracell MN, this medium is usually used in conjunction with Ficoll–Hypaque (5). Although the cells retain good viability, the yield and purity can vary considerably, depending on the volume ratio of cells:separation medium.

Protocol 2. Separation of monocytes from lymphocytes using Sepracell MN

All procedures are performed at room temperature unless otherwise stated.

1. Isolate MNC using Ficoll–Hypaque as in *Protocol 1*.
2. Wash MNC twice in HBSS. Re-suspend in 3 ml of HBSS and mix with 6.7 ml of Sepracell MN (density 1.099 g/ml) in a 15 ml centrifuge tube.
3. Centrifuge at 2000*g* for 20 min and harvest the monocytes/platelets from the opaque layer at the top of the tube.
4. Reduce platelet contamination by repeated washes in HBSS (6).

ii. Nycoprep 1.068

This medium exploits the fact that in hyperosmotic media, monocytes and lymphocytes expel water at different rates, allowing fractionation on the basis of altered buoyant densities (7). Better fractionation is achieved if EDTA is used as the anti-coagulant. Yields are also improved by using leukocyte-rich plasma, prepared by Dextran sedimentation, rather than whole blood.

Protocol 3. Isolation of monocytes from leukocyte-rich plasma

All procedures are performed at room temperature, unless otherwise stated.

1. Prepare a solution of 6% Dextran T500 (Pharmacia) in 0.9% NaCl. Filter sterilize.
2. Dilute blood with EDTA as the anti-coagulant 1:10 with 6% Dextran and allow the red blood cells (rbc) to settle for 20–40 min to form a leukocyte-rich plasma (upper layer).
3. Overlay 25 ml of this leukocyte-rich plasma on to 15 ml of Nycoprep 1.068 and centrifuge at 600*g* for 15 min.
4. Remove the leukocyte-containing layer (which will appear semi-opaque) above the pelleted rbc and wash three times in HBSS to reduce platelet contamination.

Good separation of monocytes and lymphocytes using multiple hyperosmotic Percoll gradients has also been reported (8).

3.2 Separation of mononuclear phagocytes by adherence

Monocytes can be isolated from MNC on the basis of their ability to adhere to substrates such as plastic or collagen (9, 10). Selective adherence to deplete lymphocytes followed by detachment of adherent cells allows good recovery (more than 60% of the initial population of monocytes) of pure cells (more than 90% monocytes). One disadvantage of this technique is that adherence dramatically alters the functional properties of monocytes (references (11–13) and Section 4). The detachment of adherent monocytes, usually by treatment with divalent cation chelating agents, may also affect their function.

3.2.1 Adherence to tissue-culture plastic

Mononuclear leukocytes may be prepared from whole blood using Ficoll-Hypaque (*Protocol 1*) or by Percoll density-gradient fractionation of leukocyte-rich plasma.

Protocol 4. Separation of monocytes and lymphocytes by differential adherence

1. Wash the MNC in HBSS and re-suspend them to a density of 2×10^6/ml in warm (37°C) RPMI medium containing 10% serum (FCS or autologous serum, see Section 2).
2. Seed the cell suspension on to 150 mm tissue-culture plates (7 ml/plate) and incubate at 37°C for 45 min.
3. Remove non-adherent cells by gentle pipetting. Wash the adherent cells three times in warm medium and examine the plates microscopically for the presence of non-adherent cells.
4. Add 3 ml of warm HBSS containing 10 mM EDTA (pH 7.4) and 2% serum to the plate and incubate at 37°C for 5–10 min to detach adherent cells. Although some cells detach easily, it is necessary to use vigorous pipetting to detach the majority of the cells. Mechanical detachment (rubber policemen, etc.) is not recommended as viability is reduced due to cellular damage.
5. Place detached cells in ice-cold 15 ml tubes and centrifuge at 200*g* for 6 min at 4°C. Any remaining contaminating platelets can be removed with further washes in ice-cold HBSS.

3.2.2 Adherence to other substrates

The avidity of binding of monocytes to tissue-culture plastic can result in low monocyte yields. Several methods that give a significant improvement in detachment have been described (9, 14). Essentially these methods are as described in *Protocol 5*, but the monocytes are allowed to adhere to different substrates:

- BHK-treated (micro-exudate) tissue-culture plates. Grow the baby hamster kidney cell-line BHK-21 (obtained from ECACC, UK) to confluence on 150 mm tissue-culture dishes in Glasgow's BHK-21 medium (Gibco) containing 10% tryptose phosphate broth (Gibco) and 10% FCS. Allow confluent monolayers to 'overgrow' for a further 24–48 h, then remove the cells with HBSS containing 10 mM EDTA. When treated with EDTA post-confluence, the BHK-21 cell monolayers detach easily as a sheet of cells. If the cell detachment is patchy (which can occur if the cells are not confluent or if they overgrow too much), discard the plates. The detached cell sheet, together with the HBSS/EDTA, is decanted off and the plate washed three times in HBSS. No further treatment of the plate is necessary prior to use. If not required immediately, we have stored plates at 4 °C for up to 1 month or for longer periods at −20 °C.

- Serum-coated plates. Autologous serum (or platelet-depleted plasma) can also be used to pre-coat the tissue-culture plates used for monocyte adherence. Pre-coat 150 mm tissue-culture plates with 5 ml of a 1/10 dilution of autologous serum made in HBSS. Incubate the plates for 60 min at 37 °C, remove the diluted serum and wash plates washed three times with HBSS.

These substrates are thought to promote specific adhesive interactions which are more readily reversed by EDTA.

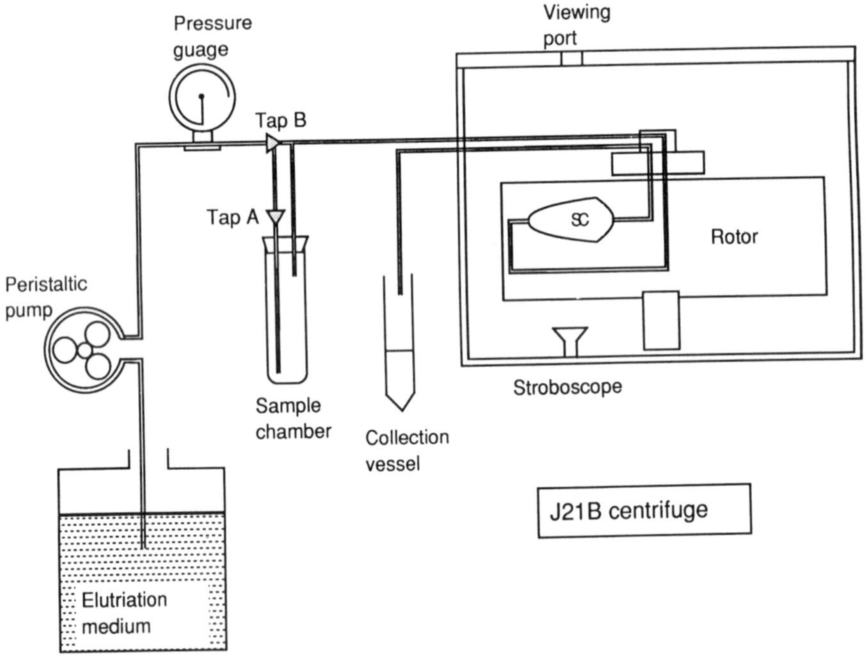

Figure 1. Apparatus for isolation of monocytes by CCE. A modified J21B centrifuge fitted with viewing port and stroboscope allows events in the separation chamber (SC) to be monitored. Elutriation medium is pumped through the rotor using a peristaltic pump for precise control of the flow rate via silicon tubing (a special rotating seal sits on top of the rotor). Undue pressure build-up is monitored using a gauge. Two three-way taps (A and B) control sample introduction into the SC.

3.3 Counterflow centrifugal elutriation (CC)

Monocytes are relatively large cells (mean cell volume (MSC) ~400 mm^3) when compared with lymphocytes (MSC ~160 mm^3) and PMN (MSC ~320 mm^3). Counterflow centrifugal elutriation (CC) allows fractionation on the basis of cell size and requires minimal manipulation of cells (reviewed in (15)). Thus, CC represents an ideal method for cell separation. Most protocols for isolation of monocytes, however, require an initial enrichment of MNC using density-gradient media and the equipment required for routine use of elutriation is expensive. Conversion of a centrifuge for use in CC requires ports to be made for inlet and outlet of medium and a stroboscope to be fitted. Additional requirements are a specialized rotor, separation chambers, and a pulse-free peripatetic pump. In our experience, without access to a cell-size analysis machine (e.g. a Coulter channelyser) CC is very labour-intensive and prone to failure due to slight variations in the separation characteristics of the cells. Another potential drawback is that separation of leukocytes from small (<100 ml) of blood is not readily achieved. CC fractionation requires:

- complete CC set-up inclusive of modified J21 centrifuge, JE6B rotor with modified 'Sanderson' separation chamber (Beckman, UK)
- Masterflex peripatetic pump
- Coulter channelyser (Coulter Electronics, Luton, UK)

Protocol 5. Fractionation of monocytes and lymphocytes by CC

1. Treat the components of the separation chamber with 'Desicote' prior to assembly to minimize cell adhesion during elutriation.
2. Assemble components as shown in *Figure 1*. Correct assembly of the elutriation chamber and removal of any trapped air from the system is essential for successful separation.
3. Prepare MNC from whole blood as described in *Protocol 1*. Wash the cells and re-suspend them in 20 ml of HBSS.
4. Flush the system with medium using the Masterflex pump (or equivalent). This pump minimizes pulse in the flow rate. Set the initial flow rate at 8 ml/min and the rotor speed to 2250 r.p.m.
5. With the medium flow by-passing the sample chamber, introduce the cells into the sample chamber via the three-way tap A (*Figure 1*).
6. Invert the chamber and direct the flow through the sample chamber via tap B (*Figure 1*).
7. After loading the cells, set the medium flow to by-pass the sample chamber using tap A. The initial flow rate/centrifuge speed allows cells to band together at the bottom of the separation chamber whilst any contaminating platelets/erythrocytes are elutriated.

Protocol 5. *Continued*

8. After collecting 2 × 5 minute fractions in 50 ml tubes gradually increase the flow rate (in 1 ml/min increments) and collect another fraction during this time.
9. Repeat step **8** to allow fractionation of the lymphocyte and monocyte populations.[a]
10. Monitor the size of the elutriated population of cells using a Coulter channelyser or by cytospin preparations.

[a] In our experience, fractions collected between 11 and 14 ml/min are almost exclusively lymphocytes by histocytochemical or immunochemical detection methods. Fractions collected at higher flow rates (17–19 ml/min) are highly purified monocytes.

3.4 Immunomagnetic isolation of monocytes

Using antibodies bound covalently to magnetic microspheres it is possible to rapidly fractionate leukocytes on the basis of cell surface molecule expression (16). When used as a negative selection procedure this is a relatively mild isolation technique that yields minimally activated cells. We have successfully used this technique to negatively select highly pure CD3+ populations from MNC by removal of monocytes, NK cells, and B cells (using a combination of CD11b+, CD16+, CD19+ MAbs — I. Dransfield, unpublished data). Recently, this technique has been used to negatively select monocytes (17). The technique requires a magnetic particle concentrator (Dynal).

Protocol 6. Separation of monocytes using magnetic beads

1. Isolate MNC as in *Protocol 1*.
2. Mix 5 × 10^8 M450 Pan T microspheres (coated with CD2-specific MAb, Dynal) and 1.5 × 10^8 M450 Pan B microspheres (coated with CD19-specific MAb, Dynal).
3. Wash the microspheres in HBSS containing 2% serum (FCS or autologous) using the magnetic particle concentrator (MPC). (Centrifugation may cause microsphere aggregation.)
4. Re-suspend 10^7 MNC in 10 ml of HBSS, add these to the magnetic microspheres and incubate at 4°C, with rotary mixing for 30 min.
5. Remove the magnetic microspheres, with bound T- and B-cells, using the MPC for 2–3 min.[a] The monocytes remain in suspension. Remove them using a pipette.[b]

[a] Improved yields may be obtained by adding fresh HBSS to the microspheres, mixing gently and repeating their removal with the MPC.

[b] Monocytes depleted of lymphocytes should be checked microscopically for the presence of microspheres. Remove these using the MPC as necessary.

One drawback of using magnetic isolation to negatively select monocytes is the high bead:cell ratios (usually 50:1) required for effective removal of the more numerous lymphocytes. Large quantities of beads are therefore needed to separate monocytes from large volumes of blood.

3.5 Isolation of mononuclear phagocytes from solid tumours

Mononuclear phagocytes may be isolated from solid tumours by mechanical or enzymatic disaggregation. A major disadvantage of this approach is that the population of cells obtained by such harsh procedures may not be representative of those originally present in the tumour. Yields are also poor. Methods for obtaining and culturing macrophages from tumours are given in reference (18). It is, however, possible to characterize mononuclear phagocytes in intact tumours using specific MAb markers (reference (19) and *Table 2*).

4. Monocyte subsets

Heterogeneity of physical and/or phenotypic properties of monocytes has been well documented. Indeed, in terms of size, density, cell surface expression, and function, there is variation within the population of circulating peripheral blood monocytes. However, it is now widely accepted that there are no stable subsets of monocytes within the circulation that ultimately give rise to macrophages of different capabilities. Rather, monocyte heterogeneity is thought to represent variation in the maturation state of circulating cells (15, 20, 21). Moreover, macrophage heterogeneity is likely to be generated by modulation of the functional repertoire of newly emigrated monocytes by the unique microenvironmental conditions present in different tissues.

This plasticity of monocyte behaviour is well illustrated by examination of data relating to 'sub-populations' of monocytes defined in terms of cell surface molecule expression. Monocytes have been divided into 'sub-populations' on the basis of expression of a number of functionally important receptors:

- Complement receptors: complement receptor type 1 (CR1, CD35); complement receptor type 3 (CR3, CD11b/CD18)
- HLA–DR/DQ
- CD4 (22)
- CD14 (23)

All of these molecules are modulated in response to external stimuli. For example, complement receptors can be readily mobilized from intracellular pools to the cell surface in response to *in vitro* temperature changes and exposure to cytokines. Isolation techniques, such as adherence, are able to up-regulate surface expression of a number of molecules including complement receptors and adhesion molecules (20, 24). Furthermore, expression of molecules involved in antigen presenting function, e.g. HLA-DR/DQ, are also up-regulated during *in vitro* culture in exposure to interferon-γ (25, 15). Similarly, although monocytes with low FcR I expression can be demonstrated (26, 21), cytokines such as interferon-γ and granulocyte–macrophage colony stimulating factor augment FcR-dependent cytotoxicity (21). Although it is possible to divide isolated monocytes upon the basis of levels of expression of different surface molecules, these differences do not remain stable in culture (compare for instance, T-lymphocyte CD4+/CD8+).

In terms of functional studies, monocytes may also be fractionated into 'sub-populations'. Observed heterogeneity is usually defined in terms of differential functional ability (see *Table 1*). When compared in terms of physical properties, monocytes that represent the smallest, or least dense, cells generally exhibit reduced functional capacity when compared with the remaining monocyte population. Although the less dense/smaller monocytes represent a small proportion of circulating cells, during cytophoresis their proportion is increased (27) indicating that such a population probably represents recently emigrated, less mature cells.

Two additional considerations apply to studies upon monocyte 'subsets'. Firstly, fractionation techniques may also differentially enrich contaminating cell types. Our studies have indicated that monocytes isolated by CC or adherence show some contamination (1–8%) with non-mononuclear cells. However, monocytes prepared by CC contain CD16+ lymphocytes or large granular lymphocytes, whereas monocytes prepared by adherence contain predominantly CD3+ T lymphocytes (28). It is therefore possible that subsequent functional studies may be affected by the presence of such contaminating cells, particularly if they are further enriched during subsequent fractionation. Secondly, a consideration of the stability of monocyte functional phenotype should be made. As discussed above, many of the molecules mediating functions which have been reported to differ on 'sub-populations' are modulated. Moreover, within the peripheral blood monocyte pool there is variation in parameters such as cell density or cell size suggestive of a continuous distribution. Arbitrary division of populations of cells on the basis of such variables may generate populations exhibiting different functional characteristics that do not represent true subpopulations as conventionally applied to cells.

5. Identification of mononuclear phagocytes

5.1 Histochemical staining

Immunochemical identification of mononuclear phagocytes using specific monoclonal antibodies has now largely superseded histochemical staining for cytoplasmic enzymes (Section 5.2). Non-specific esterase is the enzyme most

Table 1. Monocyte subsets

Capacity	**Low-density, small, 'intermediate'**	**High-density, large, 'regular'**	**Reference**
Esterase	Low	High	28
Peroxidase	Low	High	54
			26
5′ nucleotidase	Low	High	62
	Equal		26
Acid phosphatase	Low	High	26
			55
Fc receptor expression	Low	High	55
	Equal		61
C3 receptor expression	Low	High	55
	Low	High	26
Prostaglandin E_2 release	High	Low	62
	Low	High	56, 26
		Equal	15
Interleukin 1 release	Low	High	62
		Equal	15
CSF production	Low	High	63
		Equal	15
Phagocytosis	Low	High	57
ADCC	Low	High	15, 26
		Equal	61
Tumouricidal capacity	Greater	Lower	58
Activated by IFN-γ	No	Yes	15
Superoxide release in response to IFN-γ	Greater	No effect	59
Accessory cell function:			
• PWM B-cell stimulation	Low	High	55
• T-cell stimulation	High	Low	28
• PWM responses	Low	High	26
• Tetanus toxoid response		Equal	26
	High	Low	60

characteristic of mononuclear phagocytes. Ester hydrolysis is usually demonstrated using α/naphthyl acetate or α/naphthyl butyrate as a substrate. The naphthol produced is coupled to a diazonium salt to give an insoluble coloured azo dye (29). The test may be carried out on fixed cytocentrifuge preparations of cells.

Protocol 7. Staining for non-specific esterase

1. Prepare the fixative by dissolving 0.2 g Na_2PO_4 and 1 g KH_2PO_4 in distilled water. Add 450 ml acetone and 200 ml 38% formaldehyde. Make up to 1 litre with distilled water and store at 4°C.
2. Prepare a stock solution of pararosalanine hydrochloride (Hopkin and Williams, UK) by dissolving 1 g of dye in 25 ml of 2 M HCl with gentle warming. Allow the solution to cool, filter through 1 mm filter paper, and store in the dark at room temperature.
3. Prepare the counter-stain by dissolving 0.5 g of methyl green (Gurr Stains, BDH) with 50 ml distilled water.
4. The esterase substrate is prepared immediately prior to staining and should be used within 1 h:
   (a) Shake 1.2 ml of the pararosanaline stock solution with 1.2 ml of a freshly prepared 4% $NaNO_2$ solution for 1 min.
   (b) Dissolve 16 mg of α-naphthyl acetate in 2 ml ethylene glycol monomethyl ether. Add this, together with the hexazoatized pararosanaline solution, to 35.6 ml of 0.066 M sodium phosphate buffer, pH 7.6
   (c) Adjust to pH 6.1 and filter the substrate through 1 mm filter paper.
5. Prepare the cells to be stained by centrifuging 5×10^4 cells in 200 μl RPMI 10% FCS at 60*g* for 5 min on to ethanol-washed glass slides using a cytocentrifuge (Shandon).
6. Fix freshly prepared cytocentrifuge slides of cells by incubating in ice-cold fixative for 0.5 min. Rinse thoroughly in four changes of distilled water and air-dry.
7. Incubate the slides in esterase substrate solution for 45 min at 37°C. Wash three times with distilled water.
8. Counter-stain the slides by incubating for 2 min in methyl green solution (BDH). Rinse the slides three times in distilled water then air-dry.
9. Mount the slides and examine them microscopically. Esterase positive cells show diffuse red/brown staining of the cytoplasm.

Mononuclear phagocytes may be stained for other cytoplasmic enzymes such as peroxidase (30). This enzyme is not, however, lineage specific and is lost as the cells differentiate.

5.2 Monoclonal antibody staining

A wide range of MAbs directed against cell surface markers is now available (*Table 2*). Few of these are absolutely specific for mononuclear phagocytes, although the high-affinity Fc receptor for IgG (FcγRI) is almost exclusively

Table 2. Mononuclear phagocyte antigens[a]

Marker	Molecule	Mol. wt (kd)	Distribution	Function
CD4	Membrane glycoprotein	59	T helper cells, monocytes	Binds MHC class-II
CD9	Membrane protein	24	Platelets, monocytes, pre-B cells	Platelet activation?
CD11a	LFA-1α chain	180	Most leukocytes	Cell:cell adhesion. Binds ICAM-1, ICAM-2
CD11b	CR3α chain	165	Monocytes, neutrophils, NK cells	Receptor for C3bi, fibronectin, clotting factor X
CD11c	p150, 95 α chain	150	Macrophages (strong), monocytes, granulocytes (weak)	Receptor for C3bi
CD13	Aminopeptidase N	150	Monocytes, granulocytes	Membrane-bound metalloproteinase. Involved in metabolism of regulator peptides
CD14	PI-linked glycoprotein	55	Monocytes, macrophages, granulacytes (weak)	
CD15	Carbohydrate gal 1-4(Fucl-3) GINac		Granulocytes, immature monocytes	Linked to various membrane proteins. Cell:cell adhesion. Ligand for PADGEM?
CD16	FcγRIII	55–65	NK cells, granulocytes macrophages (not monocytes)	Low-affinity Fc receptor for IgG. Binds immune complexes. ADCC
CD_w17	Lactosylceramide		Granulocytes, monocytes, platelets	
CD18	Common β_2 chain of leukocyte integrins	95	Most leukocytes	Cell:cell adhesion
CD23	FcεRII	45–50	B cells, platelets, activated monocytes macrophages	Low-affinity Fc receptor for IgE
CD26	Dipeptidylpeptidase IV	120	Activated T and B cells macrophages	Serine-type exopeptidase

Table 2. *Continued*

Marker	Molecule	Mol. wt (kd)	Distribution	Function
CD31	Membrane glycoprotein	140	Platelets, monocytes, macrophages, granulocytes B cells	
CD32	FcγRII	40	Monocytes, macrophages, granulocytes, B cells	Fc receptor for aggregated IgG
CD33	Transmembrane glycoprotein	67	Monocytes, myeloid precursors	
CD35	CR1 (4 allotypes)	160c 190a 220b 250d	Granulocytes, monocytes, B cells	Receptor for C3b. Phagocytosis of opsonized particles
CD36	Platelet GPIV	90	Monocytes, macrophages, platelets	Thrombospondin receptor. Collagen binding?
CD40	Membrane glycoprotein	48–44	B cells, monocytes (weak)	Signalling/adhesion
CD43	Leukosialin	95	Leukocytes (except circulating B cells)	Activation
CD44	Transmembrane glycoprotein, 'Hermes'	80–95	Leukocytes and erythrocytes	Leukocyte homing
CD45	Membrane glycoprotein 4 isoforms	220 205 190 180	Leukocytes	Signal transduction (tyrosine phosphatase) increases with activation
CD_w49d	VLA-4 α chain	150	Monocytes, T and B cells	Adhesion
CD63	Membrane glycoprotein	30–60	Macrophages, monocytes, activated platelets	
CD64	FcγRI	72	Monocytes, macrophages. Inducible on granulocytes	Binds monomer IgG with high affinity. Increases on activation, e.g. with γIFN

CD68	Glycosylated intracellular protein	110	Monocytes, macrophages (cytoplasmic)	
CD71	Transferrin receptor	95	Activated T and B cells macrophages, proliferating cells	Binds transferrin
CD74	MHCII-associated invariant chain	41, 35, 33	B cells, monocytes/macrophages	MHCII transport
HLA-DR	MHC class-II	35, 29	Monocytes, macrophages, B cells, dendritic cells	Antigen presentation HLA-DR increases on activation
HLA-DQ	MHC class-II	35, 29		
HLA-DP	MHC class-II	35, 39		
FcαR	IgA receptor	50–70	Monocytes, macrophages	Promotes phagocytosis of IgA-coated targets

[a] The CD (clusters of differentiation) antigens described in this table were defined at the Fourth International Workshop on Leukocyte Differentiation Antigens.

expressed on monocytes and macrophages (31). Antibodies directed against CD14 and CD11c are also useful in this respect. The cytoplasmic antigen CD68 is an excellent monocyte/macrophage marker but can only be detected on permeabilized cells (32).

Some of the markers listed in *Table 2* are useful in assessing the functional or differentiation/activation status of the cells, e.g. expression of FcγRI increases on stimulation of mononuclear phagocytes with interferon-γ. Elevation in the levels of this receptor has also been reported in cancer patients (33). For a detailed description of the characteristics of activated mononuclear phagocytes, see reference (34).

Cell surface marker expression can be conveniently assessed by indirect immunofluorescence, particularly if this is used in conjunction with flow cytometry (see also Chapter 3). Since mononuclear phagocytes express Fc receptors, it is vital that appropriate isotype-matched controls for the MAbs are included in these assays. Immunoglobulins of the mouse IgG2a and IgG3 and rat IgG2b sub-classes, in particular, bind tightly to human FcγRI (35). (Note also that mouse ascitic fluid is frequently contaminated with endogenous IgG2a.) In choosing fluorescein-labelled second antibodies, intact IgG preparations raised in rabbits should be avoided for the same reason. $F(ab')_2$ fragments or antibodies raised in sheep or goats, which show no appreciable FcR binding, are preferable.

Protocol 8. Staining with specific monoclonal antibodies: indirect immunofluorescence

The assay is performed using live cells. All manipulations are carried out at 4°C to prevent capping, internalization, and shedding of antigen.

1. Use $(0.5–1.0) \times 10^6$ cells per test. The cells must be of high viability (>90%). Harvest the cells and wash twice in cold wash buffer (PBS with 0.2% bovine serum albumin, 0.1% sodium azide).
2. Re-suspend the cells to $(0.5–1.0) \times 10^6$ in wash buffer. Dispense 1 ml aliquots into LP3 tubes, and centrifuge at 400*g* for 5 min.
3. Remove the supernatants using a finely drawn Pasteur pipette attached to a suction pump. Add 50 μl of MAb (diluted in wash buffer, as necessary) to the cell pellet.
4. Re-suspend the cells by vortexing and incubate them for 45–60 min on ice.
5. Re-suspend the cells and add 1 ml of wash buffer. Centrifuge at 400*g* for 5 min. Repeat.
6. Discard the supernatants and add 50 μl of appropriately diluted FITC-labelled second antibody. Mix by inverting the tubes and incubate for 30–45 min on ice.
7. Wash the cells twice, as before.

8. For analysis by immunofluorescence microscopy, re-suspend each cell pellet in 20 μl mountant. This is PBS containing 10% glycerol and 2.5% 1,4-diazadcyclooctane (DABCO), which retards the quenching of fluorescence (36). Place the cells on a glass slide, cover with a coverslip and seal the edges with nail varnish. Examine using a microscope with appropriate illumination and filters (37).
9. For analysis by flow cytometry, re-suspend the cells with 0.5 ml of wash buffer and store on ice until sampled (see Chapter 3).

Protocol 9. Indirect immunofluorescence assay in microtitre plates

This assay is convenient when a large number of tests is required. The assay can be carried out on fewer cells ((1–2) × 10^5).

1. Harvest the cells and wash as described in *Protocol 8*. Re-suspend to (1–2) × 10^6/ml.
2. Dispense 100 μl aliquots into the wells of a flexible PVC U-bottomed microtitre plate. Centrifuge the plates at 400*g* for 1 min.
3. Remove the supernatants by flicking the plate once over a sink. Re-suspend the cells by holding the plate firmly on a vortex mixer.
4. Add 50 μl of MAb as described in *Protocol 8*. Mix by squirting back and forth using an automatic pipette and incubate for 30–45 min on ice.
5. Wash the cells three times by adding 150 μl of wash buffer to the wells, centrifuging the plate for 1 min at 400*g*, and flicking it once to remove the supernatants. Re-suspend the cell pellets between washes using a vortex mixer as described in step **3**.
6. Add 50 μl of appropriately diluted FITC-labelled second antibody and incubate for 30–45 min on ice.
7. Wash the cells twice as described in step **6** then re-suspend the cells in mountant for microscopy as described in *Protocol 8*, **OR**
8. Re-suspend the cells in wash buffer and transfer to LP3 tubes. Make up the volume to 0.4 ml for FACS analysis.

Indirect immunofluorescence can also be adapted for examination of cytoplasmic antigens.

Protocol 10. Indirect fluorescence on permeabilized cells (FACS analysis)

1. Wash the cells three times in PBS. (Use 1 × 10^6 cells per assay.)
2. Re-suspend at approximately 10^7 cells/ml in 95% ethanol/5% acetic acid. Incubate at room temperature for 5 min.

Protocol 10. *Continued*

3. Wash twice in PBS and proceed as from step **2** in *Protocol 8*. The assay may be performed at room temperature.

Protocol 11. Indirect immunofluorescence on permeabilized cells (microscopic analysis)

If the cells are to be examined microscopically, cytocentrifuge preparations can be used. Alternatively, if the mononuclear phagocytes are prepared by adherence (*Protocol 4*), the cells can be plated directly on to glass coverslips as described in steps **1–4**.

1. Sterilize round coverslips by dipping them in alcohol and flaming. Place them in square 24-well plates (Sterilin).
2. Add 1 ml of mononuclear cells (at $(2–5) \times 10^6$/ml) in RPMI 10% FCS.
3. After allowing the cells to adhere, remove unbound cells by thorough washing as described in *Protocol 4*.
4. The coverslips are now processed *in situ* as described below, taking care that the fixed cells do not dry out. At the end of the procedure, remove the coverslips from the 24-well plate using fine forceps and mount as usual.
5. Wash freshly prepared cytocentrifuge slides or coverslips with three changes of PBS.
6. Fix cells by immersing slides or coverslips in acetone at room temperature for 5 min then wash in PBS.
7. Place 50 μl of an appropriate dilution of MAb (in PBS) on the fixed cells, ensuring that the cells are completely covered with liquid. Incubate for 30 min at room temperature in a damp container.
8. Wash three times with PBS (two brief washes and one 10 min wash).
9. Add 50 μl of an appropriate dilution of FITC-labelled second antibody (in PBS). Incubate for 30 min at room temperature in a damp container.
10. Wash with three changes of PBS as in step **8**, but allowing 30 min for the final wash.
11. Mount the slides and examine as described in stage **7**, *Protocol 8*.

---

6. Functional characterization of mononuclear phagocytes

Mononuclear phagocytes are capable of a wide range of functions. Those most frequently studied include phagocytosis, chemotaxis, antigen presentation, production of superoxide, secretion of various cytokines, and cell killing. A detailed description of the many assays available for studying these functions is, however, beyond the scope of this chapter. For additional information, the reader is referred to references (38) and (39).

6.1 Tumour cell killing

Mononuclear phagocytes are able to kill tumour cells by two mechanisms. The first involves direct interaction of monocytes/macrophages with the tumour cell. The second requires Fc receptor binding of antibody-coated targets (antibody-dependent cellular cytotoxicity, or ADCC). The mechanisms of cell killing have not yet been defined but may include the secretion of neutral proteases, production of reactive oxygen intermediates (ROIs), and tumour necrosis factor (TNF). The cytotoxic functions of mononuclear phagocytes are induced by cytokines and microbial products (40, 41).

6.1.1 Spontaneous cytotoxicity

Monocytes which have been freshly isolated from peripheral blood show variable levels of spontaneous cytotoxicity towards tumour cell targets. Factors which affect spontaneous cytotoxicity include the isolation procedure used, contamination with endotoxin, the presence of non-monocytic cells, e.g. natural killer (NK) cells, and contamination of the tumour target cell-line with mycoplasma.

A number of different assay systems have been developed for measuring monocyte cytotoxicity. Long-term assays (42) are based on labelling the nuclei of tumour cell lines with radio-isotopes (e.g. [^{3}H]thymidine) and measuring the amount of label released or retained in the nucleus. Short-term assays usually involve labelling target cells with isotopes such as ^{51}Cr and measuring its release. Different assay systems may measure different tumouricidal mechanism. Short-term assays are more convenient and reduce the effects of monocyte maturation associated with *in vitro* culture. In all assays, care must be taken that contaminating cells, such as NK cells, are not contributing to the killing. Target cell-lines vary in their sensitivity to NK cells, e.g. the myeloid cell-line K562 is easily killed by NK cells, whereas actinomycin D-treated WEHI sarcoma cells are NK-resistant (see *Protocol 14*). It is also possible to deplete NK cells using specific monoclonal antibodies (43).

Protocol 13. Measurement of spontaneous cytotoxicity by ^{51}Cr release

1. Prepare an appropriate number of target cells. (Use, for example, 10^4 per test.) Centrifuge to pellet the cells.
2. Label the cells by re-suspending the pellet with 100 μCi $Na^{51}CrO_4$ (Amersham UK). Incubate for 60 min at 37°C.

Protocol 13. *Continued*

3. Wash the cells three times by re-suspending with 10 ml of PBS and centrifuging.
4. Re-suspend the cells with 10 ml RPMI–10% FCS and incubate for a further 60 min. (This reduces background contamination.)
5. Wash the cells three times with PBS.
6. Re-suspend the cells in RPMI–10% FCS, count them, and assess their viability (e.g. by trypan blue exclusion). Adjust the cell concentration to 10^5/ml in RPMI–10% FCS.
7. Count the mononuclear phagocytes and assess their viability. (Typically, a range of effector to target cell ratios of 40:1 to 5:1 is used.) Re-suspend the cells to 4×10^6/ml in RPMI–10% FCS.
8. Set up the assay plate. The assay is performed in flexible U-bottomed PVC 96-well plates. Each 'test' is performed in triplicate.
   (a) In the first well, place 100 μl of mononuclear phagocytes to give an eventual effector:target ratio of 40:1.
   (b) In the second, third, and fourth wells, titrate the cells out 1:1 with 100 μl of medium to give eventual effector:target ratios of 20:1, 10:1, and 5:1.
   (c) Include a negative control consisting of 100 μl of medium instead of effector cells.
   (d) Add 100 μl of target cell suspension to each well. Incubate the plate in a CO_2 incubator at 37°C for 6 h.
9. Centrifuge the plates at 200*g* for 5 min. Remove 100 μl supernatant from each test well and place this in a separate well.
10. Dry the plates in an oven overnight. Cut up the plates and count each well individually on a gamma counter.
11. Determine the percentage ^{51}Cr release using the formula:

$$\%\ \text{release} = \frac{(1/2\ \text{SN c.p.m.}) \times 2}{1/2\ \text{SN c.p.m.} + \text{cell pellet c.p.m.} = 1/2\ \text{SN c.p.m.}}.$$

Determine the % cytotoxicity using the formula:

$$\%\ \text{cytotoxicity} = \frac{\text{test release} - \text{spontaneous release}}{100 - \text{spontaneous release}} \times 100.$$

Treatment of some cell-lines with drugs such as actinomycin D (Act D) increases their sensitivity to mononuclear phagocyte-mediated killing (44). The mechanism of this increased sensitivity is uncertain but may relate to the drug's inhibition of protein synthesis or effects on membrane fluidity. Many workers use Act D-treated murine sarcoma WEHI 164 cells as targets for assaying mononuclear cell killing. These cells can be used in short-term cytotoxicity assays and are reported to be relatively insensitive to killing by NK cells.

Protocol 14. Treatment of WEHI 164 cells with Act D
WEHI 164 cells are grown routinely in RPMI–10% FCS

1. WEHI 164 cells are loosely adherent. Detach the cells from culture flasks by incubating them with serum-free medium containing 0.025% trypsin for 2 min.
2. Wash the cells in RPMI–10% FCS. Re-suspend the cells at approximately 10^6/ml in RPMI–10% FCS with 1 μg/ml Act D. Incubate for 3 h at 37 °C in a CO_2 incubator.
3. Wash the cells twice in PBS. Re-suspend in RPMI–10% FCS and use them in a cytotoxicity assay as described in *Protocol 13*.

6.1.2 Antibody-dependent cellular cytotoxicity (ADCC)

The ADCC activity of mononuclear phagocytes can be measured using IgG monoclonal or polyclonal antibodies which recognize antigens expressed on the surface of tumour target cell-lines. It is, of course, essential that the isotype of the antibody used is capable of binding to Fc R (35). Antibodies are included in the incubation medium in the assay described in *Protocol 13* at a concentration which gives saturating binding to the target cells (typically 10–50 μg/ml).

Alternatively, ADCC can be measured using human erythrocytes coated with anti-blood group IgG antibody (e.g. anti-A or anti-D). Such antibodies are available from the Blood Transfusion Service (UK) and the Dutch Red Cross.

Protocol 15. Measurement of ADCC using human erythrocytes

1. Use fresh human red blood cells (not more than 24 h old) bearing the appropriate blood group antigen. Collect the blood in heparin to a final concentration of 10 U/ml.
2. Wash the red blood cells (rbc) twice by re-suspending in RPMI and centrifuging at 800*g* for 3 min.
3. Incubate 0.5 ml of packed rbc with 0.5 ml RPMI containing 1% bromelain for 10 min at room temperature.[a]
4. Wash cells three times in RPMI. Re-suspend to 10 ml in the same (i.e. to give a 5% rbc suspension).
5. Dilute 100 μl of the 5% suspension with 10 ml PBS and count the cells.

Protocol 15. *Continued*

6. For labelling, use approximately 10^7 cells. Pellet the cells by centrifuging and discard the supernatant.
7. Re-suspend the rbc with 50 μCi $Na_2{}^{51}CrO_4$. Incubate at 37°C for 2 h.
8. Wash cells twice with RPMI and re-suspend to 8×10^5/ml.
9. Prepare mononuclear phagocytes as usual and re-suspend at 12×10^8/ml in RPMI–10% AB serum. (AB serum is used since FCS may cause spontaneous rbc lysis.)
10. Set up the assay plate. Sterile, U-bottomed 96-well microtitre plates are used. Each 'test' is performed in triplicate. In each test well, place, in order:
    - 50 μl of mononuclear phagocytes
    - 50 μl of anti-A1 or anti-D antibody
    - 50 μl of labelled rbc

    Set up negative control wells in which 50 μl RPMI–10% AB serum replaces the mononuclear phagocytes. To determine maximum levels of ^{51}Cr release, set up wells containing 50 μl labelled rbc and 100 μl Triton X-100 in distilled water.
11. Place a lid on the plate and incubate overnight at 37°C in a humidified CO_2 incubator.
12. Centrifuge the plate at 400*g* for 5 min to pellet the cells. Carefully remove 100 μl of supernatant from each well and transfer to an LP3 tube.
13. Count samples on a gamma counter for 90 sec.
14. Calculate % specific lysis using the following formula:

$$\%\ \text{specific lysis} = \frac{\text{test release} - \text{control release}}{\text{max. release} - \text{control release}} \times 100.$$

[a] Treatment with the enzyme bromelain promotes adhesion between effector and target cells (45).

6.1.3 Cytostasis

Inhibition of tumour growth (cytostasis) by mononuclear phagocytes has been demonstrated *in vitro*. The most reliable assays for measuring cytostasis are those which monitor a reduction in the ability of target cells to take up radiolabelled nucleosides into DNA (46).

6.2 Production of reactive oxygen intermediates

Mononuclear phagocytes produce reactive oxygen intermediates (ROIs) in response to a variety of stimuli including phagocytosis and exposure to chemoattractants. ROIs may also contribute to tumour cell killing (42). The production of ROIs results in the generation of photons, i.e. chemiluminescence. This light can be amplified and measured experimentally by using a chemiluminescent compound such as 'luminol' (5-amino-2,3-dihydro-1,4-phthalazinedione), which is converted to an excited aminophthalate ion in the presence of oxidizing species (41). The light emitted can be quantified using an instrument equipped with a photomultiplier tube. If a purpose-built photoluminometer is not available, a liquid scintillation counter can be used in 'out of coincidence' mode (47).

Mononuclear phagocyte ROI production can be stimulated by exposing the cells to opsonized particles, chemoattractants, antibodies which cross-link cell surface receptors, and phorbol esters.

Protocol 16. Measurement of mononuclear phagocyte ROI production

In this protocol chemiluminescence is measured using a liquid scintillation counter in 'out of coincidence' mode.

1. Prepare a 100 mM stock solution of luminol (Sigma) in DMSO.
2. Prepare a 2 mM stock solution of phorbol myristate acetate in DMSO. (This is one of many agents that can be used to stimulate ROI production.) Dilute to a working concentration of 100 μM in HBSS (without phenol red, containing 20 mM Hepes, pH 7.4), immediately prior to use.
3. Wash mononuclear phagocytes twice in HBSS. Re-suspend the cells at 10^6/ml in HBSS containing 0.5% (w/v) fatty-acid free BSA (Sigma).
4. Incubate the cells on ice for 30 min. Five minutes before starting the assay, transfer 1 ml aliquots of cells to scintillation vials and incubate at 37°C.
5. Add 10 μl of luminol to each vial to give a final concentration of 1 mM. Place the vials in the scintillation counter. Take readings to obtain 'background' levels of chemiluminescence.
6. Add 10 μl PMA working solution to give a final concentration of 1 μM. Swirl gently to mix.
7. Collect readings over time. Maximum chemiluminescence is taken as a measure of ROI production.

6.3 Chemotaxis

Mononuclear phagocytes are motile in response to attractants such as the complement component C5a or formyl peptides, e.g. *N*-formyl-methionyl-leucyl phenylalanine (FMLP). Defects in monocyte chemotaxis in cancer patients have been reported (48).

There are various assays for measuring monocyte chemotaxis. The following protocol, adapted from (49) and (50), has given reproducible results in our laboratory. It measures the movement of the cells through a micropore filter (a modification of a Boyden chamber) in response to a gradient of chemoattractant. Cells which migrate through the filter are stained with crystal violet and this is assayed colorimetrically rather than microscopically.

Recombinant human C5a and the peptide FMLP (Sigma) are used as potent chemoattractants.

Protocol 17. Measurement of mononuclear phagocyte chemotaxis

The apparatus used for measuring chemotaxis is shown in *Figure 2*. Perform each test in triplicate.

1. Re-suspend mononuclear phagocytes at 10^6/ml in RPMI containing 1% (w/v) BSA. For each test, place 150 μl cell suspension in an inverted LP3 tube top.
2. Spot 150 μl of 25 nM chemoattractant on to a 13 mm antibiotic assay disc (Whatman) placed in a migration plate (Sterilin). For the negative control, spot 150 μl of medium on to a disc.
3. Make a sandwich, consisting of an 0.45 μm pore size nitrocellulose filter (Sartorius) and a 5 μm pore size polycarbonate filter (Sterilin) on top of the LP3 tube top.
4. Carefully invert the LP3 tube top (containing the cells) and the filters and place it on top of the chemoattractant-soaked disc in the migration plate (*Figure 2*). The 5 μm polycarbonate filter is permeable to the cells, whereas the nitrocellulose filter is not.
5. Incubate the migration plate at 37°C for 2 h in a CO_2 incubator.
6. Remove the nitrocellulose filters and rinse thoroughly with PBS. Place each filter in the well of a 24-well tissue-culture plate containing 0.5 ml of a solution of 0.2% crystal violet (BDH) in 10% ethanol. Incubate the filters for 5 min at room temperature with shaking.
7. Remove excess dye by incubating the filters with three changes of distilled water over 30 min.
8. Elute the remaining dye by adding 1 ml of 33% acetic acid and shaking at room temperature for 10 min.
9. Aspirate the acetic acid and measure the optical density at 540 nm wavelength on a spectrophotometer.

6.4 Phagocytosis

One of the major characteristics of monocytes and macrophages is their capacity to ingest particulate matter. This process is enhanced if the particles are coated with opsonins, such as antibodies or complement C3b, since

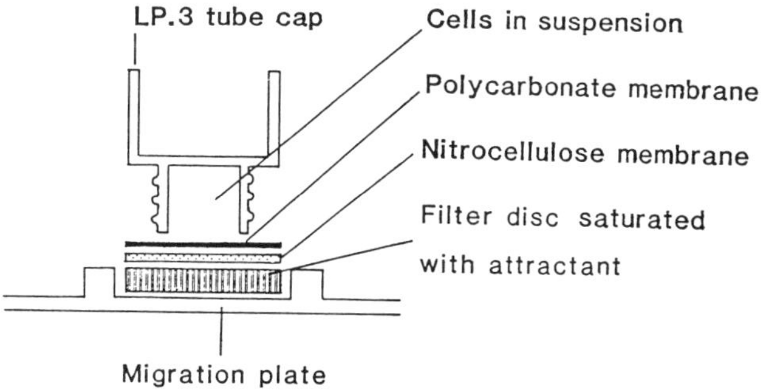

Figure 2. Apparatus for measuring chemotaxis. Each migration plate is comprised of 4 × 6 wells. The cell suspension is placed in the LP3 cap and inverted onto the attractant saturated discs.

mononuclear phagocytes have specific receptors for these molecules (*Table 2*).

There are a wide range of assays for measuring phagocytosis, differing in the use of particulate materials (e.g. red blood cells, yeast, carbon, or latex beads) and opsonins (51). The assay described here measures the phagocytosis of un-opsonized fluorescein-labelled latex beads (52). Uptake can be assessed microscopically or by flow cytometry.

Protocol 18. Measurement of phagocytosis

The assay is performed in sterile siliconized glass tubes to prevent monocyte adherence.

1. Prepare the tubes by pipetting dimethyl dichlorosilane (Sigma) over the inside surface of the tubes. Remove any excess liquid and dry in an oven. Wash the tubes with three changes of distilled water, dry, and sterilize by autoclaving.
2. Prepare mononuclear phagocytes as usual. Re-suspend at 0.5×10^6/ml in RPMI–10% FCS.
3. Transfer 2 ml of cell suspension per test to sterile, siliconized tubes. Incubate at 37°C for 5 min to equilibrate. Include a negative control in which the cells are incubated at 4°C.
4. Add 40 µl of a 2.5% suspension fluorescent 1 µM diameter microspheres (Polysciences, Warrington). Incubate for a further 60 min.
5. Carefully layer the cell suspension on to 1 ml of FCS and centrifuge at 200*g* for 5 min at 4°C.
6. Remove the supernatant containing any free beads.
7. Re-suspend the cells in PBS containing 0.1% trypsin (type IIIS, Sigma) and 5 mM EDTA. Incubate at 37°C for 10 min to remove attached beads.

Protocol 18. *Continued*

8. Layer the cells on to FCS and centrifuge as in step **5**. Wash the cells twice in PBS.
9. Analyse the cells microscopically or by flow cytometry as described in *Protocol 8*.

6.5 Antigen presentation

Mononuclear phagocytes express class-II MHC antigen and are capable of presenting antigen to T lymphocytes (53). Increased class-II expression is observed on monocyte/macrophage activation and this may correlate with increased potential for antigen presentation. Increases in expression of some class-II molecules have been reported in cancer patients.

Antigen presentation by human mononuclear phagocytes can be measured directly by assessing the cells' capacity to induce proliferation of T lymphocytes which have been exposed to antigen (e.g. tuberculin-purified protein derivative or PPD). The T lymphocytes are pulsed with radiolabelled nucleosides such as [^{3}H]thymidine, which are incorporated into the DNA of dividing cells (24).

6.6 Cytokine production

Monocytes and macrophages produce a wide range of cytokines and other soluble products, including interleukins, interferons, and complement components. Assays for measuring cytokines are described in Chapters 10 and 11.

References

1. Knapp, W., Dörken, B., Gilks, W. R., Rieber, E. P., Schmidt, R. E., Stein, H., *et al.* (ed.) (1989). *Leucocyte Typing IV. White Cell Differentiation Antigens.* Oxford University Press.
2. Wakefield, J., Gale, J. S., Berridge, M. V., Jordan, T. W., and Ford, H. C. (1982). *Biochem. J.,* **202,** 795.
3. Boyum, A. (1968). *Scand. J. Clin. Lab. Invest.,* **21** (suppl. 97), 77.
4. Dooley, D. C., Simpson, J. F., and Merryman, H. T. (1982). *Exp. Haematol.,* **10,** 591.
5. Vissers, M. C. M., Jester, S. A., and Fantone, J. C. (1988). *J. Immunol. Methods,* **110,** 203.
6. Williams, W. R., Cavolina, F., and Williams, W. J. (1983). *Br. J. Exp. Pathol.,* **64,** 451.
7. Boyum, A. (1983). *Scand. J. Immunol.,* **17,** 429.
8. Fluks, A. J. (1981). *J. Immunol. Methods,* **41,** 225.
9. Ackerman, S. K. and Douglas, S. D. (1978). *J. Immunol.,* **120,** 1372.
10. Julius, M. H., Simpson, E., and Herzenberg, L. A. (1973). *Eur. J. Immunol.,* **3,** 645.

11. Haskill, S., Johnson, C., Eierman, D., Becker, S., and Warren, K. (1988). *J. Immunol.,* **140,** 1690.
12. Kelley, J. L., Rozek, M. M., Suenram, C. A., and Schwartz, C. J. (1987). *Exp. Molec. Pathol.,* **46,** 266.
13. Fuhlbrigge, R. C., Chaplin, D. C., Kiely, J-M., and Unanue, E. R. (1987). *J. Immunol.,* **138,** 3799.
14. Treves, A. J., Yagoda, D., Haimovitz, A., Ramu, N., Rachmilewitz, D., and Fuks, Z. (1980). *J. Immunol. Methods,* **39,** 71.
15. Figdor, C. G., te Velde, A. A., Leemans, J. M. M., and Bont, W. S. (1985). In *Leukocytes and Host Defence*, (ed. J. J. Oppenheim and D. M. Jacobs), p. 283. Liss, New York.
16. Lea, T., Vartdal, F., Davies, C., and Ugelstad, J. (1985). *J. Immunol. Methods,* **22,** 207.
17. Flo, R. W., Naess, A., Lund-Johansen, F., Maele, B. O., Sjursen, H., Lehmann, V., *et al.* (1991). *J. Immunol.,* **137,** 89.
18. Russell, S. W. (1981). In *Methods for Studying Mononuclear Phagocytes*, (ed. D. O. Adams, P. J. Edelson, and H. Koren), p. 103. Academic, New York.
19. Allen, C. A. and Hogg, N. (1987). *J. Natl Cancer Inst.,* **78,** 45.
20. Dransfield, I., Corcoran, D., Partridge, L. J., Hogg, N., and Burton, D. R. (1988). *Immunology,* **63,** 491.
21. Connor, R. I., Shen, L., and Fanger, M. W. (1990). *J. Immunol.,* **145,** 1483.
22. Szabo, G., Miller, C. L., and Kodys, K. (1990). *J. Leuk. Biol.,* **47,** 111.
23. Passlick, B., Flieger, D., and Ziegler-Heitbrock, H. G. (1989). *Blood,* **74,** 2527.
24. Dougherty, G. J., Murdoch, S., and Hogg, N. (1988). *Eur. J. Immunol.,* **18,** 35.
25. Zembala, M., Uracz, W., Ruggiero, I., Mytar, B., and Pryjma, J. (1984). *J. Immunol.,* **133,** 1293.
26. Akiyama, Y., Miller, P. J., Thurman, G. B., Neubauer, R. H., and Stevenson, H. C. (1983). *J. Clin. Invest.,* **72,** 1093.
27. Dransfield, I. (1987). PhD thesis. University of Sheffield, UK.
28. Figdor, C. G., Bont, W. S., Touw, I., Roos, J. D., Roosnek, E. E., and de Vries, J. E. (1982). *Blood,* **60,** 41.
29. Yam, L. T., Li, C. Y., and Crosby, W. H. (1971). *Am. J. Clin. Path.,* **53,** 283.
30. Kaplow, L. S. (1965). *Blood,* **26,** 215.
31. Shen, L., Guyre, P. M., and Fanger, M. W. (1988). *J. Immunol.,* **139,** 534.
32. Pulford, K. A. F., Rigney, E., Micklem, K. J., Jones, M., Stross, W. P., Gatter, K. C., *et al.* (1989). *J. Clin. Pathol.,* **42,** 414.
33. Rhodes, J. (1977). *Nature,* **265,** 253.
34. Adams, D. O. and Hamilton, T. A. (1984). *Ann. Rev. Immunol.,* **2,** 283.
35. Woof, J. M., Partridge, L. J., Jefferies, R., and Burton, D. R. (1986). *Mol. Immunol.,* **23,** 319.
36. Johnson, G. D., Goddard, D. H., and Holborrow, E. J. (1982). *J. Immunol. Methods,* **50,** 277.
37. Osborn, M. and Weber, K. (1982). *Methods Cell Biol.,* **24,** 97.
38. Adams, D. O., Edelson, P. J., and Koren, H. (ed.) (1981). *Methods for Studying Mononuclear Phagocytes.* Academic, New York.
39. Zembala, M. and Asherson, G. L. (ed.) (1989). *Human Monocytes.* Academic, New York.

40. Chen, A. R., Whitaker, F. S., McKinnon, K. P., and Koren, H. S. (1986). *Cell Immunol.,* **103,** 120.
41. Kleinerman, E. S., Kurzrock, R., Wyatt, D., Quesada, J. R., Gutterman, J. U., and Fidler, L. J. (1986). *Cancer Res.,* **46,** 5401.
42. Weiss, S. J., Lobuglio, A. F., and Kessler, H. B. (1980). *Proc. Natl Acad. Sci. USA,* **77,** 584.
43. Kleinerman, E. S. and Herberman, R. B. (1984). *J. Immunol.,* **133,** 4.
44. Colotta, F., Peri, G., Villa, A., and Mantovani, A. (1984). *J. Immunol.,* **132,** 936.
45. Urbaniak, S. J. (1976). *Br. J. Haematol.,* **33,** 409.
46. Kaplan, A. M. (1981). In *Methods for Studying Mononuclear Phagocytes,* (ed. D. O. Adams, P. J. Edelson, and H. Koren), p. 755. Academic, New York.
47. Trush, M. A., Wilson, M. E., and Van Dyke, K. (1978). *Methods Enzymol.,* **57,** 462.
48. Walter, R. J., Danielson, J. R., Van Alten, P. J., and Powell, W. J. (1986). *J. Surg. Res.,* **41,** 215.
49. Barker, M. D., Jose, P. J., Williams, T. J., and Burton, D. R. (1986). *Biochem. J.,* **236,** 621.
50. Camussi, G., Tetta, C., Bussolino, F., and Baglioni, C. (1990). *J. Exp. Med.,* **171,** 913.
51. Taffeb, S. M. and Russell, S. W. (1981). In *Methods for Studying Mononuclear Phagocytes,* (ed. D. O. Adams, P. J. Edelson, and H. Koren), p. 283. Academic, New York.
52. Ito, M., Ralph, P., and Moore, M. A. S. (1979). *Cell. Immunol.,* **46,** 48.
53. Asherson, G. L. and Colizzi, V. (1989). In *Human Monocytes*, (ed. M. Zembala and G. L. Asherson), p. 313. Academic, New York.
54. Haskill, S., Johnson, C., Eierman, D., Becker, S., and Warren, K. (1988). *J. Immunol.,* **140,** 1690.
55. Schreiber, A. D., Kelley, M., Dziarski, A., and Levinson, A. I. (1983). *Immunology,* **49,** 231.
56. Elias, J. A., Ferro, T. J., Rossman, M. D., Greenberg, J. A., Daniele, R. P., Schreiber, A. D., *et al.* (1987). *J. Leuk. Biol.,* **42,** 114.
57. Chiu, K. M., McPherson, L. M., Harris, J. E., and Braun, D. P. (1984). *J. Leuk. Biol.,* **36,** 729.
58. Normann, S. J. and Weiner, R. (1983). *Cell Immunol.,* **81,** 413.
59. Turpin, J., Hersch, E. M., and Lopez-Berestein, G. (1986). *J. Immunol.,* **136,** 4194.
60. Esa, A. H., Noga, S. J., Donnenberg, A. D., and Hess, A. D. (1986). *Immunology,* **59,** 95.
61. McCartney, D. L., Shah, V. O., and Weiner, R. S. (1983). *J. Immunol.,* **131,** 1780.
62. Picker, L. J., Raff, H. V., Goldyne, M. E., and Stobo, J. D. (1980). *J. Immunol.,* **124,** 2557.
63. Yasaka, T., Mantich, N. M., Boxer, L. A., and Boehner, R. L. (1981). *J. Immunol.,* **127,** 1515.

7

T cells: proliferative and cytotoxic responses

R. ADRIAN ROBINS

1. Introduction

In many experimental tumour models, T cells have been shown to play a critical role in the effector phase of immunologically mediated tumour rejection (1) and of course, T cells play a vital role in the regulation of many aspects of the immune response, including final effector mechanisms of broad specificity. The characterization of T cells involved in these varied roles in the immune responses to tumours is central to tumour immunobiology. There have been rapid developments in the techniques available to identify T cells, analyse the cytokines they produce, and to monitor their interactions with tumour cells as well as other cells of the immune system. This chapter will describe methods for the separation of lymphocytes from tissues including tumours; for purification of T cells from these populations; and for measuring the reactivity of these T cells in terms of proliferation and cytotoxicity. Associated technologies, for example relating to T-cell markers, cloning, and cytokines, are discussed in detail in other chapters of this book, and cross-references will be made where appropriate.

Many of the methods described are generally applicable to a wide range of tumour types, and in principle are usable in human and experimental systems. Attention will be drawn, however, to variations suitable for particular systems, or to approaches for optimization of a technique for novel applications.

2. Media for lymphocyte preparation and assay

2.1 Salt base, buffer, and nutrients

The media used for lymphocyte preparation should provide an appropriate pH in vessels exposed to normal atmospheric concentrations of CO_2, and an osmolarity appropriate to the species being studied. For the mouse, this will be 310 mOsmol, and for the human, 272 mOsmol. We find it convenient to check the osmotic strength of media and density gradients (see below) using a freezing-point osmometer; the osmolarities given are the values we determine with reference to the manufacturer's 300 mOsmol standard. The control of osmolarity is particularly important when using density gradients, for example with Percoll (see below).

Buffering of media with up to 25 mM Hepes can be advantageous, but care must be taken to ensure that the optimum osmolarity of the medium is not exceeded. For human cultures especially, it may be necessary to use a medium base with a reduced NaCl concentration to accomplish this. Also, for media to be used to culture cells for more than a few hours, the initial pH of Hepes buffer must be above 7.4, otherwise the buffering capacity of the medium will easily be exceeded.

A balanced salt solution buffered with a low concentration of bicarbonate, such as Hanks' balanced salt solution (HBSS) is appropriate for dissociation and washing of lymphocyte suspensions, although it is important to include a protein supplement. For most studies, 2% serum is adequate.

For human studies, RPMI 1640 is a standard culture medium, and we have found Dulbecco's modified Eagle's minimal essential medium (DMEM) good for mouse T-cell studies. In both cases, supplementation with additional non-essential amino acids, sodium pyruvate and 2-mercaptoethanol (5×10^{-5} M) is required. Glutamine is a labile essential ingredient of culture medium, and fresh glutamine should be added (to 2 mM final concentration) after media have been stored at 4°C for more than two weeks.

2.2 Serum or protein supplements

2.2.1 Bovine serum

Foetal bovine serum (FBS) is the most frequently used serum supplement for lymphocyte separation and assay. The product should be clear and straw coloured, with no haemoglobin contamination. It may be necessary to test batches of serum to select suitable material. 10% serum is included in culture medium.

2.2.2 Species-compatible serum

For some assays it is desirable to use serum from the same species as the lymphocytes under study. Rat and mouse serum can be toxic, but low concentrations (1–2%) will support blastogenesis and cytotoxicity assays. Batches of human AB serum should be checked for good support of cell growth and lack of inhibitory activity.

3. Dissociation and separation of lymphocytes

The first step in the process of examining T cells for their recognition of tumour-associated antigens is to obtain those cells in suspension; further purification and analysis can then proceed. Separation of lymphoid cells from blood and lymphoid tissues is so well established that detailed descriptions are not necessary. Attention will be drawn, however, to points which we have found to be of particular importance.

3.1 Sources for lymphocyte isolation

3.1.1 Blood

Centrifugation over Ficoll–metrizoate mixtures with a density of 1.077 is widely used to prepare mononuclear cells from whole blood (2), and prepared solutions for this method are readily available (e.g. Lymphoprep, from Flow Laboratories). Particular care should be taken to ensure that the separation medium and blood are at room temperature before separation is undertaken. If blood cannot be separated immediately after being drawn, it is best stored at room temperature. Similarly, transport of unseparated blood samples is best done in insulated containers to prevent the blood cooling below approximately 20°C. Recovery of lymphocytes in good yield and without selective loss of major sub-populations defined by CD3, CD4, CD8, and CD19 markers can be obtained from blood stored overnight at room temperature.

3.1.2 Lymphoid tissues

Lymphocytes are easily liberated into suspension from lymph node or spleen tissue by gentle teasing and pressing against stainless steel mesh in a petri dish containing 5–10 ml of HBSS + 2% serum. After washing by centrifugation with HBSS + 2% serum, cells are re-suspended in culture medium.

3.1.3 Peritoneal cavity

Induced peritoneal exudates can be a good source of specific T cells in experimental systems; for example, we have been able to detect anti-tumour cytotoxicity (3) and transfer-delayed hypersensitivity (4) using these cells. Peritoneal lavage is performed by injecting HBSS + 2% FBS, gently massaging the abdomen, then carefully withdrawing medium back into the syringe.

3.1.4 Tumour tissue

Methods used for dissociation of tumour tissue vary depending on the tumour type under study. Indeed, with human tumours, the technique may need to be tailored to each individual tumour. Tumour material should be suspended in sterile medium (RPMI + 2% FBS), and transferred to the laboratory as promptly as possible. Refrigerate at 4°C before processing the tumour. With tumours from non-sterile sites such as the colon, it is necessary to include a cocktail of antibiotics in the medium, including a fungicide such as amphotericin B.

The most frequently used enzymes for tumour dissociation are collagenase and trypsin. Collagenase-based enzymes are least destructive to cell surface structures, and are effective on a wide range of tumours. Trypsin is effective, particularly with some murine tumours, and has the property of digesting dead tumour cells, giving highly viable tumour cell suspensions; however, some cell surface structures are sensitive to trypsin (e.g. rat CD4). DNase is a useful addition to dissociation mixtures, digesting DNA released from damaged cells which otherwise aggregates cells into large stringy clumps. Any dissociation protocol should of course be checked for effects on the markers or functions of interest.

- *Collagenase*: the suitability of the enzyme source used should be checked both for effective dissociation and lack of toxicity for the cells being analysed. We have found that Boehringer Mannheim collagenase that has been screened for hepatocyte dissociation is good for 'difficult' cells. Use a solution containing 0.1% collagenase in RPMI 1640.
- *Trypsin*: 0.25% trypsin in serum-free RPMI is used for dissociation. This may be made from sterile stock solutions (e.g. Flow Laboratories), but ensure that enzyme solutions are stored frozen and kept on ice when thawed, as the enzyme autodigests, and rapidly loses activity, even at room temperature.
- *DNase*: stock solution of 0.025% DNase (Sigma type I) in RPMI-1640.

Protocol 1. Enzymatic dissociation of tumour tissue[a]

1. Place the tumour sample in a petri dish and dissect the tumour tissue from any associated normal tissue or tumour capsule; separate and discard any necrotic tissue. Cut the tumour tissue into small fragments using a sharp scalpel.
2. Transfer the tissue to a universal container, and remove any debris by washing the tumour fragments by decantation with HBSS + 2% FCS. If the amount of tumour tissue is limited, or a quantitative recovery of cells is required, the tumour cells released mechanically during dissection of the tumour can be recovered by centrifugation. Note also that some tumour types can be dissociated to a large extent by mechanical means.
3. Add the dissociating enzyme solution plus a few drops of DNase, and agitate the mixture gently. A magnetic stirrer must be run as slowly as possible, to minimize damage to released cells, and stirrers should be checked to ensure that they do not overheat the tumour suspension.
4. Incubate at 37°C for 15–45 min, monitoring the dissociation of tumour fragments. Decant the released cell suspension from any remaining tumour tissue, and add fresh enzyme solution to continue the digestion process. Alternatively, the enzyme solution may be incubated with tumour for longer time periods at room temperature.
5. Recover the released cells by centrifugation. Centrifugation conditions should be tailored to the aims of the experiment: if both malignant and infiltrating inflammatory cells are required, an initial slow-speed spin to pellet malignant cells should be performed, allowing ready re-suspension

of these large and often fragile cells. The supernatant from this initial centrifugation can then be centrifuged at higher speed to recover those lymphocytes remaining in suspension. Centrifugation times and *g* forces should be optimized for the equipment and cell types being studied.

6. Wash cells twice by centrifugation with HBSS + 2% FCS, and finally resuspend in a suitable culture medium such as RPMI 1640 + 10% serum.

[a] See also Chapter 1.

---

4. Purification of lymphocytes and T cells

A range of methods exists to separate lymphocytes and T cells or their subsets from tumour cell suspensions. Fluorescence-activated cell sorting (FACS) is a valuable method for selecting specific cell populations using combinations of physical characteristics and monoclonal antibody-defined phenotype, particularly when relatively small numbers of specific cells are required for subsequent assays. The analytical use of flow cytometry is of course recommended to confirm the identity and purity of cell populations purified by other means. These approaches are covered in Chapter 4.

Separation methods based on cell size, such as velocity sedimentation, can provide excellent purification of lymphocytes and tumour cells under very gentle conditions (5), but this approach ideally requires a reorientating sedimentation chamber to separate large numbers of cells, and is a time-consuming procedure. With some experimental tumours, the differential adherence properties of tumour cells and infiltrating T cells can be exploited to provide a rapid single-step purification of tumour-infiltrating T cells (6).

Two methods for separating T cells from tumours of more general applicability are: to use differences in cell density, separating cells by isopycnic centrifugation on Percoll gradients; and to identify cell surface markers to selectively bind magnetic beads, allowing separation of cells in a magnetic field. These methods are discussed in more detail below.

4.1 Density gradients

PVP-coated colloidal silica (Percoll, Pharmacia Ltd) is a valuable medium for density separations, as density and osmolarity can be controlled independently, and separation solutions are of low viscosity and non-toxic to cells. Osmolarity is important for density separations (7) and in our experience, dilution of Percoll with 10× strength PBS results in solutions with higher osmolarity than expected (Percoll itself has a very low osmolarity). Dilution with distilled water may be necessary to achieve the desired osmolarity, and further dilution to make solutions of required density can then be made using culture medium. For consistent results, the density of diluted Percoll solutions should be checked using a specific-gravity bottle, to allow for batch to batch variations in Percoll and diluting solutions.

A density of 1.080 will support most mononuclear cells and tumour cells, but polymorphs and erythrocytes will pellet through this density. Erythrocytes may be removed from small volumes of tumour cell suspension rapidly and with quantitative recovery of malignant cells using 1.080 density Percoll. 1 ml of Percoll is layered under the tumour cell suspension with a Pasteur pipette, and the tube centrifuged for 10 min at 500*g*; purified tumour cells may then be collected from the interface.

The optimal densities of Percoll for separation of lymphocytes from malignant cells may need to be determined for the tumour type under study. Many tumour cell types will accumulate at an interface of Percoll with a density of 1.050–1.055, through which most mononuclear cells will pass, at an osmolarity of 300 mOsmol.

4.2 Magnetic beads

For tumours where cell surface markers are available for the malignant cells, the magnetic bead separation method can be used rapidly and effectively to separate infiltrating host cells. The tumour cell suspension is treated with saturating amounts of anti-marker antibody and washed to remove unbound antibody. A panel of antibodies may be necessary to achieve staining of all the malignant cells in the suspension (8). Magnetic beads coated with appropriate anti-immunoglobulin antibody are then mixed with the cell suspension, using the ratio of beads to cells recommended by the manufacturer (Dynal Ltd). Cells with magnetic beads attached are then retained in the tube by a magnet, and the purified cell suspension removed.

This type of separation is particularly effective for depletion (negative selection), although positively selected cells can also be recovered. The growth of tumour cells is not markedly affected by the presence of magnetic beads.

5. Cryopreservation of lymphocytes

A good cryopreservation technique allows the time course of an immune response to be studied in a single experiment (9), as well as overcoming logistic difficulties that are often encountered when measuring responses against autologous tumour cells. Preservation of some effector cells, particularly NK cells, is difficult, but cytotoxic precursors and proliferative responses are usually recoverd quantitatively.

- *Dimethyl sulphoxide (DMSO)*: DMSO is unstable, building up by-products in storage, and should therefore be bought in small quantities. Sealed glass ampoules containing cell-culture-screened DMSO are available (Sigma Chemical Co.).

Protocol 2. Cryopreservation and recovery

1. Re-suspend cells in a 'freezing mixture' consisting of 5% DMSO in bovine serum, and dispense in aliquots in plastic vials designed for low-temperature storage.
2. Freeze vials under controlled conditions. A programmable controlled-rate freezing apparatus is ideal, but excellent results can be obtained using a −70°C freezer. The vials are placed in a box with cardboard or polystyrene divisions which is at room temperature, and then put in the freezer. Avoid direct contact with metal parts, which will result in a too rapid a rate of cooling.
3. After 24 h, transfer the vials to the vapour phase over liquid nitrogen for long-term storage.
4. For recovery of cells, rapidly thaw the vial by shaking in a 37°C waterbath, removing the vial from the waterbath as the last ice melts.
5. Without delay, dilute the cell suspension, but add culture medium gradually (one or two drops at a time at first) to minimize osmotic shock caused by differential concentrations of DMSO inside and outside the cell.
6. Wash the cells twice by centrifugation and re-suspend in culture medium.

6. Proliferation assays

The proliferative response that follows effective triggering of T cells by antigen can be used to detect and characterize T cells responsive to tumour-associated antigens. Replicate cultures of lymphocytes in microwells are stimulated with tumour cells and appropriate antigen-presenting cells, and the resulting lymphocyte proliferation monitored. The incorporation of [^{3}H]thymidine is the standard method by which this proliferation is evaluated, but the conditions required for this incorporation to reflect proliferation accurately are not always appreciated.

The specific activity of the [^{3}H]thymidine used is particularly important, as this usually reflects the total thymidine concentration in the well. Thus, at very high specific activities, the thymidine concentration is low, and uptake can be limited by the availability of thymidine. The total concentration of thymidine should be saturating over the pulse time chosen, so that incorporation is uniformly related to DNA synthesis throughout. Further problems with high-specific-activity [^{3}H]thymidine are that:

(a) incorporation may be reduced by radiotoxicity

(b) uptake may be into intracellular pools, rather than into DNA synthesis and

(c) unlabelled thymidine released by cells in the assay will have a marked effect on the specific activity and thus the uptake of [^{3}H]thymidine

For all these reasons, a maximum specific activity of around 6 Ci/mMol is recommended for a 6 h pulse (10), with lower concentrations (0.5–1 Ci/mMol) for longer pulse periods.

A protocol for blastogenesis assays using 96-well Microtest II plates is given, as the equipment for this approach is more frequently available than that required for alternative methods using hanging cultures in 10 μl wells (11). However, the latter method is economical of cells and is therefore particularly suitable for detailed analysis of dose responses and time courses.

Where tumour cell-lines are used as stimulator cells, care should be taken to ensure that the cells are mycoplasma free. Lines should be obtained where possible from culture collections, and subsequently tested regularly to ensure that they remain uninfected. Mycoplasma infection can be detected by staining with Hoescht dye 33258, or by using ^{3}H-labelled probe (Genprobe Ltd) to detect mycoplasma DNA. The chance of mycoplasma contamination can be reduced by culturing established cell-lines without use of antibiotics, so that a mishap causing contamination is not obscured (see also Chapter 1).

Protocol 3. Proliferation assay

1. Dilute responder cells to (0.5–2) × 10^6 cells/ml, and dispense 100 μl per well (5 × 10^4 to 2 × 10^5 cells per well).
2. Stimulator tumour cells are irradiated with 6000 rads to prevent their proliferation, and added to the wells in 100 μl medium. The number of cells added must be optimized; a starting point of 3000 cells per well is recommended. Similarly, the concentration of a soluble tumour antigen preparation will need to be determined by experiment.
3. Incubate the plates for 2–4 days at 37°C.
4. Pulse the wells with [^{3}H]thymidine. We find it convenient to add 10 μl per well of a thymidine solution containing 1 μCi at a specific activity of 1 Ci/mMol (see our comments on specific activity above).
5. Incubate for a further 24 h, and then collect and wash cells using a multiple automated sample harvestor, which deposits the cells on to a glass-fibre disc.
6. Add the discs to counting vials with suitable scintillant, and count the [^{3}H]thymidine in a β-counter.

Results of proliferation assays are conventionally expressed either as a proliferation index, which is the *ratio* of the [^{3}H]thymidine incorporation in stimulated wells to that in medium controls, or a delta index, which is the *difference* between stimulated and control incorporation of [^{3}H]thymidine.

Background incorporation by stimulator cells alone and residual counts in pulsed empty wells should be subtracted before making these calculations. A lectin such as phytohaemaglutinin is a useful positive control, especially when a number of cryopreserved lymphocyte preparations are being compared.

7. Cytotoxicity assays

Assays to measure the impact of effector cells on target tumour cell growth and/or survival can be divided into different groups according to the type of damage that can be revealed, and the time-scale over which that damage is inflicted. For short-term damage (up to 24 h), ^{51}Cr release methods have been used extensively, and this remains a standard approach. The survival of tumour cells after longer-term interactions between effector and target cells can be evaluated by the using pre-labelled target cells, or using a label added at the end of the assay which is taken up quantitatively by surviving target cells (post-label assay). These longer-term assays are usually performed with carcinoma and sarcoma target cells, which grow in monolayer culture and remain adherent whilst viable.

The time-scale of pre-labelling assays is limited by the stability of the label in the target cells; pre-labelling methods also require that this stable incorporation of the label does not affect the viability of the target cell, and that label is released and not reincorporated on target cell damage (12). Post-label assays have the potential for longer assay times, but the conditions for label incorporation must accurately reflect the number of surviving target cells.

7.1 ^{51}Cr release

In addition to specific targets of interest, control target cells with known high and low NK sensitivity may usefully be included in assays of mixed populations of effector cells. In the human system, K562 erythroleukaemia and Daudi Burkitt's lymphoma respectively are suitable cell-lines.

Protocol 4. ^{51}Cr release assay

1. Harvest the cultured target cells from logarithmic growth, wash them and perform a cell count. Freshly derived target cells should be similarly washed and counted.
2. Centrifuge an aliquot of $(1–5) \times 10^6$ target cells in a conical-bottomed 10 ml tube, and re-suspend the pellet in 200 μl of culture medium. Some target cells may label more satisfactorily in 200 μl FCS.
3. Add 100 μCi $Na^{51}CrO_4$, diluted to 100 μl in PBS and incubate for 45–90 min at 37 °C in a CO_2 incubator. The tube will reach 37 °C rapidly if placed in a beaker containing water previously equilibrated to 37 °C. Re-suspend the cells frequently during the labelling period.

Protocol 4. *Continued*

4. Wash the cells three to four times with 10 ml of medium, then re-incubate at 37°C for 30–60 minutes.
5. Add effector cells in 100 μl aliquots to 96-well microtest II plates, in triplicate, with a range of effector cell numbers usually in doubling dilutions. Include wells containing medium alone.
6. Wash the target cells once more, re-suspend them, count, and dilute to 5×10^4 cells/ml; add 100 μl of target cells per well. Aliquots of target cells are also added to tubes for counting to determine the total radioactivity per well.
7. Incubate at 37°C and remove 100 μl of supernatant to determine released ^{51}Cr. This is usually done after 4 h, but 6 and 8 h have been used successfully.

---

^{51}Cr activity released into supernatant is determined from the proportion of supernatant removed for counting, and this is calculated as a percentage of the total counts per well. Percentage cytotoxicity is calculated according to:

$$\%cyto = 100 \frac{e - m}{t - m}$$

where e is % release with effector cells, m is % release with medium, and t = 100, or maximum counts released by 0.1 M HCl.

Comparison of different effector cell populations is a complex issue, which has been approached in a variety of ways. With some effector cell/target cell combinations, a linear relationship between percentage cytotoxicity and effector cell number is apparent, particularly at cytotoxicities below 25% where target cells are not limiting. Linear regression can then be used to estimate this relationship, and the relative activity can be expressed as the ratio of slopes (13). Where the relationship between percentage cytotoxicity and effector cell number is non-linear, curve-fitting methods can be used (14). In this case, a convenient measure of cytotoxic activity is the lytic unit, that is the number of effector cells required to achieve a given level of cytotoxicity, although it should be borne in mind that for this comparison to be valid, the shape of the dose–response curve should be the same for the effector populations being compared. To express this activity on a scale which increases with increased lysis, lytic units per 10^6 effector cells is usually calculated.

7.2 Post-label cytotoxicity assays

Considerations discussed with respect to uptake of [^{3}H]thymidine by lymphocytes (Section 6) also apply to the use of precursors whose uptake is used to quantitate target cell survival. A DNA precursor such as [^{3}H]thymidine is often used for this purpose, and if appropriate conditions of saturation are observed, accurate quantitation can be obtained. It should be noted that some precursors, such as [^{125}I]iododeoxyuridine, require higher concentrations to achieve saturation, and toxicity can then limit the pulse length over which uptake is quantitative (15).

A problem with some types of target cells is their limited utilization of DNA precursors supplied externally. We have observed this phenomenon particularly with human colorectal tumour cells. An effective solution to this problem is to use an amino acid precursor, and [^{75}Se]selenomethionine is a particularly convenient gamma-emitting analogue of methionine suitable for this purpose (15). It is essential to ensure by control cell-counting experiments that whichever precursor is selected, it is being used under conditions where uptake accurately reflects cell survival.

Protocol 5. Post-label cytotoxicity assay

1. Dispense target cells (in 100 μl of complete culture medium) into microtest II plates with flat-bottomed wells, selecting an inoculum which will not be fully confluent in untreated wells by the end of the assay.
2. Add graded numbers of effector cells to replicate wells, and medium alone to control wells. It is essential to control for incorporation of precursor by effector cells alone, especially when these are tumour-derived, and could contain malignant cells.
3. After 2–4 days' incubation, add isotope labelled precursor. [^{3}H]thymidine can usually be used at similar concentrations to those used in blastogenesis assays. [^{75}Se]selenomethionine is usually used at 0.1 μCi per well; additional unlabelled methionine may be required to ensure saturation, although with some target cells, methionine present in the medium may still be present at an adequate concentration.
4. After a further 16 h of incubation, wash away unincorporated precursor and process the wells appropriately to allow counting of the incorporated isotope. Washing conditions may need to be tailored to the adherence properties of the target cell being studied. Very gentle but effective washing can be achieved by completely immersing the plate in three successive baths of phosphate-buffered saline.

References

1. Robins, R. A. (1986). *Biochim. Biophys. Acta,* **856,** 289.
2. Boyum, A. (1968). *Scand. J. Clin. Lab. Invest.,* **21** (suppl. 97), 9.
3. Baldwin, R. W., Britten, V., Ferry, B., Kays, S., and Robins, R. A. (1985). In *Immunity to Cancer*, p. 149. Academic, New York.
4. Austin, E. B., Robins, R. A., Baldwin, R. W., and Durrant, L. G. (1991). *J. Natl Cancer Inst.,* **83,** 1245.

5. Ferry, B. L., Flannery, G. R., Robins, R. A., Lawry, J., and Baldwin, R. W. (1984). *Immunology,* **53,** 243.
6. Robins, R. A., Flannery, G. R., and Baldwin, R. W. (1979). *Br. J. Cancer,* **40,** 946.
7. Braide, M. and Bjursten, L. M. (1986). *J. Immunol. Meth.,* **93,** 183.
8. Durrant, L. G., Robins, R. A., Byers, V. S., Ballantyne, K. C., Marksman, R., Hardcastle, J. D., *et al.* (1989). *Br. J. Cancer,* **60,** 855.
9. Robins, R. A., Denton, G. W. L., Hardcastle, J. D., Austin, E. B., Baldwin, R. W., and Durrant, L. G. (1991). *Cancer Res.,* **51,** 5425.
10. O'Leary, J. J., Mehta, C., Hall, D. J., and Rosenberg, A. (1980). *Cell Tissue Kinetics,* **13,** 21.
11. Knight, S. C. (1987). In *Lymphocytes,* (ed. G. G. B. Klaus), p. 189. IRL Press, Oxford.
12. Brooks, C. G. (1978). *J. Immunol. Meth.,* **22,** 23.
13. Brooks, C. G. and Flannery, G. R. (1980). *Immunology,* **39,** 187.
14. Pross, H. F., Baines, M. G., Rubin, P., Schragge, P., and Patterson, M. S. (1980). *J. Clin. Immunol.,* **1,** 51.
15. Brooks, C. G., Rees, R. C., and Robins, R. A. (1978). *J. Immunol. Meth.,* **21,** 111.

8

Cloning and propagation of human T lymphocytes

GRAHAM PAWELEC

1. Introduction

The utilization of T-cell clones (TCC) has proved of critical importance in understanding the role of T cells as the central control elements of the immune system. The enigma of the nature of the T-cell receptor for antigen (TCR) was first resolved by the production of monoclonal antibodies against the unique 'clonotypic' determinants of human TCC (1), followed by cloning of TCR genes from monoclonal populations (2). TCC constitute vital probes for the recognition of specific antigen determinants, enabling for example, the demonstration of TCR recognition of peptide fragments in association with MHC molecules (3). Additionally, reductionist studies of T-cell function have benefited from the use of TCC, so much so that the apparent difficulty in generating TCC with a particular function has even been cited as evidence against the very existence of cells with that particular function (4).

The generation of TCC necessarily requires the application of long-term tissue-culture methodologies (since 21 population doublings (PD) are needed even to generate 10^6 cells from a single progenitor). Usable numbers of cells (10^8–10^9) require 28–31 PD, which remains significantly less than the Hayflick number of 50 PD, at which point normal cells are thought to begin to senesce and die (5). The present chapter will therefore concern itself only with the techniques required for propagating human TCC up to an age of about 35 PD, representing nearly 10^{10} cells, which are sufficient for most immunological investigations of antigen recognition, T-cell regulation, cytokine gene transcription, and even possibly for their eventual utilization for adoptive immunotherapy. The behaviour of human TCC after this time point, which is of interest to researchers in ageing, tumour biology, immunophysiology, etc. is controversial (6), and beyond the scope of this chapter.

Note that there are no universally agreed protocols for producing human TCC; rather, each laboratory uses its own modifications of a similar consensus methodology. In this chapter, I present our methods, and point out various differences known to be in use in others' laboratories. The procedures for the production and propagation of human TCC will be treated in the following steps:

- tissue-culture medium and growth factors required
- source of T cells for cloning, and their activation
- cloning methodologies and long-term culture of TCC
- cryopreservation
- assurance of monoclonality

2. Tissue-culture medium and growth factors

The proliferation of human T lymphocytes in long-term culture is, like that of other mammalian cells, governed by the requirement for factors found in serum, in addition to simple nutrients. Furthermore, T lymphocytes require additional sources of specialized growth factors, as well as those found in serum. The medium of choice for the propagation of human TCC is RPMI 1640, but, particularly when attempting to use serum-free formulations, Dulbecco's modified Eagle's medium (DMEM) is often used. Although human TCC can be grown in medium supplemented with either human serum (HS) or foetal calf serum (FCS), the well known disadvantages of serum (batch-to-batch variability, micro-organism contamination, presence of undefined factors influencing what you want to measure) suggest that a serum substitute would be beneficial. Unfortunately, the formulation of a serum-free medium (SFM) suitable for long-term culture of human TCC has been problematic. We find that the best SFM is our modification of Yssel's medium (7); although in our hands this does *not* allow cloning, it is possible to propagate established clones for several PD in this formula, which can be useful for certain purposes. Although Yssel *et al.* originally suggested that their SF medium alone was sufficient for long-term human T-cell growth, the same group later modified their culture technique by adding back a small amount of plasma to the SFM (8).

Protocol 1. Formulation of modified Yssel's SFM (YSFM) for human TCC

1. Make stock solutions of the basic additives with which to supplement Iscove's modified DMEM (IDMEM):
   - fatty acid-free bovine serum albumin (Cohn Fraction V) at 2.5 mg/ml in IDMEM
   - human insulin at 5 mg/ml in 0.01 M HCl
   - human transferrin (with iron) at 35 mg/ml in PBS
   - ethanolamine at 20 mM in IDMEM

- linoleic acid at 1 mg/ml in ethanol
- palmitic acid at 1 mg/ml in ethanol
- oleic acid at 1 mg/ml in ethanol

2. Add 1 ml of each of the above to 1 litre of IDMEM, being sure to add the BSA **first**. This is standard YSFM, to which should be added (freshly, for long-term culture):
   - 250 μg/ml of β-cyclodextrin
   - 20 ng/ml low-density lipoprotein
   - 2 μM L-putrescine
   - 2 mM L-glutamine
   - and, if desired, 20 mM HEPES and antibiotics.
3. All media must be sterile filtered through membranes selected for low protein absorbing capacity.

Because of the difficulties with SFM, TCC are routinely cultured in serum-containing medium. Human serum must be from non-transfused males, not necessarily only of blood group AB. It is regularly heat-inactivated, although some claim a growth advantage of using serum which has not been inactivated (9). We have not found this. Human serum with intact complement components is a potent anti-mycoplasmatic (10), which could explain better growth of (mycoplasma-contaminated) cultures in non-inactivated serum. Each individual human serum must be pretested for its ability to support growth of T cells, before pooling to create a large batch for use over a long period. Similarly, each batch of FCS must be pre-screened. We find that more than 95% of human sera are acceptable, but less than 10% of FCS batches are suitable for long-term T-cell culture.

The other vital component of the TCM for T-lymphocyte propagation is the T-cell growth factor(s) (TCGF). Although the major TCGF remains interleukin (IL) 2, at least four other factors are now known to function as direct TCGF (direct in contrast to facilitative). These are IL-4, IL-7, IL-9, and IL-12, all of which are present in the conditioned medium (CM) of normal peripheral blood mononuclear cells (PBMC) activated with T-cell mitogens (such as phytohaemagglutinin, PHA). CM also contains facilitative factors such as IL-6, interferon-γ, and probably other not yet defined factors. For cloning certain types of T cell, it may therefore be advisable to use not only IL-2 as the TCGF, but to set up parallel cloning experiments using CM as a source of TCGF. In this way, TCC can be obtained which are dependent on not-yet identified factors other than IL-2 alone. The identification of the factors required can then be approached by repeating experiments in mixtures of known recombinant cytokines.

3. Source of T cells for cloning, and their activation

3.1 T-cell source

The most convenient common source of human T cells for cloning is peripheral blood. Mononuclear cells (PBMC) are usually isolated by centrifugation over a density-gradient separation medium, such as a mixture of Ficoll and sodium Hypaque with a specific gravity of 1.077. Erythrocytes are agglutinated by the Ficoll, and they and the polymorphs transit through the separation medium to leave PBMC (usually about 20% monocytes, 10% B cells, and 70% T cells) at the interface. These PBMC may be further fractionated into sub-sets, most commonly by a variety of antibody-based techniques such as sorting or panning. For example, we and many investigators find that the isolation of $CD8^+$ or TCR1 $(\gamma/\delta)^+$ TCC is a rare event unless the population of cells to be cloned is first enriched for that particular sub-population.

A second important source of human T cells for cloning is tissue infiltrating lymphocytes (TIL). Particularly for studies on tumour immunity, rejection of transplanted organs, or in autoimmune diseases one assumes that lymphocytes within the target tissue may be more relevant to the disease process than those in the peripheral blood. There are two main approaches to cloning and culturing TIL:

(a) Cut the tissue into small pieces (1 mm^3) and place individually into wells of cluster plates with medium containing T-cell growth factors (usually IL-2, but there may be advantages to investigating mixtures of TCGF). Inspect the plates regularly and observe T cells emigrating from the tissue. Transfer these to new culture vessels for propagation (see Section 4). Usually, T cells emigrate quite rapidly (< 1 week), but this varies according to tissue; for example, T cells may first emigrate from inflamed synovial membrane as long as four weeks after initiation of culture, so don't give up too early.

(b) Cut the tissue into small pieces and subject to enzymatic digestion (5 mg/ml collagenase type-IV with 0.15 mg/ml DNase type-I for 4 h at 37°C). Then pass through a 250 μm nylon mesh, wash and separate viable lymphocytes over Ficoll–Hypaque gradients.

3.2 Activation

T lymphocytes must be activated before they will proliferate and allow themselves to be cloned. According to the aims of the experimenter and the source of the cells to clone, this may be achieved (a) by isolating pre-activated cells *ex vivo*, (b) by stimulating non-specifically with the aim of activating all of the T cells (e.g. for 'repertoire' analysis), and (c) by stimulating with selected antigen to activate only the relevant antigen-specific cells.

(a) Clone the cells directly after isolation or after pre-culture in medium without antigen or mitogen but containing TCGF.

(b) Stimulate the cells with mitogens such as PHA, which seems to trigger proliferation of all competent cells. When using human serum in the culture medium, higher concentrations of the mitogen are required (use 1 μg/ml pure PHA in SFM, but use at least 10 μg/ml in medium with 10% HS). Wash cells well after 48 h and clone.

(c) Stimulate *in vitro* with the antigen of choice. T lymphocytes respond to alloantigens but to little else without prior *in vivo* sensitization. Protocols for *in vivo* and *in vitro* sensitization to foreign antigens are uncommon and beyond the scope of this chapter. In tumour immunology it is common to 'boost' responding cells *in vitro* by co-culturing them with autologous tumour cells. These protocols differ according to tumour and laboratory, but always consist of co-culturing responder cells with proliferation-inactivated (usually irradiated) purified or enriched tumour cells, sometimes in the presence of exogenous TCGF from the beginning of culture. I give an example of a variant of the 'mixed lymphocyte tumour culture' (MLTC) employed in our laboratory (11, 12):

Protocol 2. MLTC using PBMC from chronic myelogenous leukaemia (CML) patients

1. Select chronic-phase patients with more than 75% tumour cells in PBMC, irradiate with 20 Gy and re-suspend at 1×10^6/ml in RPMI 1640 with 10% HS.
2. Treat 1×10^6/ml cells from the same patients with 100 μg/ml cytosine arabinoside (Ara-C) for 60 min at 37 °C and wash well (this simply results in destruction of tumour cells, which are otherwise difficult to remove in CML).
3. Set up (a) diagnostic and (b) sensitization MLTC.
   (a) Mix 5×10^4 Ara-C-treated cells with an equal number of irradiated untreated cells from the same donors, in triplicate in 200 μl medium per round-bottom well microtitre plate. Controls should include normal donors' lymphocytes to assure adequate stimulating and responding capability of the patients' cells, and, if possible, HLA-identical siblings of the patient (to check autologous leukaemia specificity). After 5 days, add 37 kBq of tritiated thymidine (specific activity 185 GBq/mmol) to each well, and harvest cell nuclei between 6 and 18 h later. Assess incorporated radioactivity in the usual way (most often by liquid scintillation spectroscopy). The expected results are that the responses of the patients', but not their HLA-identical siblings', cells to the untreated leukaemic PBMC are markedly increased.

Protocol 2. *Continued*

(b) Mix 1×10^6 Ara-C-treated cells with the same number of irradiated untreated cells from the same donors in 2 ml RPMI + 10% HS in 16 mm diameter cluster plate wells. Incubate for 6 days, then harvest surviving cells for culture and cloning (if the results from experiment (a) have confirmed anti-leukaemic activity).

4. Cloning and propagation of human T lymphocytes

Monoclonal populations are simply those derived from a single progenitor. The isolation of this single cell by micromanipulation, FACS deposition, or agar colony formation can be attempted. However, the most common procedure for cloning is the limiting dilution (LD) approach. Here, high dilutions of cells are made, so that the probability of plating only one cell per culture well is high. The LD technique offers rapid plating of large numbers of wells, advantageous when a low cloning efficiency is expected, but suffers the disadvantage of only assuring a statistically defined probability of monoclonality for any particular clone. Thus, even when an average of fewer than 0.5 cells/well are plated, the Poisson statistic still predicts that the probability of the occurrence of wells containing two or more cells is 0.08. However, cloning efficiencies are rarely 100% and in practice almost all lines derived from wells seeded with, for example, 0.45 cells are in fact found to be monoclonal (see Section 6). Again, cloning protocols vary between different laboratories, and I therefore restrict myself to presenting a generalized cloning protocol from my own laboratory in the following:

Protocol 3. Generalized human T lymphocyte cloning protocol

1. Assess blastoid cell fraction of T cells to be cloned. If necessary (e.g. for populations with fewer than 10% blasts), purify blasts by centrifugation over 15–38% Percoll gradients, or by positive selection of CD25+ cells. In general, alloactivated or mitogen-activated PBMC will already be more than 75% blasts, whereas TIL may contain very few such cells.
2. Dilute cells in three steps in selected growth medium so that 10 μl contain 45, 4.5, or 0.45 cells. Set up a test culture plate to check acceptability of dilution. Use 1 mm diameter 60-well microculture ('Terasaki') plates, adding 10 μl medium per well, leaving plates for 1 h before microscopically determining the percentage of wells containing at least one cell. If this exceeds 37%, the cells must be rediluted and the procedure repeated. If between 30 and 37%, plate at least 5 (×60) wells at 0.45 cells/well as well as one plate with 4.5 and one with 45 cells per well.

3. Add an excess of feeder cells to each well. These are most usually PBMC after irradiation at 30 Gy. Use (1–2) $\times$ 10^4 per well. They must be matched to the cloned cells according to the nature of the experiment. For example, generation of antigen-specific cells will require autologous or HLA-matched antigen presenting cells as well as antigen; alloreactive cells will require stimulator-type feeder, etc. A useful general source of feeder cells is a pool of PBMC from about 20 random normal donors which can be frozen pre-irradiated in appropriate aliquots. Some laboratories cite improved results using mixtures of PBMC and B-lymphoblastoid cell-line (B-LCL) cells; we do not observe this. Some laboratories add mitogens at this point; we find this to be inhibitory, at least for alloreactive cells.
4. Establish clones by serial transfer into 7 mm diameter flat bottom microtitre plates and then into 16 mm diameter cluster plates. Further transfer into culture flasks rarely succeeds, but a minority of clones can be adapted to growth in flasks. Clones are ready for the first transfer from Terasaki plates after about one week, when wells more than one third full must be transferred. However, retain the Terasaki plates and continue to observe 'latecomers' for up to two weeks. New medium and feeder cells ((1–2) $\times$ 10^5 per well) must be added on transfer. Transfer to cluster plates generally occurs before 7 days, obviating the requirement for feeding most clones in the flat-bottom microtitre plates. Cluster plate wells should be seeded with (2–5) $\times$ 10^5 feeder cells in 2 ml of fresh medium.
5. Propagate clones in cluster plates by sub-cultivating when wells are full, or at fortnightly intervals, whichever occurs first. However, add fresh feeder cells only at sub-culture, and then only if the interval between fillers was at least seven days. When clones are established, and some have been cryopreserved (see Section 5), it can be tested whether they will grow on B-LCL feeders (at (1–2) $\times$ 10^5 per well). Most, but not all, clones can, since B-LCL are good antigen presenters and allostimulators. Some laboratories state that they must mix PBMC with B-LCL for long-term growth; we do not find this an advantage over LCL alone once the clones have been established. It is also at this stage of clonal expansion that the addition of PHA along with the feeder cells appears to confer a growth advantage (13), and for this purpose one-fifth of a maximally mitogenic concentration (e.g. 0.2%) can be employed.

5. Cryopreservation

Human T-cell clones generated as described above manifest finite lifespans and cannot be maintained in culture indefinitely. In experiments involving the concurrent use of a large number of different TCC, it would also be very impractical to maintain all the necessary lines continuously in culture. For these reasons, human TCC are routinely cryopreserved, so that supplies of young clones can be grown up when required, and so that many clones cultured at different times can be used concurrently.

Protocol 4. Cryopreservation of human TCC

1. Re-suspend washed cells in RPMI 1640 with 40% FCS at twice the concentration desired for freezing (between 2 and 10×10^6 per ml) at room temperature.
2. Make up cryoprotectant stock solution by mixing cold protein-free RPMI with sterile dimethylsulphoxide (DMSO) to give 20% final concentration.
3. To one volume of cell suspension, add one-half volume of DMSO stock solution in one aliquot at room temperature and mix rapidly. Wait 5 min for the DMSO to equilibrate across the cell membrane (to avoid osmotic damage), and then add a second one-half volume aliquot of DMSO stock to give a final concentration of 10%. Transfer cells to freezing vials, put in a cardboard honeycomb box and place in −70°C freezer as fast as possible.
4. Allow to freeze for at least 4 h, but do not leave at −70°C for longer than a week. For long-term storage, transfer to −196°C liquid-nitrogen tanks.
5. To thaw, place in 37°C water bath, transfer vial contents to centrifugation tubes and add an equal volume of RPMI 1640 at room temperature. Wait 5 min to equilibrate, then add another equal volume of RPMI, immediately centrifuge, and re-suspend in culture medium

6. Assurance of monoclonality

Since the limiting dilution technique must compromise between aiming for a high probability of monoclonality (by using a high dilution of cells) and the practical requirements for limited numbers of seeded plates per cloning experiment (low dilutions of cells increasing the number of positive wells and thus decreasing the number of plates required), there is no guarantee that any particular TCC is in fact monoclonal. This can usually be established, however, by examining whether the rearrangement patterns of the genes encoding the antigen receptor (TCR) are characteristic of a homogeneous population. Normal polyclonal T cells (e.g. from peripheral blood) possess numerous different TCR gene rearrangements, but none is visible as a single non-germ-line band on a Southern blot because they are below the threshold of sensitivity for this method. In most cases, it will be sufficient to examine the TCRβ chain gene rearrangement in *Eco*RI and *Bam*HI (or *Hind*III) DNA digestions. The rearrangement of the TCRγ chain genes, which occurs in both

TCR1 (γ/δ) and TCR2 (α/β) cells, provides further information on both types of T cell.

Protocol 5. Southern blot analysis for TCR gene rearrangements

1. Prepare high molecular weight genomic DNA from T-cell clones by standard techniques. Include DNA from B-LCL and from leukaemic T cell-lines as controls for germ-line and rearranged TCR genes respectively. Digest the cell lysates (in 100 mM Tris–HCl, pH 7.5, 25 mM EDTA, 10 mM β-mercaptoethanol, 0.5% SDS) with proteinase K (250 μg/ml, 1–2 h at 65 °C), purify the DNA by extraction with phenol/chloroform (2:1) and chloroform/isoamylalcohol (24:1) and, after the addition of 1/10 volume of 4 M LiCl, precipitate with ethanol.
2. Digest DNA (5–7.5 μg) of each sample with *Eco*RI, *Bam*HI, or *Hind*III (5 U/μg DNA) for at least 2 h at 37 °C and size-fractionate, together with a molecular weight standard, on 0.5–0.7% agarose gel. After pre-treatment of the gel and blotting according to Southern, fix the DNA (by alkali (0.4 M NaOH) if using positively charged nylon membrane, e.g. Hybond N+, Amersham).
3. Label human TCR-specific cDNA probes with α[^{32}P]dATP (110 TBq/mM, Amersham) by the random primer method as described by Feinberg and Vogelstein (14) to a specific activity of about 10^9 c.p.m./μg. Use, for example, pCβREX, a cDNA probe for constant (C) region sequences ($C_\beta1$ and $C_\beta2$) of the TCR β chain (800 bp *Eco*RI × *Bgl*II, subcloned into pBR322 (15)). For the TCR γ chain, use, for example, the pH60 J-region-specific probe (700 bp *Hind*III × *Eco*RI, isolated from the genomic clone M13H60 subcloned into pUC 8 (16)). This fragment contains the $J_\gamma1$ region but cross-hybridizes with the $J_\gamma2$ region located upstream of $C_\gamma2$ and detects all possible rearrangements.
4. Hybridize overnight at 65 °C in a solution containing 1% BSA, 1 mM Na_2-EDTA, 0.5 M Na_2HPO_4 at pH 7.2 with 7% SDS (according to a method first described by Church and Gilbert). Autoradiograph (e.g. on Kodak X-OMAT XAR5) for 24–36 h at −70 °C using Dupont 'lightning-plus' intensifying screens.

Figure 1 interprets an example of such a TCR rearrangement analysis performed according to *Protocol 5*. The TCRβ pattern for TCC1 shows that both alleles of $C_\beta1$ have been deleted (loss of the 11 kb germ-line band, but no new band, *Figure 1A*) and productive rearrangements into the $C_\beta2$ region have occurred on both alleles (two new bands, *Figure 1B*). TCC2 represents rearrangement events involving both the $C_\beta1$ and $C_\beta2$ regions of the TCRβ gene. Further, both clones are characterized by rearrangements involving the J regions of the TCRγ chain gene (*Figure 1C*).

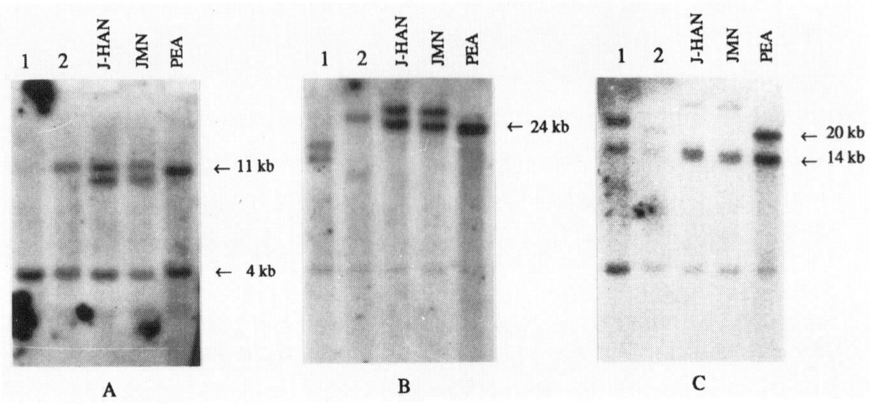

Figure 1. Southern blot of *Eco*RI (A)- and *Bam*HI (B)-digested genomic DNA isolated from two TCC, hybridized with the cDNA probe pC_βREX, specific for the constant region of the TCRβ chain gene. The B-LCL (PEA) represents the germ-line configuration: 11 kb ($C_\beta1$ region), 4 kb ($C_\beta2$ region) for the *Eco*RI digest, and 24 kb for the *Bam*HI digest. The Jurkat T cell-lines J-HAN and JMN are the positive controls for rearrangement, in this case of $C_\beta1$, indicated by the loss of the 11 kb band and the appearance of two new bands in the *Eco*RI digest. C additionally shows a genomic *Bam*HI-digest hybridized with the J_γ-region probe pH60. The germ-line bands are indicated: 20 kb ($J_\gamma1$) and 14 kb ($J_\gamma2$).

Acknowledgements

The author's work is funded by the Deutsche Forschungsgemeinschaft through grants SFB 120 (A1) and Pa 361/1-1, and the Deutsche Krebshilfe through grant W 2/91/Pa 1. The essential contributions of H. Pohla, A. Rehbein, M. Adibzadeh, A. Schenk, and E. Schlotz are gratefully acknowledged.

References

1. Reinherz, E. L., Meuer, S. C., and Schlossman, S. F. (1983). *Immunol. Rev.,* **74,** 83.
2. Hedrick, S. M., Cohen, D. I., Nielsen, E. A., and Davis, M. M. (1984). *Nature,* **308,** 149.
3. Townsend, A. R. M. and Skehel, J. J. (1982). *Nature,* **300,** 655.
4. Moller, G. (1988). *Scand. J. Immunol.,* **27,** 247.
5. Hayflick, L. (1965). *Exp. Cell Res.,* **37,** 614.
6. Effros, R. B. and Walford, R. L. (1984). *Human Immunology,* **9,** 49.
7. Yssel, H., De Vries, J. E., Koken, M., Van Blitterswijk, W., and Spits, H. (1984). *J. Immunol. Methods,* **72,** 219.
8. Spits, H., Yssel, H., Takebe, Y., Arai, N., Yokota, T., Lee, F., *et al.* (1987). *J. Immunol.,* **139,** 1142.

9. Van de Griend, R. J., Van Krimpen, B. A., Bol, S. J. L., Thompson, A., and Bolhuis, R. L. H. (1984). *J. Immunol. Methods,* **66,** 285.
10. Ziegler-Heitbrock, H. W. L. and Burger, R. (1987). *Exp. Cell Res.,* **173,** 388.
11. Pawelec, G., Schmidt, H., Rehbein, A., and Busch, F. (1989). *Cancer Immunol. Immunother.,* **29,** 242.
12. Pawelec, G., Reutter, M., Owsianowsky, M., Rehbein, A., and Busch, F. W. (1991). *Cancer Immunol. Immunother.,* **33,** 54.
13. Pawelec, G., Schwuléra, U., Blaurock, M., Busch, F. W., Rehbein, A., Balko, I., *et al.* (1987). *Immunobiology,* **174,** 67.
14. Feinberg, A. P. and Vogelstein, B. (1983). *Anal. Biochem.,* **132,** 6.
15. Acuto, O., Campen, T. J., Royer, H.-D., Hussey, R. E., Poole, C. B., and Reinherz, E. L. (1985). *J. Exp. Med.,* **161,** 1326.
16. Hata, S., Brenner, M. B., and Krangel, M. S. (1987). *Science,* **238,** 678.

9

Association of TCR expression with MHC recognition

SUSAN L. HAND, BRUCE LEE HALL, and OLIVERA J. FINN

1. Introduction

The T-cell receptor (TCR) for antigen and major histocompatibility complex (MHC) is a disulphide-linked heterodimeter composed of an α chain and a β chain, each of which has a variable (V) and a constant (C) region. The V regions are made up of two (*V*α and *J*α) or three (*V*β, *D*β, and *J*β) discrete gene segments which are separated in the germ-line DNA and are rearranged during T-cell development to form a continuous sequence. TCR diversity is generated by the combination of one of the at least 50 *V*α segments with one of about 50 *J*α segments and of the 57 known *V*β segments with one of two *D*β and 13 *J*β segments. Additional diversity is obtained through junctional variations, the addition of non-germ-line-encoded nucleotides at the junctions, and the association of the different α and β chains with each other. All of the variable elements of both the α chain and the β chain are thought to be involved in forming the contact site of the TCR with its ligand. TCR recognize foreign antigenic peptides bound to self-class-I or class-II MHC molecules on the surface of antigen-presenting cells. In addition, many TCR recognize allogeneic MHC molecules (alloreactivity), though the extent to which MHC-bound peptides are involved in allorecognition is not yet understood.

Examination of the known TCR α and β sequences has led to the identification of three hypervariable or complementarity determining regions (CDR) in each chain. CDR1 and CDR2 are encoded by V-region gene segments, while CDR3 is encoded by the junctional regions (*VJ*α and *VDJ*β) and has the greatest concentration of sequence polymorphism. The prevailing model for TCR–MHC interaction predicts that the highly variable CDR3 contacts the antigenic peptide bound in the MHC groove and that the less variable CDR1 and CDR2 contact the α-helices of the MHC molecule. Based on this model, it has been postulated that the composition of CDR3 might determine the antigen specificity of a TCR, while CDR1 and CDR2 (hence the germ-line-encoded V segments) might be most involved in recognition of the MHC molecule. If this is the case, then it stands to reason that there would be structural correlations between MHC molecules and the V regions of the TCR used in their recognition, as well as correlations between specific antigenic peptides (e.g. tumour-associated antigens) and certain segments of the TCR used in their recognition.

Differences in V-region frequencies have been observed in murine T-cell populations responding to various alloantigens, although no simple, direct correlations have been made between MHC type and V region used (1–3). In humans, the diversity of *V*β utilized by a group of 11 HLA-B27-specific T-cell clones was shown to be limited (4); and a study of TCR gene segment usage by 10 HLA-DR1-reactive T-cell clones demonstrated heterogeneity in TCR gene utilization, although some segments were used more than once, and some similarities were found among CDR (5). Another study of a human alloreactive response reported that *V*β14 was used predominantly in a bulk tertiary anti-DPw2 MLR and by DPw2-reactive T-cell clones derived from this MLR (6). Similarly, our laboratory has shown that both an anti-DR1, long-term MLR, and a DR1-reactive renal allograft-derived T cell-line show predominant usage of *V*β8 (7). Restricted expression of *V*α7 has been found in tumour-infiltrating lymphocytes of uveal melanomas (8), suggesting that a specific antigen may be eliciting a response.

Until recently, the determination of TCR V-region gene usage was labour-intensive, and usually required cloning and sequencing the low abundance TCR message. If one wished to determine relative levels of *V* gene expression in polyclonal populations of T cells, this method was even less efficient. In addition, very few anti-human TCR *V*β or *V*α monoclonal antibodies are available.

Recently, several laboratories have applied a semiquantitative polymerase chain reaction (PCR) technique to the analysis of V-region gene expression in human T-cell populations (9–12). This technique has the advantages of being sensitive, comprehensive, reproducible, semiquantitative, and relatively quick; complete analysis of V-region gene expression by a population of T cells can be accomplished in a matter of days. Our laboratory has applied this method to the analysis of TCR *V*β gene usage in human alloreactive T-cell populations and is beginning to use it to study the TCR repertoire in human tumour-reactive T-cell populations. In this chapter we describe the generation and maintenance of alloreactive cultures of human T cells. This same approach can be used to expand tumour-specific T cells from peripheral blood lymphocytes (PBL), lymph nodes, or tumour-infiltrating cells. We also describe the protocols for RNA isolation, cDNA synthesis, and semiquantitative PCR used in our laboratory. Some practical and theoretical considerations of the approach are also addressed. All the examples given here will deal with *V*β repertoire analysis, although this approach may certainly be applied to the analysis of the *V*α repertoire with *V*α-specific primers.

2. Growth of human alloreactive T-cell cultures

Alloreactive T-cell cultures may be grown from biopsies of several types of human allografts. In most cases, the resulting T cell-lines are specifically reactive for alloantigens present on the donor graft. Our laboratory has generated numerous alloreactive T cell-lines from biopsies of human renal allografts and has examined their *V*β gene utilization, previously by Southern blot analysis, use of the available *V*β-specific monoclonal antibodies, and sequencing clones from cDNA libraries, and more recently by *V*β-specific, semiquantitative PCR. In the majority of long-term lines studied, one or more *V*β genes is predominantly expressed (13, 14). A disadvantage of using allograft-derived T cell-lines for these studies is that it is difficult to examine a significant number of cultures with the same alloreactivity, which would be desirable in order to make correlations between TCR V-region usage and MHC recognition. In addition, in the vast majority of cases, there are a number of HLA mismatches between the donor and the recipient, and, in some cases, HLA typing is incomplete. To circumvent these problems, we have recently begun to establish mixed lymphocyte cultures (MLC) in which the responding and stimulating lymphocytes are chosen to have maximum sharing of all HLA alleles, except for the allele to be studied. Using MLC, one can examine the responses of different individuals to the same alloantigen and of the same individual to the same alloantigen, presented by different stimulator cells. We are now using this approach to generate alloreactive T-cell populations which may then be examined for TCR *V*β gene expression. The generation of both types of alloreactive T-cell cultures is described below.

2.1 Renal allograft-derived T-cell cultures

Renal needle biopsies are teased apart into small fragments and plated in 2 ml of growth medium per well in several wells of a 24-well tissue culture plate (Flow Laboratories). Growth medium consists of RPMI 1640 medium containing 2 mM glutamine, 10% (v/v) heat-inactivated human serum (Gemini Bioproducts), 5 U/ml recombinant interleukin-2 (IL-2) (DuPont), 100 U/ml penicillin, and 100 μg/ml streptomycin. The cultures are grown in a 5% CO_2 humidified incubator at 37°C. Every two to three days the cultures are either split in half, or half of the medium is removed and replaced with fresh medium. Approximately 10^5 irradiated (6000 rad=60 Gy) Epstein–Barr virus (EBV)-transformed donor B cells per well are added to the cultures every 7–10 days as an antigenic stimulus.

2.2 Mixed lymphocyte cultures

Responder and stimulator PBL are separated from whole blood using Ficoll density-gradient centrifugation (LSM, Organon Teknika Corp.). 10^6 responder cells and 10^6 irradiated stimulator cells, in 2 ml of complete T-cell growth medium, are added per well of a 24-well plate. Cultures are grown and maintained as described above for allograft derived T-cell cultures. Antigen stimulation of the MLC is repeated every 7 to 10 days by the addition of either 10^6 irradiated (2000 rad=20 Gy) stimulator PBL or 10^5 irradiated (6000 rad= 60 Gy) EBV-transformed stimulator B cells per well. Immediately prior to the addition of antigen, the MLC are split, and half of the cells are taken for use in *V*β-specific PCR analyses.

3. Preparation of total cellular RNA from T-cell cultures

In order to analyse the TCR *V*β repertoires of the alloreactive cultures, total cellular RNA is prepared for use in cDNA synthesis and subsequent *V*β-specific, semiquantitative PCR analysis. There are a number of methods for isolation of high-quality RNA, and any of these should be fine to use at this step. However, in our hands, protocols that use vanadyl ribonuclease complexes as inhibitors of ribonucleases (RNases) have not worked well. As always when working with RNA, care should be taken to avoid contaminating the samples with RNases (e.g. all solutions should be DEPC-prepared, gloves should be worn, and disposable or DEPC-treated tubes and reagent bottles should be used). The method used in our laboratory to prepare total cellular RNA is a modification of a published technique (15) and is described in *Protocol 1* (a number of techniques for RNA preparation are described in Chapter 10).

Protocol 1. Isolation of total cellular RNA

1. Harvest 10^7 or fewer cells and wash them twice with ice cold phosphate-buffered saline (PBS); drain as much of the supernatant as possible from the final pellet.
2. Re-suspend the cell pellet in 200 μl of a solution of 10 mM Tris–HCl pH 8, 1 mM EDTA pH 8, and 100 mM NaCl and transfer to a 1.5 ml microcentrifuge tube.
3. Add 400 μl of urea lysis buffer (4.7 M urea, 1.3% sodium dodecyl sulphate, 230 mM NaCl, 6.7 mM Tris–HCl pH 8, 0.67 mM EDTA pH 8) and vortex the mixture for 60 sec.
4. Shear the DNA by numerous passages through 19-gauge, then 22-gauge, then 27-gauge needles, until the viscosity of the solution is sufficiently reduced for organic extraction.
5. Extract the sample with an equal volume of phenol:chloroform:isoamyl alcohol (50:49:1) three times and with an equal volume of chloroform: isoamyl alcohol (49:1) once.

6. Precipitate the nucleic acids by adding 40 μl of 5 M NaCl and 900 μl 100% ethanol and storing at −70°C for more than 30 min or at −20°C overnight or longer.
7. Centrifuge the sample at 16 000*g* for 30 min, wash the pellet twice with 80% ethanol, and vacuum dry.
8. Treat the sample with RNase-free deoxyribonuclease (DNase) (Boehringer Mannheim) to remove the DNA.
   (a) Re-suspend the dried pellet in 100 μl of a solution of 10 mM Tris–HCl pH 7.4, 10 mM $MgCl_2$.
   (b) Add 250 units of RNase-free DNase (less enzyme can be used for fewer cells).
   (c) Incubate the reaction at 37°C for one hour.
9. Add 300 μl of DEPC-treated H_2O to the sample.
10. Extract once with an equal volume of phenol:chloroform:isoamyl alcohol (50:49:1) and once with chloroform:isoamyl alcohol (49:1). If 300 000 or fewer cells were used initially, add no more than several micrograms of yeast tRNA as carrier at this point.[a]
11. Precipitate the RNA by adding 40 μl 3M NaOAc pH 5.2 and 1 ml ethanol and incubating at −70°C for more than 30 min or at −20°C overnight or longer.
12. Centrifuge, wash, and dry the RNA as in step **7**.
13. Re-suspend the dried RNA in no more than 20–25 μl of DEPC-treated H_2O, depending on the size of the pellet.
14. Evaluate and quantitate total RNA by ethidium bromide visualization of 1 μl of the RNA solution in an agarose gel and comparison to known RNA standards run in the same gel.
15. If present, remove residual genomic DNA by repetition of DNase treatment (repeat steps **8–14**).

[a] Before this point the DNA present in the sample acts as a carrier, and if the yeast tRNA is added before this step, it can inhibit the DNase.

4. Synthesis of cDNA from total cellular RNA

Total cellular RNA is used to synthesize cDNA for the PCR. There are a number of different protocols for synthesizing cDNA from RNA. The method used in our laboratory is given in *Protocol 2*. The advantages of using random hexamers and Moloney murine leukaemia virus (MMLV) reverse transcriptase have been described (16, 17). cDNA synthesis can also be performed using avian myeloblastosis virus (AMV) reverse transcriptase

(Gibco BRL) if no yeast tRNA is used during RNA isolation, since yeast tRNA inhibits AMV reverse transcriptase. We generally use 3 μg of total RNA in each reverse transcription reaction. This makes enough cDNA for about 30 PCR reactions (100 ng RNA equivalent cDNA per reaction), which is the size of our *V*β-specific PCR primer panel. As for RNA isolation, all solutions used in cDNA synthesis are DEPC-prepared and precautions are taken to avoid contamination of the samples with RNAses.

Protocol 2. Reverse transcription of cDNA from total cellular RNA

1. Aliquot 3 μg, or less if necessary, of total RNA for each reverse transcription reaction.
2. Combine the following in a 50 μl reaction mixture:
   - 3 μg total RNA
   - 10 μl reverse transcriptase buffer (5 × stock buffer, Gibco BRL: 250 mM Tris–HCl, pH 8.3, 375 mM KCl, 15 mM $MgCl_2$)
   - 5 μl (10 mM) dithiothreitol (0.1 M stock solution, Gibco BRL)
   - 100 mOD random hexamers[a]
   - 1 mM each of dATP, dCTP, dGTP, and dTTP[a]
   - 500 units MMLV reverse transcriptase (Gibco BRL)[b]
   - DEPC H_2O to bring the volume to 50 μl
3. Incubate the reaction at 37°C for 60 min, then at 65°C for 5 min (to inactivate the enzyme).
4. Store cDNAs at 4°C (short term) or at −20°C (long term).

[a] Random hexamers and dNTPs may be purchased from Boehringer Mannheim or another source, and stock solutions of each may be prepared in advance, aliquoted in small volumes, and stored frozen.

[b] Mock cDNA syntheses, leaving out reverse transcriptase, may be performed and used as controls for DNA contamination in PCR analyses.

5. Vβ specific, semiquantitative PCR analysis

The semiquantitative PCR analysis of TCR *V*β gene usage performed in our laboratory (10) (*Protocol 3*) is similar to one previously described, in which amplifications for specific *V*βs are performed in a number of separate reaction tubes (9). The semiquantitative nature of this approach has been discussed in detail elsewhere (10) and will be addressed, in part, below. PCR is performed in a Perkin-Elmer Cetus DNA thermal cycler, using Taq polymerase (Perkin Elmer Cetus) in a 50 μl volume of the manufacturer's recommended buffer: 10 mM Tris–HCl, pH 8.3, 50 mM KCl, 1.5 mM $MgCl_2$, 0.001% (w/v) gelatin.

The use of DEPC-treated H_2O is not necessary at this point and, in fact, any residual DEPC present in the reaction might inhibit Taq polymerase and/or cause pH changes during PCR. For panel analysis, all components are combined in a master mix and aliquoted, except the 5′Vβ region-specific primer for each reaction and the 5′Cβ region-specific primer for the constant region amplification. These 5′ primers are individually added to each of 31 separate tubes (GeneAmp tubes, Perkin Elmer Cetus). Since we very carefully selected our primer panel to ensure comparability, sensitivity, and specificity, we have provided their sequence in *Table 1*. Note, however, that different *V*β, as well as *V*α, primer panels have been published and utilized by other investigators (4, 9, 18, 19).

Protocol 3. *V*β-specific PCR

1. Aliquot 25 pmol (in a 2 μl volume of H_2O) of 5′Vβ- or 5′Cβ-specific primers into each of 31 separate GenAmp (Perkin Elmer Cetus) PCR tubes.[a]
2. Combine the following components into a master mix (the volumes and amounts given are for **one** 50 μl reaction mixture and should be multiplied by the appropriate number of reactions for panel analyses):
   - 100 μM each of dATP, dCTP, dGTP, and dTTP[b]
   - 500 nM (25 pmol per reaction) of the 3′Cβ primer (TCRCβ5-329)
   - 2.5 units of Taq polymerase (5 U/μl, Perkin Elmer Cetus)
   - about 5 μCi [^{32}P]dCTP (Amersham, >3000 Ci/mmol, 10 μCi/μl) for quantitation (20)
   - 100 ng RNA-equivalent cDNA (cDNA reverse transcribed from 3 μg total RNA is included in a master mix for 31 reactions, unless RNA is limiting)
   - 1 × PCR buffer (from 10× stock buffer prepared as above)
   - H_2O to bring the volume to 48 μl
3. Vortex master mix well to mix components.
4. Aliquot 48 μl of master mix to each of the tubes containing 25 pmol (in 2 μl) of 5′ primer.
5. Vortex tubes to mix reactants.
6. Add an equal volume of light mineral oil (three or four drops, Sigma) to each tube and centrifuge briefly.
7. Perform PCR with an initial three minute denaturation at 94°C, followed by 22–24 cycles of the profile: 30 sec at 94°C, 30 sec at 65°C, 60 sec at 72°C.

Protocol 3. *Continued*

8. Incubate at 72°C for 7 min to allow complete extension of products.
9. Maintain at 4°C until analysis by gel electrophoresis.

[a] The number of tubes will vary depending on the size of the primer panel used.
[b] dNTPs may be purchased from Boehringer Mannheim or another source, and stock solutions may be prepared in advance, aliquoted in small volumes, and frozen.

Table 1. Sequences of Vβ oligonucleotide primers

Designation[a]	Sequence, 5′→3′
TCR Cβ 5–329	TGTGCACCTCCTTCCCATTCACC
TCR Cβ 3–195	CCGAGGTCGCTGTGTTTGAG
*V*β 1.12 (all)	CACAACAGTTCCCTGACTTGCA
*V*β 2.123 (all)	ATACGAGCAAGGCGTCGAGAAG
*V*β 3.12 (all)	ACAGTGTCTCTAGAGAGAAG
*V*β 4.123 (all)	CAACCTGGACAGAGCCTGACA
*V*β 5.14 (half)	AGTGAGACACAGAGAAACAA
*V*β 5.23 (half)	GCCCCAGTTTATCTTTCAGT
*V*β 6.1–9 (all)[b]	TCAGGTGTGATCCAATTTC
*V*β 6.167	AATTTACTTCCAAGGCA
*V*β 6.1	CGGGTGCGGCAGATG
*V*β 6.67	CAAGGCAACAGTGCAC
*V*β 6.23589	CAGAATGAAGCTCAACT
*V*β 6.4	AATTATGAAGCCCAACA
*V*β 7.12 (all)[c]	CCTGAATGCCCCAACAGCTCTC
*V*β 8.1234 (all)	TCTGGTACAGACAGACCATGAT
*V*β 9.1 (all)	ACCTAAATCTCCAGACAAAGCT
*V*β 10.12 (all)	GCTCCAAAAACTCATCCTGTAC
*V*β 11.12 (all)	AGAGAAGGGAGATCTTTCCTC
*V*β 12.12 (all)	GACAGAGGATTTCCTCCTCACT
*V*β 12.3(13.1) (half)[d]	GACCAAGGAGAAGTCCCCAA
*V*β 12.4(13.2) (half)[d]	TGGTGAGGGTACAACTGCCA
*V*β 14.1(3.3) (all)[d]	TCTCTCGAAAAGAGAAGAGGAA
*V*β 15.1 (all)	CTCGACAGGCACAGGCTAAA
*V*β 16.1 (all)	AGAGTCTAAACAGGATGAGTCC
*V*β 17.1 (all)	ACTGTGACATCGGCCCAAAA
*V*β 18.12 (all)	TGAGTCAGGAATGCCAAAGGAA
*V*β 19.1 (all)	CTCAATGCCCCAAGAACGCAC
*V*β 20.1 (all)	CCTCCAGCTGCTCTTCTACTC
*V*β 12ALL[e]	CTGGTATCGACAAGACCC
*V*β 21.123 (all)	GATTCACAGTTGCCTAAGGA

[a] For *V*βs, primer designations indicate *V*β family before the period, and all members specifically primed after the period. If amplified members represent the entire family, this is indicated as (all).
[b] This primer matches all members of *V*β6, except that the sequence of *V*β6.2 is not published at this site.
[c] Identical to the *V*β7 primer previously published (9).
[d] There is an inconsistency in the nomenclature. These designations represent a single V region.
[e] This primer serves as a useful control, matching *V*βs 12.1234, 3.1, 14.1, and 15.1.

6. Gel electrophoresis and quantitation of PCR products

In order to quantitate the products of PCR, 9 μl of each sample are analysed by 3% wide-range agarose (Sigma)/1% regular agarose (Sigma) gel electrophoresis at 5–6 V/cm. pBR322 DNA digested with *Hae*III is used as a size marker. Ethidium bromide is used for visualization of the markers and abundant products. Gels are run until the bromophenol blue dye front is 4 to 5 cm from the wells, and the gels are rinsed in H_2O to remove residual radioactive gel buffer. Gels are photographed, completely dried, and exposed to film (Kodak XAR-5) for several hours to overnight. An example of an autoradiograph of a dried gel, is depicted in *Figure 1*. The radioactivity incorporated into the PCR products can then be quantitated in one of two ways. The simpler of the two is to scan the dried gel on an Ambis radioanalytic image system (Ambis Systems, San Diego, California) and to select and quantitate (in c.p.m.) the desired bands using this system. If one does not have access to this or a similar system, the desired products may be located on the dried gel using the autoradiograph as a guide, then excised, and counted in a beta counter in scintillation fluid. In both cases, background counts for

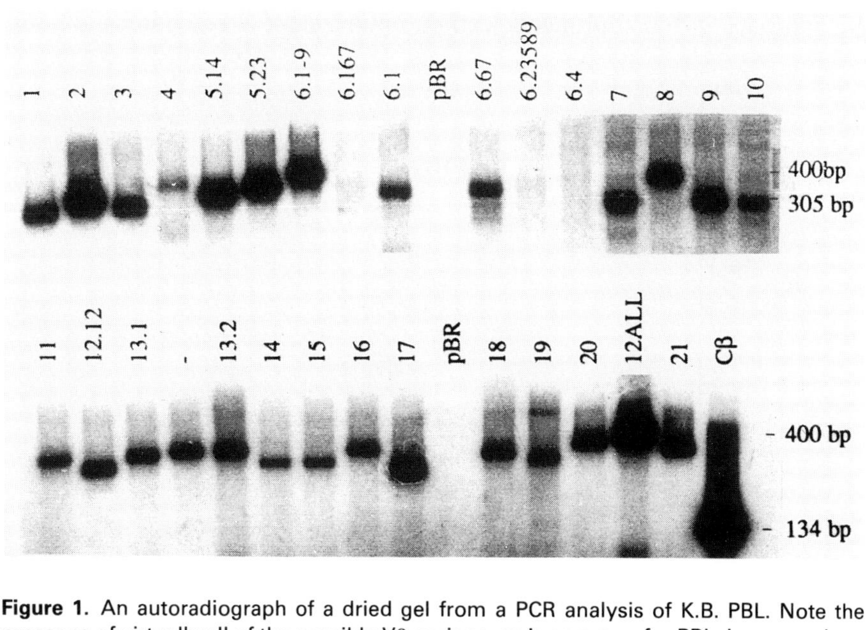

Figure 1. An autoradiograph of a dried gel from a PCR analysis of K.B. PBL. Note the presence of virtually all of the possible Vβ regions, as is common for PBL. Lane numbers correspond to *V*β primers. pBR is a marker lane containing *Hae*III-digested pBR322 plasmid DNA. 400 bp and 305 bp indicate the sizes of several of the amplified fragments. The constant-region amplification (Cβ) is indicated by the 134 bp size marker. Lane '–' contains an amplified product of a primer no longer included in the panel.

each lane are obtained and subtracted from the specific product signals. The resulting counts (c.p.m.) are corrected for product incorporation of radio-labelled dCTP by dividing by a factor which represents the actual number of cytosine residues in each product, excluding primers, assuming an average contribution of 35 cytosine by DJ, and based on use of the constant-region primer TCRCβ5-329 ((10, 14), *Table 1*). Data for particular *V*β signals are expressed as relative signal strength, R, calculated as: R = % of total signal generated = specific signal/sum of all signals ×100.

Control experiments in which identical gels were quantitated using both methods demonstrated no significant differences in R values between the two procedures (S. L. Hand, unpublished data). An example of the final results, expressed as R values, derived from quantitation of the gel in *Figure 1* is shown in *Figure 2*.

7. Practical and theoretical considerations of the technique

The validity of using this semiquantitative, PCR-based technique to analyse gene expression within the human TCR *V*β multigene family has previously been investigated (10). The considerations addressed in the development of the approach included primer selection, optimization of reaction conditions,

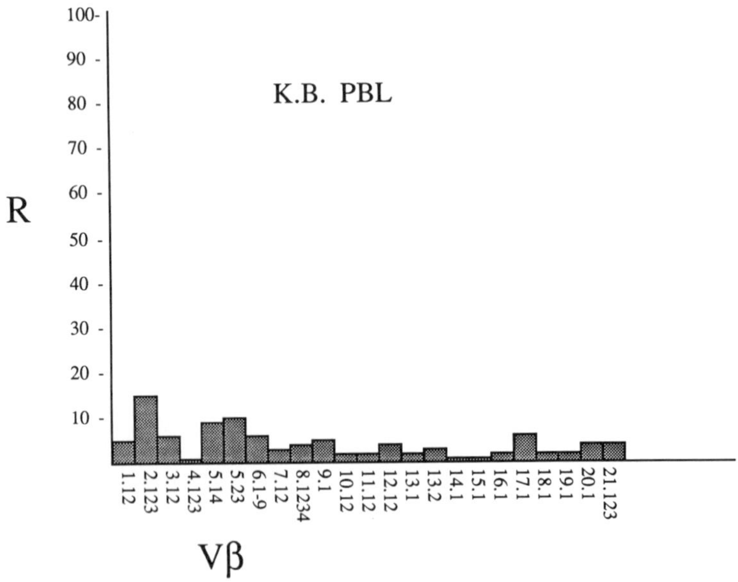

Figure 2. PCR analyses of TCR *V*β gene expression in K.B. PBL. Primer designations indicate *V*β family before period, and all members specifically primed after the period. R = % of total signal generated = specific signal/sum of all signals × 100.

the precision and accuracy of the technique, and the relationship between target prevalence and PCR signal. These are addressed briefly below.

7.1 Primer selection

The panel of *V*β-specific PCR primers used for these analyses was chosen with three major concerns in mind: amplification efficiency, coverage of known *V*β sequences, and match and mismatch to target and non-target sequences.

7.1.1 Amplification efficiency

A panel of PCR primers designed for use in semiquantitative comparisons of different messages must have comparable amplification efficiencies in order for comparisons to be valid. The amplification efficiency of a given primer pair depends on many factors including target prevalence, number of cycles of amplification, and reaction conditions (e.g. concentration of reactants). Since we are interested in semiquantitative comparisons, rather than rigorously quantitative results, we did not attempt to prove equivalent efficiencies of amplification for each of our primer pairs at each possible target abundance. Instead, we considered two factors affecting hybridization behaviour and amplification efficiency: primer hybridization temperature (T_{hyb}) and size of the amplified fragment. We chose primers which are comparable with regard to these properties.

A major determinant of the hybridization efficiency of any two complementary nucleic acid sequences, including PCR primers and their targets, is specific hybridization temperature. We therefore chose all primers to have T_{hyb}s grouped within a narrow range (between 50 and 55°C). The T_{hyb} parameter we used has been described previously (21) and was derived from the mean stacking temperature of each oligomer (22). This parameter has been shown to be an improvement over other parameters such as GC content and to accurately reflect actual hybridization behaviour for 20mers in a PCR-type buffer (21). Therefore, all the primers in this panel were chosen to be 20, 21, or 22mers (with exceptions in the *V*β6 family (see below)). To further improve comparability, we use a relatively high annealing temperature of 65°C. At this annealing temperature our primers are predicted to behave quite similarly based on hypothetical hybridization curves (10).

The second factor we considered with regard to amplification efficiency was the size of the amplified fragment, since it has been reported that smaller products can amplify more efficiently than larger ones (20, 23). This appears to be much more evident for very small or large fragments; and, in fact, it has been shown that two fragments of 308 and 420 bp, amplified with the same primers, amplify equally efficiently (24). Therefore, our targets were chosen to be approximately within this size range (295–400 bp), and we believe that size differences among the amplified fragments do not affect the results obtained with this panel. Control PCR amplifications have been performed on PBL, and the results are compatible with other published reports (9) and demonstrate that no obvious primer biases exist (10) (*Figure 2*).

7.1.2 Coverage of known *V*β sequences

Our primer panel covers 21 of the 24 known *V*β gene families, with only the three recently reported *V*β22, *V*β23, and *V*β24 genes being omitted (25). As new *V*β genes are reported, new primers can be designed to cover these. It has been estimated that the *V*β1–20 family sequences account for more than 90% of peripheral blood T cells, so we are confident that our panel covers the vast majority of the *V*β segments utilized by human T-cell populations.

Each of the primers was also designed to have a relatively small number of target sequences so that no one oligo would have a large stochastic bias. Most of the primers amplify one or two sequences, while none amplifies more than four sequences. The *V*β6 family is the only exception. It is the largest family, encompassing nine members. One oligo was chosen which amplifies all of the members, and then the family was subdivided into three groups, each having a separate primer, with one subgroup being further subdivided into two (*Table 1*). This allows detailed analysis of *V*β6 gene utilization if desired. Because of the difficulty in choosing primers to subdivide this family, some of the above-mentioned primer characteristics, such as size and T_{hyb}, had to be sacrificed. This is discussed in detail elsewhere (10); however, when performing refined analyses of the *V*β6 family using these primers, we have found that an annealing temperature of 55 °C gives the best results, rather than the 65 °C annealing temperature used for the rest of the panel.

7.1.3 Match and mismatch to target and non-target sequences

To favour high specificity of priming, all of the primers were chosen to match their targets perfectly and to have sufficient mismatches to non-target sequences. This was done with the aid of computer homology analyses. Mismatches and gaps between primers and their most nearly identical non-targets were maximized. In addition, since badly matched 3′ ends are a poor substrate for Taq polymerase, we emphasized mismatches in the last four or five 3′ nucleotides of the most nearly identical non-targets whenever possible. (See reference (10) for examples and discussion.)

7.2 Reaction conditions

The reaction conditions for this experimental system were chosen to maximize the specificity of the PCR amplifications, while maintaining acceptable sensitivity. In general, conditions that increase specificity tend to decrease sensitivity and vice versa. Therefore, for any given PCR application, conditions must be carefully chosen to give acceptable levels of both. To increase the specificity of our system, we decreased the concentrations of primers and nucleotides, used fairly short annealing times (30 sec), and limited the extension period to one minute. To increase sensitivity we use increased concentrations of enzyme, which helps maintain high efficiencies of amplification. We optimized the number of cycles to achieve the desired sensitivity yet minimize non-specific amplification products. Results using this panel indicate that the desired specificity is achieved: products of the correct size for each *V*β are amplified; all of the amplified products which have been sequenced have been shown to be the appropriate *V*β region (10, 14); oligo extension reactions, using a nested constant-region primer on the reaction products from an analysis of PBL, produced labelled products of the expected size (10), confirming their identity as *V*β region amplifications; and no primer in the panel reacted with B-cell cDNAs. Sufficient sensitivity is achieved under the chosen conditions when 18–26 cycles of PCR are performed. In control studies, a signal was easily detected from a target at 1% prevalence after 22 cycles of PCR (10). This level of detection is suitable for studies such as ours since most of the *V*β genes in heterogeneous populations of T cells (such as PBL) are expressed on average at about 2%; and in restricted populations of T cells, such as those selected after repeated alloantigenic stimulation, the selected *V*βs are generally represented at prevalences of 10% or greater. For a more detailed discussion of these considerations see (10).

7.3 Precision and accuracy

The precision of this technique has been examined in two ways: (a) identical samples were taken through the steps of gel sample preparation, gel loading, band localization, excision and counting, and (b) duplicate aliquots of total RNA have been carried through the whole procedure separately (10). When identical gel samples were prepared and quantitated, the maximal variation seen was about 4% from the mean value, with the mean variation being about 2%. It should be noted that this is operator dependent, and it is important that these steps be performed as carefully as possible. When duplicate aliquots of total RNA were evaluated, it was found that, at low target prevalences ($R = 0$–3), the experimental variation can be several R points (as high as 50% or more of the assigned value). However, in most instances the difference between an assigned value of $R = 1$ and $R = 3$ will not qualitatively change the nature of the conclusions. At higher target prevalences ($R = 5$–40) the absolute value of the experimental variation is greater, but the relative error is less than it is at low target prevalences. The maximal variation seen was ±12% of the mean value, with the standard deviation of the mean value generally 4–9%. This variation includes the 2–4% seen for gel sample preparation and quantitation described above.

To examine the relationship between input RNA and signal strength, inverse titration experiments were performed in which cDNAs derived from two clonal T cell-lines were mixed, based on the weight of total RNA reverse transcribed (10). The results demonstrated that as the amount of input RNA increases, signal strength increases, but the *rate* of the increase declines in a smooth, continuous manner. Due to this, it is difficult to distinguish between high target prevalences based on signal strength, because the differences between the signals approaches the experimental variation (4–9%). This plateau effect is eventually observed in all PCR reactions. For our system, this means that no valid distinctions can be made for estimated prevalences above about 50%, and at these prevalences underestimation may easily occur. At prevalence of 5–40%, however, the accuracy is much greater since the efficiency remains higher, and better distinctions between prevalences can be made given the 4–9% experimental variation. Considering the limits of the precision and accuracy described above, it is possible to make meaningful distinctions between sufficiently separated target ranges, i.e. 0–1%, 3–5%, 10%, 30%, and more than 50%. This is in agreement with a number of other semiquantitative PCR systems that have demonstrated discrimination of smaller than three-fold differences in mRNA target levels (15, 26–28).

8. Representativeness of the message pool

The PCR data obtained in these analyses reflect the message pool of the initial cell population. The composition of the message pool is determined by the number of cells expressing a given message and the level of message expressed by each cell. Thus, the PCR signal obtained from a given message is not always directly proportional to the actual percentage of cells expressing that message. Despite this, at least one group has determined that it is generally valid to correlate PCR signal data with cell surface expression data obtained by immunofluorescence analyses (9). One factor that could potentially affect correlations of this sort is the presence of non-functional transcripts in the message pool. The results of several groups indicate that the majority of T-cell clones express only one functional *VDJ* transcript and that the presence of non-functional transcripts probably does not interfere with analyses of this type. However, it should be remembered that the importance of these transcripts will depend on the population or clone being studied, and the presence or level of a particular PCR signal is most directly related to the message pool, rather than to cell surface expression.

The sensitivity of PCR has made possible the analysis of the message pools from very small numbers of cells. When a large panel of primers is being used, however, a lower limit must be set on the number of cells to be used so that there are enough cells both to be representative of the whole population and to reach the limit of detection after the cDNA is divided among the different reactions. Statistical analysis demonstrates that, at the very least, 130 000 cells are needed to represent a 1% target as between 0.5 and 1.5% with 99.9% confidence using a panel of 30 primers (10). We recommend that the lower limit be drawn at approximately 250 000 cells.

Acknowledgements

This work was supported by National Institutes of Health grant 5R01-AI26935 to O.J.F. and training grants 5T32-AI19386 to S.L.H. and 5T32-GM07171 to B.L.H.

References

1. Garman, R. D., Ko, J.-L., Vulpe, C. D., and Raulet, D. H. (1986). *Proc. Natl Acad. Sci. USA,* **83,** 3987.
2. Borst, J., De Vries, E., Spits, H., De Vries, J. E., Boylston, A. W., and Matthews, E. A. (1987). *J. Immunol.,* **139,** 1952.
3. Bill, J., Yagüe, J., Appel, V. B., White, J., Horn, G., Ehrlich, H. A., *et al.* (1989). *J. Exp. Med.,* **169,** 115.
4. Bragado, R., Lauzurica, P., Lopez, D., and Lopez de Castro, J. A. (1990). *J. Exp. Med.,* **171,** 1189.
5. Geiger, M. J., Gorski, J., and Eckels, D. D. (1991). *J. Immunol.,* **147,** 2082.
6. Beall, S. S., Lawrence, J. V., Bradley, D. A., Mattson, D. H., Singer, D. S., and Biddison, W. E. (1987). *J. Immunol.,* **139,** 1320.
7. Hand, S. L., Hall, B. L., and Finn, O. J. (1992). *Transplantation,* **54,** 357.
8. Nitta, T., Oksenberg, J. R., Rao, N. A., and Steinman, L. (1990). *Science,* **249,** 672.
9. Choi, Y., Kotzin, B., Herron, L., Callahan, J., Marrack, P., and Kappler, J. (1989). *Proc. Natl Acad. Sci. USA,* **86,** 8941.
10. Hall, B. L. and Finn, O. J. (1992). *Biotechniques,* **13,** 248.
11. Paliard, X., West, S. G., Lafferty, J. A., Clements, J. R., Kappler, J. W., Marrack, P., *et al.* (1991). *Science,* **253,** 325.
12. Davies, T. F., Martin, A., Concepcion, E. S., Graves, P., Cohen, L., and Ben-Nun, A. (1991). *New Engl. J. Med.,* **325,** 238.
13. Miceli, M. C. and Finn, O. J. (1989). *J. Immunol.,* **142,** 81.
14. Hall, B. L. and Finn, O. J. (1992). *Transplantation,* **53,** 1088.
15. Arrigo, S. J., Weitsman, S., Rosenblatt, J. D., and Chen, I. S. Y. (1989). *J. Virol.,* **63,** 4875.
16. Noonan, K. E. and Roninson, I. B. (1988). *Nucl. Ac. Res.,* **16,** 10366.
17. Witsell, A. L. and Schook, L. B. (1990). *Biotechniques,* **9,** 318.
18. Oksenberg, J. R., Stuart, S., Begovich, A. B., Bell, R. B., Erlich, H. A., Steinman, L., *et al.* (1990). *Nature,* **345,** 344.
19. Wucherpfennig, K. W., Ota, K., Endo, N., Seidman, J. G., Rosenzweig, A., Weiner, H. L., *et al.* (1990). *Science,* **248,** 1016.
20. Schowalter, D. B. and Sommer, S. S. (1989). *Anal. Biochem.,* **177,** 90.
21. McGraw, R. A., Steffe, E. K., and Baxter, S. M. (1990). *Biotechniques,* **8,** 674.
22. Gotoh, O. and Tagashira, Y. (1981). *Biopolymers,* **20,** 1033.
23. Saiki, R. K., Gelfand, D. H., Stoffel, S., Scharf, S. J., Higuchi, R., Horn, G. T., *et al.* (1988). *Science,* **239,** 487.
24. Wang, A. M., Doyle, M. V., and Mark, D. F. (1989). *Proc. Natl Acad. Sci. USA,* **86,** 9717.
25. Robinson, M. A. (1991). *J. Immunol.,* **146,** 4392.

26. Chelly, J., Kaplan, J.-C., Maire, P., Gautron, S., and Kahn, A. (1988). *Nature,* **333,** 858.
27. Syvänen, A.-C., Bengtström, M., Tenhunen, J., and Söderlund, H. (1988). *Nucl. Ac. Res.,* **16,** 11327.
28. Rappolee, D. A., Wang, A., Mark, D., and Werb, Z. (1989). *J. Cell. Biochem.,* **39,** 1.

10

Cytokines: identification and measurement of gene activation

F. S. DI GIOVINE, S. STONES, D. WOJTACHA, and G. W. DUFF

1. Introduction

Cytokines are inducible peptide mediators with actions in cell growth, differentiation, and function. Altered rates of cytokine production have been implicated in the pathophysiology of many infectious, inflammatory, and neoplastic diseases, hence the growing interest in mechanisms of cytokine gene expression and its detection *in vivo*. In general, the rate of production of a cytokine is determined by the rate of synthesis and the stability of its mRNA. Most analytical techniques are therefore aimed at detecting and measuring accumulated mRNA, mRNA transcription rate, or mRNA half-life. Because of the high sensitivity of cytokine production to exogenous agents, such as bacterial products, coagulation products, etc., and the lability of mRNA, the handling of samples should be minimal and planned carefully in advance. Clearly, a more reliable picture of cytokine expression will be obtained if cells or tissue samples can be fixed or frozen immediately (e.g. within the operating theatre).

The induction pathways for cytokine gene expression are complex. Triggering of cellular receptors during immune response or inflammation is followed by cytoplasmic signalling, synthesis, and/or activation of transcriptional factors, and their binding to DNA. The RNA that is transcribed from the gene is spliced and processed near the nuclear membrane, transported to the cytoplasm, and translated at the endoplasmic reticulum. The levels of cytokine subsequently released to the extracellular environment will depend also on translation rate, processing, and secretion of the protein. The analysis of all these mechanisms is beyond the scope of this chapter. We will focus specifically on techniques to study steady-state mRNA expression, mRNA transcription rate, and half-life. These provide evidence of gene activation, but should be supplemented by cytokine protein immunodetection for a complete picture of cytokine involvement in a homeostatic or pathogenic process.

2. Measurement of steady-state mRNA levels

The preparation of undegraded RNA from a number of cell types is often made difficult by the presence of active nucleases (RNases). RNases can be introduced from many external sources in the laboratory, and are liberated during cell lysis (including normal epidermis). Therefore special precautions are required when handling RNA and during sample extraction.

All areas used for RNA work should be kept clear of potential sources of contamination and, ideally, designated solely for that purpose. Glassware, plasticware, and electrophoresis tanks that are to be used for experiments with RNA should be marked distinctly and stored in a designated, enclosed place. Gloves should be worn throughout the extraction procedure and changed frequently. Sterile disposable plasticware should be used wherever possible; Pyrex glassware should be cleaned thoroughly in mild detergent, rinsed several times in double-distilled H_2O and then covered in foil before baking at 250°C for at least two hours. Spatulas, magnetic bars, etc. for preparation of solutions should be baked in the same way (PTFE-coated bars will withstand high temperatures). Solutions should be prepared in advance from unopened chemicals which are then kept solely for RNA work and clearly labelled as such. Autoclaving does not remove RNase activity, therefore 'sterile' is not synonymous with RNase-free. Ultrapure sterile water, HPLC grade (18 MΩ/cm, 10 KDa ultrafiltered) is RNase-free and can be used safely. Water of lesser quality (double distilled) can be treated with diethylpyrocarbonate (DEPC; overnight, 0.1%, 37°C), which is then released by autoclaving for 30 min (this is important as DEPC will interfere with nucleic acid hybridization and with other chemicals, such as Tris). Particular caution should be taken when ordering your stocks, as many of the chemicals, including DEPC, are very labile. General plasticware should be soaked in 0.1% DEPC overnight, covered with aluminium foil, and autoclaved. Pipette tips should be taken from a fresh unopened bag, handled at all times using gloves, and autoclaved (remember to use the dry cycle after autoclaving). Electrophoresis apparatus (typically a 21 × 16 horizontal gel tank) should be cleaned with detergent solution, rinsed copiously with DEPC–water, then soaked overnight in 3% H_2O_2 at room temperature. Before use, rinse thoroughly with ultrapure water. A fume hood is essential for most procedures involving the manipulation of RNA, particularly those involving the use of formaldehyde, formamide, phenol, guanidinium isothyocyanate, and concentrated DEPC.

2.1 Northern analysis

This is the equivalent of Southern hybridization, applied to RNA. RNA is fractionated on agarose, transferred to a membrane, and hybridized to a cDNA (or other probe) specific for the mRNA of interest. The position of the labelled probe on the membrane should correspond to the predicted molecular size of the transcript of interest, and the intensity of signal proportional to its amount.

2.1.1 Isolation of total RNA

There are several useful methods for the separation of total RNA from tissue or cells. These include the lithium–urea method (1) which is particularly useful for large amounts of tissue, the caesium chloride–guanidinium method (2), and phenol–chloroform one-step extraction (3). For limited amounts of tissue we would use one of the latter two methods.

Protocol 1. Lithium–urea extraction

1. Tissue is homogenized in a 50 ml polypropylene tube, adding 10 ml of 6 M urea 3 M LiCl. We use a hand-held homogenizer (Omni 2000), full speed at pulses of 10 min each. Cellular preparations can be directly lysed in the solution with no need for homogenization. Shear the suspension with a 10 ml syringe fitted with a 23-gauge needle, and transfer to a pre-cooled 30 ml Corex tube. Large amounts of tissue can be pulverized in a mortar at −70 °C, or cut in ultrathin cryotome sections, collected directly in a 30 ml Corex tube and sheared as described.
2. Leave the extracted tissue overnight at 4 °C.
3. Centrifuge the tubes for 20 min at 10 000*g*, at 4 °C in a swing-out rotor.
4. Add to the supernatant an additional 10 ml of urea–LiCl mixture. Repeat step **3**.
5. Aspirate and discard the supernatant, add 15 ml of pre-cooled urea/LiCl mixture, mix vigorously, and allow the RNA to precipitate at −70 °C for 20 min. Centrifuge as in step **3**.
6. Repeat step **5**.
7. Dissolve the precipitate in 6 ml 10 mM Tris–HCl pH 7.5, 0.5% SDS at room temperature and transfer to a 15 ml polypropylene tube. Add proteinase K (50 μg/ml final) or Pronase E (final: 500 μg/ml). Incubate at 37 °C for 30–120 min.
8. Phenol-extract with 6 ml per tube of Tris-saturated phenol (pH 7.6). Aqueous phase and interphase are extracted with 1:1 phenol–chloroform mix. The resulting aqueous phase is then extracted with chloroform–isoamyl alcohol mix (24:1).
9. Transfer the aqueous phase to a pre-cooled 30 ml Corex tube. Add 0.1× volume of 2 M sodium acetate (pH 5.5) and 2.5 volumes of pre-cooled ethanol. Mix gently and in a few seconds a fibrous material (DNA) will precipitate. Spool it out with a heat-sealed and bent Pasteur pipette. Transfer the tube at −20 °C overnight or at −70 °C for 2 h.

Protocol 1. *Continued*

10. Centrifuge as in step **3**. Aspirate supernatant and drain the precipitate well. Add 10 ml 80% ethanol, precipitate at −70°C for 2 h, and repeat the centrifugation.
11. Vacuum-dry the precipitate, re-suspend the pellet in 2 mM EDTA (pH 7.5), heat at 65°C for 10 min. Take an O.D. at 260 and 280 nm. If the 260/280 ratio is nearly 2.0, you can trust that 1 O.D. is equal to 40 μg RNA. Store at −70°C.

Protocol 2. Guanidinium–caesium chloride extraction

1. Homogenize tissue in a 15 ml polypropylene tube, adding 5 ml of homogenization buffer[a] (HB) with a hand-held homogenizer (as described above).
2. Add Sarcosyl to a final concentration of 0.5%, vortex, and centrifuge at room temperature for 10 min at 5000*g*.
3. Transfer the supernatant into a fresh centrifuge tube using a 1 ml syringe fitted with a 23-gauge needle. Use the same syringe to shear genomic DNA by aspirating and delivering a few times, and later to layer the sample on to a CsCl/EDTA cushion in a clear ultracentrifuge tube.
4. The CsCl/EDTA mix is prepared with 96 g of CsCl and 90 ml of 0.01% EDTA (pH 7.5) and DEPC up to a final 0.1%. After 30 min at room temperature, the solution is autoclaved (20 min, liquid cycle) and ultrapure water added up to 100 ml. We have used several different ultracentrifuges with this technique, with different swing-out rotors (see reference (4)). There are several suitable choices, for example a Beckman TL-100 centrifuge with a TL55 rotor. In this case 1 ml of sample is layered on the top of 0.8 ml CsCl mix. Use homogenization buffer to balance the tubes, and spin for 2.5 h at 200 000*g*.
5. Gently remove all supernatant up to 0.5 cm from the bottom of the tube. Using a red-hot blade held in a haemostat, cut off the bottom of the tubes, just above the level of the remaining fluid. Remove excess fluid with a sterile tip. Wash with 70% ethanol, spin at 12 000*g*, and allow the pellet to dry. Dissolve the pellet in 30 μl TE buffer[b] (pH 7.6)/0.1% SDS by pipetting back and forth.
6. Transfer RNA to a microfuge tube, with 50 μl TE (pH 7.6)/0.1% SDS, 10 μl 3 M sodium acetate (pH 5.2), and 300 μl ice-cold ethanol. Wash the bottom of the tube with 20 μl TE buffer. Mix well and store at −20°C for 30 min.

7. Spin at 12 000*g* for 10 min at 4°C. Re-suspend the pellet in 100 μl 2 mM EDTA (pH 7.5), and assess the extraction as in the urea/LiCl method.

[a] Homogenization buffer = 4 M guanidinium isothyocyanate, 0.1 M Tris–HCl (pH 7.5); added before use of 1% β-mercaptoethanol.
[b] TE buffer = 0.01 M Tris–HCl (pH 7.4), 1 mM EDTA pH 8.0.

Protocol 3. Acid guanidinium–phenol–chloroform extraction

This method is particularly useful for processing a large number of small samples, and does not require the use of an ultracentrifuge. The recovery is usually excellent even for minute specimens, particularly if the samples are supplemented with 20–40 μg rRNA as carrier.

1. Homogenize tissue in 1 ml of denaturing solution.[a,b]
2. Sequentially add 0.1 ml of 2 M sodium acetate, pH 4.0, and 0.2 ml of chloroform–isoamyl alcohol mix (49:1). Shake vigorously for 15 sec and cool on ice for 15 min.
3. Spin at 10 000*g* for 20 min at 5°C. Transfer the aqueous phase (for best results, aspirate 50 μl less, rather than disturbing the interphase) to a fresh tube, mix with ice-cold isopropanol, and leave at −20°C for 1 h.
4. Spin at 4°C for 10 min at 10 000*g* and re-suspend the pellet (containing the RNA) in 75% ice-cold ethanol. Pipette back and forth, keep on ice for 10 min and spin at 10 000*g* for 15 min. The pellet is semi-dried and re-suspended in 2 mM EDTA. Store at −70°C until used.

[a] Denaturing solution = 4 M guanidinium isothiocyanate, 25 mM sodium citrate, pH 7.0; 0.5% Sarcosyl. This is stable for three months at room temperature. Before use, add 0.36 ml β-mercaptoethanol/50 ml stock.
[b] A very convenient, pre-mixed solution which allows a single-step extraction is commercially available ('*RNAzol*', Biogenesis Ltd, Biotecx Laboratories Inc.). This has proved very useful and yields reproducible results, i.e. efficient extraction of good-quality RNA (O.D. ratio > 1.90).

2.1.2 Isolation of mRNA

This is based on the affinity separation of poly-A RNA (mRNA) on a solid support with immobilized poly-dT oligonucleotides. Poly-dT columns are used conventionally but poly-dT-coated magnetic beads are particularly suitable for a large number of smaller samples (Dynal, UK; Promega Ltd).

Protocol 4. Affinity separation of mRNA with magnetic beads

1. Add ultrapure water to about 75 μg total RNA, to reach a volume of 100 μl. Mix gently by pipetting and heat at 65°C for 2 min.

Protocol 4. *Continued*

2. Wash 100 μl of magnetic beads (0.5 mg) with 100 μl 2× binding buffer.[a] To separate the beads, use a dedicated 1.5 ml magnetic separator that can be purchased from the manufacturers of the beads.
3. Add 100 μl of 2× binding buffer to the beads. Add the RNA solution, mix gently, and leave at room temperature for 5 min.
4. Separate the beads, discard the supernatant, and wash the beads twice with 200 μl washing buffer.[b]
5. Add the desired amount (typically 20 μl) of 2 mM EDTA, heat at 65 °C for 2 min (to dissociate poly-dA from poly-dT), quickly separate using the magnet, and transfer the poly-A RNA to a fresh tube. Store at −70 °C until used.

[a] 2× binding buffer = 20 mM Tris–HCl, 1 M LiCl, 2 mM EDTA (pH 7.6).
[b] Washing buffer = 10 mM Tris–HCl, 0.15 M LiCl, 1 mM EDTA (pH 7.6).

2.1.3 Gel electrophoresis and transfer

The RNA preparation and the ssRNA size markers are size-fractionated in a denaturing gel, i.e. in presence of agents such as formaldehyde that will reduce formation of secondary structures or re-association, factors that would alter electrophoretic mobility.

Protocol 5. Gel electrophoresis and blotting of RNA

1. For a 21 × 16 agarose gel, prepare a denaturing gel using 2.2 g ultrapure agarose, 180 ml ultrapure water, and 20 ml of 10 × MOPS buffer.[a] Reagents are added in a flask and melted in a microwave oven on medium for approximately 3 min, then allowed to cool to 60 °C. In a fume cupboard add 10.2 ml formaldehyde (37%), mix well, and pour the gel on a levelled tray. Once the gel is set, it can be submerged in the gel tank with 1 × MOPS buffer.
2. To a sterile 1.5 ml tube, add 8 μl poly-A and 8 μl FSB.[b] Heat at 65 °C for 5 min, then cool on ice. Add 4 μl loading dye[c] and load immediately.
3. Similarly in one of the outer lanes run 3–5 μl of a low-molecular-weight RNA ladder (240–9690 bp ladder, BRL). Run the gel overnight on 30 V, or during the day, at 60–120 V.
4. When the dye marker has run 10–16 cm into the gel, cut the excess gel with a scalpel, and cut a nylon membrane (Hybond N, Amersham; Zeta-probe, Biorad) to the same size. Cut one of the corners to identify orientation.
5. Assemble a capillary transfer as in *Figure 1*. The sponge should be very

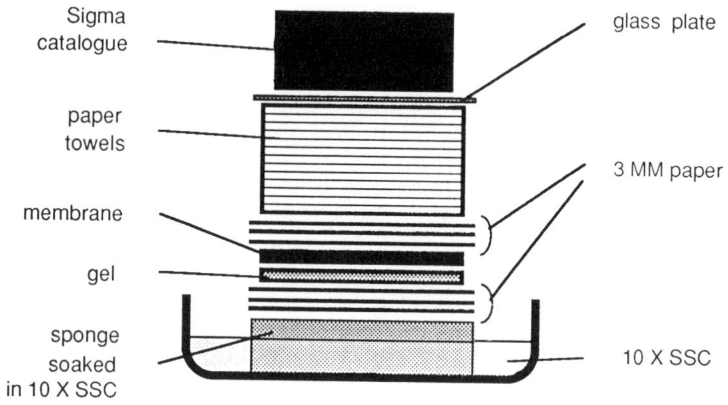

Figure 1. Northern blot.

firm, but still capable of a good capillary action. RNA is transferred for 6–18 h in 10 × SSC.[d] Very good, fast transfers can be obtained with vacuum or positive-pressure blotters (Appligene, Hybaid, Stratagene, Pharmacia).

6. After blotting, air-dry the membrane for 10 min. Then expose the membrane to UV for 3–5 min to cross-link the RNA, cut the strip containing the markers, and stain the latter in 1 M acetic acid (10 min) and in staining solution.[e] Destain in water for 10 min.

[a] 10 × MOPS = 0.2 M MOPS sodium salt, 50 mM Na acetate, 10 mM EDTA (pH 7.0).
[b] Formamide sample buffer = 100 μl 10× MOPS, 200 μl deionized formamide (99%), 120 μl formaldehyde.
[c] Loading dye = 500 μl EDTA 0.2 M, pH 7.0; 0.3 g Ficoll 400; traces of bromophenol blue; ultrapure water up to a final 1 ml.
[d] 10 × SSC = 0.15 M sodium citrate, 1.5 M NaCl.
[e] Staining solution = 0.4 M acetic acid, 0.4 M sodium acetate, 0.2% (w/v) methylene blue.

2.1.4 Preparation of probe

Depending on the application, a wide choice of probe types as well as different labelling procedures are now available. Non-radioactive detection systems have been developed and seem to provide a viable alternative to radiolabelled probes (British Biotechnology, Amersham, Boehringer, Pharmacia, Biorad). The cDNA or RNA probe can be labelled with biotin and detected colorimetrically with anti-biotin antibodies or streptavidin-associated alkaline phosphatase or horseradish peroxidase. Alternatively, the cDNA could be synthesized to incorporate digoxygenin, becoming detectable with suitable antibodies, or it is sulphonated and detected with antibodies to sulphonated DNA. Random-primed oligolabelling is still, however, widely used, often because of the very high specific activity obtainable, which is useful when dealing with low-copy mRNAs:

Protocol 6. Preparation of radiolabelled cDNA probes[a]

1. cDNA to be used as the template is prepared in advance (for details of subcloning plasmid preparation and restriction see reference (4)), fractionated on low-melting-point (LMP) agarose, and divided in aliquots of LMP each containing 50 ng cDNA.
2. Prepare the reaction mix.[b]
3. Heat the DNA/LMP agarose aliquot at 65 °C, and make up the volume to 34 μl with ultrapure water. Incubate at 65 °C for 2 min, at 95 °C for 7 min, and at 37 °C for 10 min.
4. Add sequentially:
   - 10 μl reaction mix
   - 50 μCi [^{32}P]dCTP (3000 Ci/mmol)
   - water up to 49 μl
   - 1 μl (= 8 U) of T7 DNA polymerase
5. Incubate at 37 °C for 15–30 min.
6. Fractionate the probe on a Sephadex G50 column (15 × 0.8 cm). Incorporated label will run in the void volume, free nucleotides will be retarded. A mini-counter with a narrow probe allows easy detection of the fractions. Incorporation can be monitored by Cerenkov radiation, i.e. by dotting 5 μl from each fraction on a glass-fibre disc in a scintillation vial, and β-counted with a program for ^{3}H. Calibration is needed to convert c.p.m. into d.p.m. and finally into specific activity of the probe. A typical incorporation should be of 70–95%, with a specific activity of up to 1×10^9 d.p.m./μg DNA. The probe can only be stored for up to 36 h because of radiolysis. We usually label probes while pre-hybridizing the blots, then use them immediately.

[a] A number of random-labelling kits using Klenow, Taq, or T7 polymerase are commercially available (Amersham, USB, Pharmacia, BRL), and all perform satisfactorily.

[b] Reaction mix = 7 parts of solution 'C', 25 parts of solution 'B', and 25 parts of 1 M Hepes (pH 6.6):

- 'A' = 250 mM Tris–HCl (pH 8.0); 50 mM 2-mercaptoethanol; 25 mM $MgCl_2$
- 'B' = dissolve 100 μM of each dNTP in solution A.
- 'C' = 1 mM Tris, 1 mM EDTA, pH 7.5; add 90 O.D./ml of random hexamers.

2.1.5 Hybridization

The following protocol describes hybridization.

Protocol 7. Hybridization of cDNA probes to blotted mRNA

1. Make a plastic bag containing the membrane and 50 ml of hybridization solution.[a] Seal the bag, carefully squeezing out the air bubbles.[b]
2. Secure the bag flat on the platform of a shaking incubator at 37 °C for 2–16 h.
3. Transfer the membrane to a second bag. Heat the labelled probe and an amount of salmon testes DNA (enough for a final 50 μg/ml) at 98 °C for 10 min. Quickly add them to 15–30 ml of fresh hybridization mix, and pour into the bag containing the membrane. Seal the bag with particular attention to avoid bubble or froth formation, secure it on the platform avoiding kinks, and shake overnight at 40–60 °C (depending on stringency needed).
4. Then, carefully transfer the membrane to a fresh bag with 2 × SSC and 0.1% SDS. Shake for 15 min at 40 °C, change the solution, and repeat twice. Successive washes can be in a lunch box: in 1 × SSC, 0.1% SDS (once, 15 min, 40 °C); in 0.2 × SSC, 0.1% SDS (once, 15 min, 40 °C); in 0.1 × SSC, 0.1% SDS (once, 15 min, 40 °C). If needed, washes can be done at higher temperatures for higher stringency. If the membrane is to be re-used with a different probe, it should not be allowed to dry completely.
5. Label the membrane with radioactive ink at the edges, and wrap it in Saran.

[a] Hybridization mix should be prepared in advance: 50 ml deionized formamide, 20 ml 20 × SSCP, 2 ml 50× Denhart's solution, 25 ml water. Store on ice. 20 × SSCP = 2.4 M NaCl; 0.3 M Na citrate; 0.4 M sodium phosphate dihydrate; pH 7.4. 50 × Denhart's = 1% bovine serum albumin; 1% Ficoll (400 KDa); 1% polyvinyl pyrrolidine (40 KDa).

[b] Hybridization in glass bottles is increasing in popularity because it allows maximum containment and hybridization at very high temperatures. This allows the use of very simple (and stable) hybridization buffers, without any loss of stringency. Hybridization ovens have been on the market now for several years (Hybaid, Biometra, Robbins, Appligene, Techne).

2.1.6 Detection

Membranes are exposed in X-ray cassettes with intensifying screens and double-coated film (Amersham Hyperfilm-MP; Dupont NDT; Kodak X-OMAT) for 12 h at 70 °C. This first exposure allows a better calculation of the time needed for a sharp autoradiographic image. Allow the cassette to reach room temperature before developing. A new film can be exposed for as long as needed. The membrane can be re-used with a different probe, provided that it has not dried and has been stored in the dark at −70 °C. To 'strip' the membrane of existing probe, wash for 2 h at 65 °C at low stringency (low-stringency wash = 0.5 mM Tris–HCl, pH 8.0; 0.2 mM EDTA, 1× Denhart's). Remember to re-expose the membrane after stripping to check efficiency of washes.

2.2 Slot/dot-blot analysis

This technique is particularly useful when large numbers of samples need to be processed, when a relatively small number of cells is available, or when quantitative analysis of hybridization is required. The RNA is transferred by using a manifold that allows the deposition of the RNA at regular intervals on the membrane (in the shape of dots or slots depending on the apparatus). The membrane is then treated as in a Northern hybridization, and hybridization can be quantified by scanning densitometry of the autoradiography. No information is obtained about the size of the transcript, hence the requirement to check specificity and stringency of hybridization by a full Northern analysis.

Protocol 8. Preparation of dot or slot-blots

1. Denature the RNA by adding to 50 μl of aqueous solution of RNA, 20 μl of 20 × SSC and 20 μl of formaldehyde. Heat at 65 °C for 15 min, then let it cool on ice. Prepare dilutions and load.
2. For each slot use RNA from a minimum of 4×10^4 cells per slot. For most cytokines typical dilutions (in 15 × SSC) should be 4×10^5 cells per slot followed by two or three 1:5 dilutions. Dot blots can accept up to 10 times more.
3. Assemble the apparatus according to the manufacturers' instruction. We have satisfactorily used manifolds from Schleier and Schuell, Millipore, and Biorad. Cut the nylon membrane to the size required, making sure to cut a corner to identify the orientation. The membrane should be wetted in ultrapure water, then 10 × SSC, for 15 min each.
4. Load the samples. If the dilutions have been performed in a microtitre plate, it will be possible to use a multichannel pipette to load the samples. Apply gentle vacuum after the samples have been loaded, and once they have been deposited, add an extra 300 μl of 10 × SSC per well.
5. Dry the membrane in air for 10 min (RNA side facing upwards), wrap in Saran and expose to UV for about 4 min. Store flat in the dark until used.
6. The membrane can now be hybridized as in the Northern protocol (*Protocols* 6 and 7).

Manifolds for this application are usually very delicate (and expensive!), treat them accordingly. Surfaces should be carefully cleaned with mild detergent, soaked in ultrapure water, and stored wrapped in their container.

2.3 Nuclease protection assay

Nuclease protection assays are based on the liquid-phase hybridization between mRNA and single-stranded, radiolabelled complementary probes.

After nuclease digestion the hybrid will be intact and can be easily visualized by autoradiography after electrophoresis. An alternative protocol to the one that follows, which also gives low background and high sensitivity, is based on S1 nuclease digestion (6).

Protocol 9. RNase protection assay

1. Synthesize a strand-specific RNA probe, by labelling with α-[^{32}P]dCTP the transcript from a Riboprobe vector containing the cDNA of interest (7). At the end of *in vitro* transcription, digest with DNase (RNase-free) for 15 min, followed by heating at 95°C for 20 min. Store at −70°C until used (within 36 h). It is important to monitor the size of the probe on an agarose/formaldehyde gel (Section 2.1.3) followed by transfer on to nylon membrane and methylene blue staining. If needed, a preparative gel should be used for purification. A standard reaction yields enough probe for 50–80 hybridizations.
2. Extract target RNA as in Section 2.1.1. Dissolve it in 50 μl ultrapure water, read the O.D. and transfer the equivalent of 30 μg total RNA to a fresh 1.5 ml tube. Dry in a vacuum desiccator until nearly dry. Control yeast tRNA should be similarly prepared.
3. Add the hybridization mixture (30 μl),[a] containing about 5×10^5 c.p.m. of probe. The ratio of cellular RNA to labelled RNA should be determined empirically in advance to achieve optimal background and sensitivity. A slight excess of probe is usually necessary.
4. Incubate the mixture at 90°C for 10 min, then incubate in a dry-block for 10–16 h at a temperature usually between 40°C and 60°C. The stringency needed should be assessed in pilot experiments with the RNA probe to be used.
5. Let the tubes cool at room temperature, then add 300 μl of digestion mixture.[b] Incubate at 30°C for 1 h.
6. Digest RNase by adding 20 μl of 10% SDS and 10 μl of Proteinase K (10 mg/ml stock). Incubate at 37°C for 30 min.
7. Phenol-chloroform extract. Precipitate the upper phase in 75% ice-cold ethanol, for 15 min at −70°C. Spin at 12 000*g* for 15 min at 4°C. Aspirate the supernatant, wash the pellet with ice-cold 75% ethanol and spin again. Aspirate the supernatant and heat at 50°C for 5 min to evaporate all traces of ethanol.
8. Add 10 μl of sample-loading buffer,[c] mix very well, heat at 95°C for 5 min, then quickly cool on ice.
9. Prepare and load a polyacrylamide/7 M urea gel (4). Samples are loaded to include a negative control (yeast tRNA) and the radiolabelled probe

Protocol 9. *Continued*

alone. The molecular size of the protected probe should match the free probe and its intensity expresses the amount of specific transcript; the yeast tRNA should fail to protect the probe, which should be digested.

[a] Hybridization buffer = 40 mM Pipes (pH 6.4); 1 mM EDTA, pH 8.0; 0.4 M NaCl; 80% deionized formamide.
[b] Digestion mixture = 4 μg/ml RNase T1, 50 μg/ml RNase A, 5 mM EDTA, pH 7.5; 10 mM Tris–HCl pH 7.4; 300 mM NaCl.
[c] Sample-loading buffer = 10 mM EDTA, pH 8.0; 1 mg/ml xylene cyanol; 1 mg/ml bromophenol blue; 80% formamide.

The major advantage of this method over a Northern blot is specificity, in that it is possible to see exactly how much of the probe is protected (i.e. hybridizes to) the target mRNA.

2.4 Reverse-transcription PCR analysis (RTPCR)

Polymerase chain reaction (PCR) has been established in the last 5–7 years as a major tool in molecular biology. Extension of oligonucleotide primers on native or cloned DNA templates is achieved through repeated cycles of melting, annealing, and extension. Through 30–40 such cycles of duplication, PCR allows a high yield of target DNA copies. It is assumed here that the reader is familiar with the technique of PCR, for which several good protocols are available (8, 9). In order to use PCR to amplify RNA sequences, the RNA must first be converted to DNA. The conversion of RNA to cDNA is performed using reverse transcriptase (RT). We perform all steps of the procedure in a dedicated suite, with precautions taken to avoid cross-contamination by previously amplified templates, including the use of class-II cabinets, UV lights, positive displacement pipettes, or resin-protected tips on dedicated air-displacement pipettes. The single most important factor is probably physical containment and, of course, the careful planning of each single step.

Apart from cross-contamination giving false positive results, there are other dangers related to the extraordinary sensitivity of this technique. A sub-microlitre mistake in delivery of reagents, an incompletely homogeneous sample, a different purity of RNA can all result in gross differences in the outcome. However, if the handling and the quality of the reagents are very consistent, the results can be semi-quantitative, i.e. allowing comparison within the same experiment.

Protocol 10. Analysis of mRNA by RTPCR

1. Design and synthesize suitable oligonucleotide primers.[a]
2. Extract total RNA from samples (see Section 2.1.1). Total purity is not needed, but should be constant between samples. If required, store at −70°C.

3. Prepare stock solutions in advance:
   - each dNTP is diluted to 10 mM using 10 mM Tris–HCl, pH 7.5 (neutralized 100 mM solutions; Promega, Pharmacia)
   - RNasin (RNase inhibitor), 20 U/μl (Promega)
   - random hexamers at 50 μM (Pharmacia)
   - 10 × buffer : 500 mM KCl; 100 mM Tris–HCl pH 8.8; 1% Triton X-100; 15 mM $MgCl_2$
   - AMV reverse transcriptase HC (Promega, Boehringer) at 25 U/μl.
4. For reverse transcription, prepare in a 0.5 ml tube the following reaction mix:

Reagent	**Volume per reaction**	**Final conc.**
H_2O	4 μl	
dNTP	2 μl of each	1 mM each
RNasin	1 μl	1 U/μl
Hexamers	1 μl	2.5 μM
10× buffer	2 μl	1 ×
Total	16 μl	

   Templates should include a negative control, and for each sample a series of dilutions is needed for quantitative interpretation (see step **12**).
5. Deliver a 16 μl aliquot of the mix in each tube.
6. Heat 1 μl of RNA template at 90°C, then cool on ice for 15 min. This should contain 1 μg total RNA (equivalent to 5×10^4 mammalian cells). Mix gently, pulse-spin in a microcentrifuge, and add 3 μl of RT enzyme to each tube (75 U). Remember to change tips.
7. Overlay with 50 μl of light white mineral oil (Sigma).
8. In a thermocycler, incubate the tubes at 20°C for 10 min, 42°C for 60 min, and 95°C for 10 min; chill on ice.
9. Use 10 μl as template in a 50 μl PCR reaction. Using the Perkin-Elmer Cetus PCR kit for each tube you should add 4 μl 10 × PCR buffer (containing 15 mM $MgCl_2$), 0.25 μl of Taq polymerase, 2 μl of oligonucleotide primer mix (15 μM), and up to 50 μl with ultrapure water. Mix well and overlay with mineral oil.
10. PCR cycles should be optimized for the different primer/template combinations. A good start could be: (95°C, 2 min; 55°C, 1 min; 74°C, 1 min) ×3; followed by (95°C, 1 min; 55°C, 1 min; 74°C, 1 min) ×30; and (95°C, 1 min; 55°C, 1 min; 74°C, 5 min) ×3. The software mentioned previously can give the annealing temperature in pilot experiments.

Protocol 10. *Continued*

11. Run the PCR products in a high-sieving agarose gel (3% agarose in TBE (Sigma, BRL) or 3% Nusieve/1% agarose (FMC Bioproducts)).
12. For semi-quantitation of the initial transcript, each sample should have been prepared in two series of four dilutions each (1:1; 1:10; 1:100; 1:1000). One series is amplified with the primers for the mRNA being tested, the other with control (we use β-actin) primers. Samples should be compared by the amplification in two lanes from dilutions with similar β-actin product. Remember to run a 'no-RT' control for plasmid pseudogenes.
13. The efficiency of RT can be easily checked by running in two of the outer lanes the initial amount of template RNA contained in 10 μl (usually 0.5 μg), and the 10 μl of RT product that has not been used in the PCR. Ethidium staining should show a higher intensity in the RT sample, because of the newly synthesized DNA.

[a] Primers should be directed to regions which are within 200–600 bp on the mRNA, but on different exons on the gene; this will allow easy recognition of an RNA sample contaminated with genomic DNA or nuclear RNA. Traditionally, primers of 22–24 bp containing 45–55% G/C are preferred. It is very important to check for secondary structures of the regions and of the primers, the likelihood of self-annealing, and energy state of the region to be amplified. We also screen primers for their specificity using the FIND program (10) at the SERC facility Seqnet VAX 3600 on node DLVH (janet.000001009302). The program should be run as a batch file if all human sequences are being searched allowing 10% mismatches. On the same line the program PRIMER can be used to check primer suitability for PCR use. Several good programs are available commercially (*OLIGO*, National Biosciences; *Primer Detector*, Cambridge Bioscience). Make sure that primers have been deprotected (in ammonia at 55°C overnight) and purified by cartridge, butanol, or HPLC.

2.5 *In situ* hybridization

This technique is used to detect nucleic acids in intact tissue or cells, using a complementary nucleic acid probe. When combined with immunocytochemistry it offers a powerful tool to study the histology of gene activation in disease. It is, therefore, a popular RNA detection method, despite its technical difficulties and non-quantitative results.

The following protocol has been successful in our laboratory to identify cytokine mRNA in inflammatory tissue (*Figure 2*) (11). We use random-primed, α-[^{32}P]dCTP-labelled cDNA probes for ease of detection (12).

Protocol 11. *In situ* hybridization of mRNA, in conjunction with immunophenotype

1. Rapidly freeze tissue in liquid N_2 immediately after excision and keep at −70°C.
2. To preserve RNA, and improve adherence of tissue to the slide, bake good-quality glass slides at 240°C for 4 h, and coat them with a solution

of 0.5% gelatine, 0.25% $CrK(SO_4)_2$, and 0.02% DEPC in ultrapure water. The blade of the cryotome should be prepared by treatment with NaOH 0.5 M at 65 °C for 30 min; set the cryotome at −25 °C, and leave the blade to equilibrate at −25 °C, and deposit two tissue sections on each slide.

3. Go to step **6** if immunophenotyping is not required.
4. Fix for 5 min in cold acetone, and air dry.
5. Before immunophenotyping, incubate antibodies and serum with 0.08% DEPC for 30 min at 37 °C. We have used mouse primary antibody, biotinylated horse antimouse secondary antibody, and block with normal horse serum. Detect biotin using a commercially available alkaline phosphatase/horseradish peroxidase detection kit (Vector ABC, Vector UK). Wash finally in DEPC water for 5 min after final reaction.
6. Dip for 15 sec in ice-cold Carnoys fixative (1 part acetic acid; 6 parts ethanol; 3 parts chloroform).
7. Re-hydrate in PBS/5 mM $MgCl_2$ for 10 min at room temperature then 0.1 M glycine/0.2 M Tris–HCl, pH 7.4, for 10 min.
8. Pre-hybridize for 30 min at room temperature in pre-hybridization mix: 4 × SSCP, 50% deionized formamide, 1 × Denhart's solution,[a] and 400 μg yeast tRNA/ml.
9. Hybridize overnight at 37 °C in about 20 μl pre-hybridization mix with the addition of vacuum-concentrated ^{32}P-labelled probe, 10 mM vanadyl sulphate, and 150 μg/ml denatured sheared calf thymus DNA covered with a salinized coverslip.
10. Wash once in 2 × SSC for 30 min; then 1 × SSC, 50% formamide for 30 min; and last 1 × SSC for 30 min. Air dry.
11. Dip slides vertically once in Ilford K5 emulsion which has been diluted 1:2 with warm ultrapure water. Dry them for 2 h at room temperature in a (locked!) darkroom, then in a light-proof box with silica for 3–14 days. Develop slides with Kodak D170 and fix in F24. Typically 5–7 slides with consecutive section are prepared, and developed at different time points.
12. Counterstain with 2% Giemsa for 7 min, wash, dry, and mount in 'histomount'.
13. Using the high-power lens, positive cells will appear covered in black grains, not necessarily directly over the cytoplasm, because of the high energy of ^{32}P.

[a] Hybridization mix should be prepared in advance: 50 ml deionized formamide, 20 ml 20 × SSCP, 2 ml 50× Denhart's solution, 25 ml water. Store on ice. 20 × SSCP = 2.4 M NaCl; 0.3 M Na citrate; 0.4 M sodium phosphate dihydrate; pH 7.4. 50 × Denhart's = 1% bovine serum albumin; 1% Ficoll (400 kD); 1% polyvinyl pyrrolidine (40 kD).

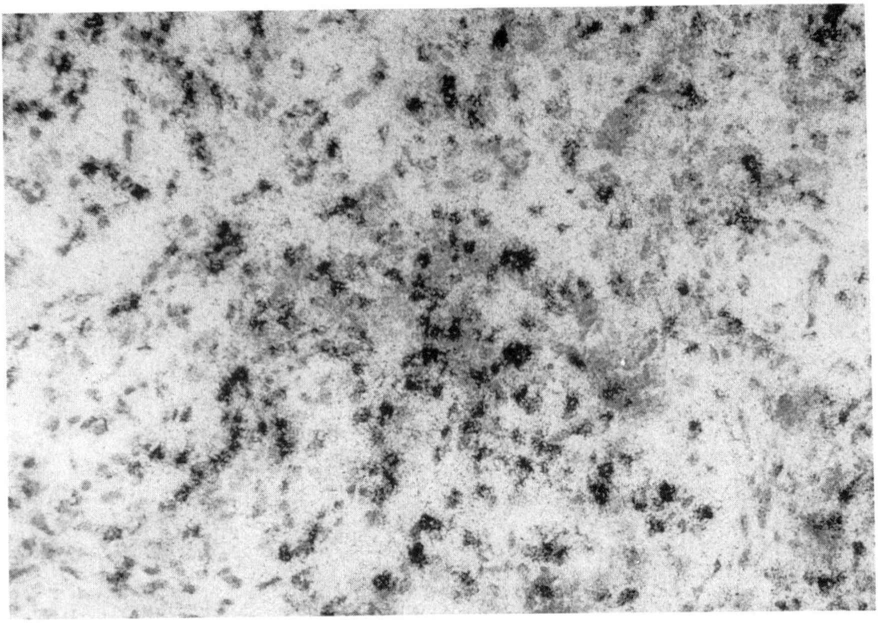

Figure 2. *In situ* hybridization. Rheumatoid arthritis synovial tissue, hybridized to ^{32}P-labelled IL-1β cDNA probe.

As previously mentioned (Section 2.1.4), alternatives to isotopic detection are available. Apart from safety considerations, advantages would include the avoidance of lengthy multiple exposures and the stability of the labelled probe (>6 months at −20°C). High sensitivity and excellent localization can be obtained with immunogold reagents, i.e. anti-biotin antibodies conjugated to gold particles, which are visible at confocal laser microscopy.

3. Transcription rate analysis (nuclear run-on assay)

This method (13, 14) measures the amount of specific transcript produced in a defined period of time after stimulation *in vitro* or in tissue that is presumed to be activated.

3.1 Preparation of nuclei

Protocol 12. Preparation of nuclei

1. Culture cells as required. Typical lengths of culture would be 15 min, 30 min, 1 h, 2 h, 4 h, 6 h, 8 h after stimulation.
2. Wash the cells twice with ice-cold RSB.[a]

3. Re-suspend each different cell preparation in 5 ml RSB at a concentration between 1×10^6 and 1×10^7/ml.
4. Add 10 μl Nonidet (NP-40; Sigma). Gently pipette back and forth a few times to break the cytoplasmic membranes.
5. Layer carefully on 7.5 ml of 2 M sucrose (BDH, 68.46 g/100 ml), in a 15 ml Corex tube.
6. Spin on Sorvall HB4 rotor or Beckman JS 13.1 rotor at 10 000 r.p.m. for 15 min.
7. Aspirate the supernatant and re-suspend the pellet in 5 ml RSB. Spin at 10 000 r.p.m. for 5 min.
8. Re-suspend whole nuclei in 100 μl NFM (nuclear freezing medium = 50 mM Tris–HCl, pH 8.3; 40% glycerol; 5 mM $MgCl_2$; 0.1 mM EDTA), and freeze in liquid N_2 by leaving in the gas phase for 6 h and then quickly transferring to the liquid phase.

[a] Reticulocyte standard buffer = (RSB) 10 mM Tris–HCl, pH 7.4; 10 mM NaCl; 5 mM $MgCl_2$; 1 mM DTT.

3.2 Labelling of nascent RNA; preparation of probe

In the previous protocol, the nuclei have been metabolically arrested by placing in liquid N_2, and contain all the hardware and instructions to start producing primary transcript. They are incubated in presence of radiolabelled UTP for 30 min, and subsequently stopped and the RNA extracted.

Protocol 13. Labelling of nascent RNA; preparation of probe

1. Pre-incubate reaction buffer[a] for 5 min at 30°C.
2. Add each nuclear preparation to 100 μl RB and incubate at 30°C for 30 min. Stop by adding 20 U DNaseI and 40 μg tRNA, and incubate for 20 min at 37°C.
3. Extract RNA as previously described (Section 2.1.1). Before the last ethanol precipitation the RNA is treated with 0.24 M NaOH on ice for 10 min.
4. Add acid-free HEPES to a final 0.24 M and ethanol-precipitate. Count activity by Cerenkov radiation (see Section 2.1.4). If at the end of extraction the RNA is not used immediately, store at −70°C (but use within 20 h to avoid radiolysis).

[a] Reaction buffer (RB) = 10 mM Tris–HCl, pH 8.0; 5 mM $MgCl_2$; 300 mM KCl; 0.5 mM ATP; 0.5 mM CTP; 0.5 mM GTP; 100 μCi α-[^{32}P]UTP, 760 Ci/mmol.

3.3 Membrane hybridization

A nylon membrane is prepared on which several cDNAs of interest have been slotted. One of the advantages of this method is that the radiolabelled nuclear RNA preparation contains all RNA types activated by that stimulus, and many genes can be screened at the same time.

Protocol 14. Membrane hybridization

1. Transfer the cDNAs of interest to several membranes (typically 10 μg DNA/slot) with a dot or slot-blot apparatus, as detailed in Section 2.2. Before slotting, the cDNA is boiled (98°C, 15 min). Ideally, probes from bidirectional *in vitro* transcription vectors (such as from the SP6 or T7 promoters of pGEM series) should be used, as they can provide the two strands for test and control.
2. Cross-link the membrane with UV light.
3. Re-suspend RNA in buffer A[a] at about 5×10^6 c.p.m./ml. Add to an equal volume of buffer B.[a] Hybridize in bags or a hybridization oven at 65°C for 36 h.
4. Wash twice in 2 × SSC for 2 h at 65°C. Treat with 10 μg/ml RNase A for 30 min at 37°C in 2 × SSC.
5. Wash twice in 2 × SSC at 37°C for 1 h. Leave to dry for 1 h and expose with intensifying screens.

[a] Buffer A = 10 mM TES, pH 7.4; 0.2% SDS, 10 mM EDTA. Buffer B = 10 mM TES pH 7.4; 0.2% SDS, 10 mM EDTA, 600 mM NaCl.

---

4. mRNA transport into cytoplasm

Processing of RNA and/or its transport into cytoplasm are also stages where protein production can be regulated. This can be studied by extracting mRNA from nuclear and cytoplasmic fractions of cells at different time points, and probing it with the cDNA of interest.

Protocol 15. Assessing the rate of mRNA transport into the cytoplasm

1. Wash cells with ice-cold PBS. Spin at 500*g* for 5 min. Re-suspend at 1×10^7/ml in lysis buffer.[a] Leave for 5 min on ice.
2. Spin at 1000*g* for 10 min. The supernatant contains the cytoplasmic extract; the nuclei are in the pellet.

3. Extract both fractions as in Section 2.1.1. To analyse processing, Northern analysis should be performed; in all other cases, slot or dot-blotting will be sufficient to assess rate of transport in cytoplasm.

[a] Lysis buffer = 10 mM Tris–HCl, pH 7.4; 10 mM NaCl; 3 mM $MgCl_2$; 0.5% NP40.

5. Cytoplasmic mRNA half-life

An effective way to measure mRNA half-life consists of making serial extractions of mRNA and performing Northern blots following treatment with an inhibitor of RNA synthesis (e.g. actinomycin-D at 10 μg/ml). This 'inhibitor-chase' technique (*Figure 3*) is particularly useful for short-half-life transcripts, although it has been pointed out that the introduction of such a potent inhibitor would affect cell metabolic processes in other ways, and validation is required by 'steady-state labelling' analysis (15).

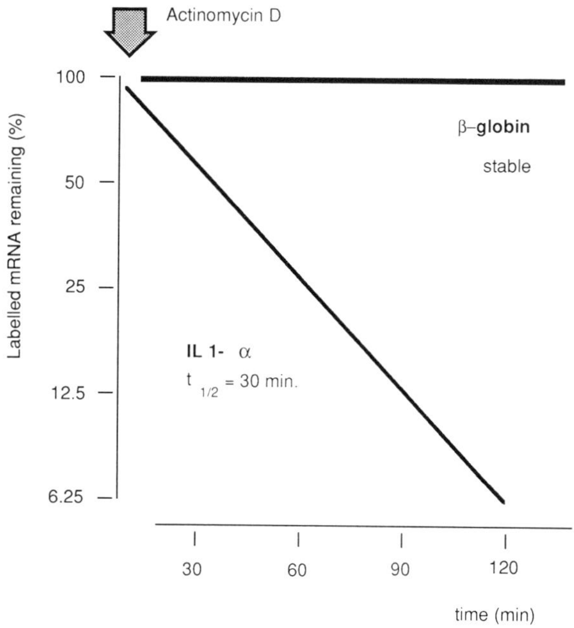

Figure 3. Inhibitor-chase method.

Acknowledgements

This work has been funded by the Arthritis and Rheumatism Council for Research (UK), The Nuffield Foundation (Oliver Bird Fund), and the National Kidney Research Fund.

References

1. Lovell-Badge, R. H. (1987). In *Teratocarcinomas and Embryonic Stem Cells: A Practical Approach*, (ed. E. J. Robertson), pp. 132–3. IRL Press, Oxford.
2. Chirgwin, J. M., Przybyla, A. E., McDonald, R. J., and Rutter, W. J. (1979). *Biochemistry,* **18,** 5294–9.
3. Chomczynsky, P. and Sacchi, N. (1987). *Anal. Biochem.,* **162,** 156–9.
4. Maniatis, T., Fritsch, E. F., and Sambrook, J. (ed.) (1989). *Molecular Cloning*, 2nd edn. Cold Spring Harbor Laboratory, Cold Spring Harbor, NY.
5. Feinberg, A. P. and Vogelstein, B. (1984). *Anal. Biochem.,* **137,** 266–8.
6. Davis, L. G., Dibner, M. D., and Battey, J. F. (ed.) (1986). *Basic Methods in Molecular Biology*, pp. 276–84. Elsevier, New York.
7. *Promega Protocols and Application Guide*, 2nd edn, pp. 58–63.
8. McPherson, M. J., Quirke, P., and Taylor, G. R. (ed.) (1991). *PCR, a Practical Approach*. IRL Press, Oxford.
9. Innis, M. A., Gelfand, D. H., Sminsky, J. I., and White, T. J. (ed.) (1990). *PCR Protocols*. Academic, New York.
10. Devereux, M., Haeberli, F., and Smithes, J. (1984). *Nucl. Acids Res.,* **12,** 387–95.
11. Wood, N. C., Symons, J. A., Dickens, E., and Duff, G. W. (1992). *Clin. Exp. Immunol.,* **87,** 183–9.
12. Ogilvie, A. D., Woods, N. C., Dickens, E., Wojtacha, D., and Duff, G. W. (1990). *Ann. Rheum. Dis.,* **49,** 434–9.
13. Greenberg, M. E. and Ziff, E. B. (1984). *Nature,* **31,** 433–7.
14. Turner, M., Chantry, D., Buchan, G., Barrett, K., and Feldman, M. (1989). *J. Immunol.,* **143,** 3556–61.
15. Harpold, M. M., Wilson, M., and Darnell, J. E. (1981). *Mol. Cell Biol.,* **1,** 188–94.

11

Cytokine bioassay

F. P. WINSTANLEY

1. Introduction

Bioassays quantitate analytes by the magnitude of the effect that they provoke in sensitive organisms, tissues, or isolated cells. These assays can be used for both detection of the bioactive material (e.g. in a purification procedure) and for determining the potency of the preparation, both in absolute terms and in relation to a standard. The term 'potency' is used rather than 'quantity' or 'amount', since only the biologically active form of the analyte is being determined. Other assay types, such as immunoassays, do not necessarily distinguish between bio-active and bio-inactive forms of analytes. However, the corollary of this is that bioassays may not perform adequately in situations in which the preparation contains a mixture of substances each with biological activity (stimulatory or inhibitory) affecting the test tissue. Nevertheless, by careful examination of the dose–response curves and by the use of neutralizing antibodies, such pitfalls may be avoided.

The general method of cytokine bioassay is as follows:

- make serial dilutions of the unknown and standard preparations
- add sensitive cells and measure the response
- compare the dose–response curves for the unknown and standard preparations and calculate the potency of each preparation and the relative potency of the unknown in terms of the standard

The relationship between the response and the log dose (or log dilution) is generally sigmoid, but sometimes a 'hook' is observed at high doses. The potency of a cytokine preparation can be described in terms of arbitrary units, where 1 U/ml is generally taken to be the concentration required to stimulate a half-maximal response in the test system. The potency of the unknown preparation can also be described relative to a standard preparation if the two are analysed simultaneously. The relative potency of the unknown is the ratio of concentrations (standard:unknown) giving equal responses. This is essentially the horizontal distance between the linear portions of the sigmoid dose–response curves on a semilogarithmic plot. Transforming the sigmoid to near-linearity in many cases facilitates the estimation of relative potency. The assumptions underlying this kind of comparative dilution bioassay are:

(a) that the diluent is neutral in the assay system, with the response being proportional solely to the analyte concentration, and
(b) the bioactive substance in the unknown and standard preparations being identical

To test the first assumption there should be no (or negligible) response to the diluent alone, and an assay of the diluent spiked with a range of concentrations of the test substance should yield a series of parallel dose–response curves. The second assumption is more difficult to test, but reasonable confidence in the identical nature of the bioactive substance in both unknown and standard preparations can be held if the dose–response curves have similar upper and lower asymptotes and similar, parallel slopes. Further confidence can be placed in the specificity of the comparative bioassay if the responses provoked by both the unknown and standard can be abolished by neutralization with monoclonal antibodies against the standard.

The bioassays described in this chapter fall into three main categories on the basis of the responses of the stimulated cells. The assays for IL-1, IL-2, and IL-6 are cell proliferation assays, whilst the assay for TNF/LT is a cytotoxicity assay. The assay for IL-8 is based on quantitation of cytokine-stimulated degranulation. The cell proliferation and cytotoxicity assays require a system of determining viable cell numbers. Tetrazolium salt reduction using MTT provides a rapid and inexpensive colorimetric method for obtaining an index of viable cell numbers (*Protocol 1*). This method is based on those published by Mossman (1) and by Hansen *et al.* (2). The original methods used acidified isopropanol as a solvent for the reduced formazan. Unfortunately, this precipitated highly proteinaceous samples such as serum and plasma. The use of sodium dodecyl sulphate/dimethylformamide (SDS/DMF) as a solvent prevents this interference in the assay.

Protocol 1. Determination of an index of viable cell numbers

Reagents required

- MTT (3-[4,5-Dimethylthiazol-2-yl]-2,5-diphenyltetrazolium bromide; Sigma No. M 2128) dissolved at 5 mg/ml in saline, then filtered through a 0.22 μm filter
- SDS/DMF solvent: dissolve SDS (20% w/v) in 50% (v/v) aqueous N,N′-dimethylformamide at 37°C. Adjust pH to 4.7 with HCl. Keep at 37°C to retain the SDS in solution
- microtitre plate reader with filters for either 540 and 630 nm, or 570 and 690 nm

Method

1. Add 10 μl MTT solution to flat-bottomed microtitre plate wells containing cells in 100 μl culture medium. Incubate at 37°C for 2 h. Viable cells will reduce the soluble tetrazolium salt to give a purple precipitate.
2. Add 100 μl SDS/DMF solvent to each well. Mix gently for 2–3 min on a microtitre plate shaker. The purple precipitate will slowly dissolve. The formazan may be fully dissolved within a few minutes, otherwise the plate can be left overnight at room temperature. Three to four minutes' sonication in an ultrasonic water bath has also been used to hasten this step.
3. Read optical density when the reduced formazan is fully dissolved. Suitable wavelengths include 540 nm with a reference at 630 nm, and 570 nm with a reference at 690 nm.

2. Cell proliferation bioassays

Interleukins 1, 2, and 6 can be determined using bioassays based on the proliferative response of cell-lines that have absolute dependency on the individual cytokine as a growth factor. The IL-1 bioassay is based on the D10(N4)M cell-line which has been shown to be much more sensitive than the original thymocyte proliferation assay, responding to as low as femtomolar concentrations of recombinant IL-1 (3). The dose–response curve of the D10(N4)M cells to IL-1 is made much steeper by the incorporation of IL-2 into the assay. The addition of a saturating dose of IL-2 to this assay increases the specificity of the assay for IL-1 by neutralizing any effect of IL-2 in the test sample.

Several cell-lines including CTLL, HT-2, and MT-1 have been reported as being dependent on IL-2 as a growth factor. The assay described here uses the CTLL cell-line (4).

IL-6 can be determined using a variety of cell-lines including 7TD1 and B9. Details of the B9 assay (5) are given here.

The conditions for maintenance of the cell lines are given in *Protocol 2*. The assay procedures all follow the same basic plan. This, together with any special recommendations for individual cytokine assays, is presented in *Protocol 3*.

Protocol 2. Maintenance of cell-lines

1. D10(N4)M (for IL-1 bioassay)
   (a) Source: Dr S. J. Hopkins, Rheumatic Diseases Centre, Hope Hospital, Salford M6 8HD, UK.
   (b) Culture medium: RPMI 1640 buffered with bicarbonate and 20 mM Hepes + 10% FCS, 2 mM glutamine, 50 μM 2-mercaptoethanol and 3

Protocol 2. *Continued*

μg/ml Concanavalin A (Con A). Add rhIL-2 (20–50 U/ml), and IL-1 (20–40 pg/ml) to this basal medium before use. rhIL-1 can be used, but a crude IL-1 preparation from silica- or LPS-stimulated monocytes is a more economical alternative.

(c) Culture conditions: grow the cells in 5–10 ml of medium in 25 cm^2 flasks. Sub-culture every 3–4 days by suspending the cells using a Pasteur pipette and diluting this suspension 1:5–1:10 in fresh medium.

2. CTLL (for IL-2 bioassay)

(a) Source: European Collection of Animal Cell Cultures, Porton Down SP4 0JG, UK, or American Type Culture Collection, 12301 Park Lawn Drive, Rockville, MD 20852–1776, USA.

(b) Culture medium: RPMI 1640 buffered with bicarbonate and 20 mM Hepes + 10% FCS and 2 mM glutamine. 10–20 U/ml of rhIL-2 are added to the medium to maintain cell growth.

(c) Culture conditions: grow the cells in 5–10 ml of medium in 25 cm^2 flasks. Sub-culture every 3–4 days by suspending the cells using a Pasteur pipette and diluting this suspension 1:5–1:10 in fresh medium. The cell density prior to subculture is approximately (3–5) × 10^5/ml.

3. B9 (for IL-6 bioassay)

(a) Source: Dr L. A. Aarden, Central Laboratory Blood Transfusion Service, PO Box 9406, 1006 AK Amsterdam, The Netherlands.

(b) Culture medium: RPMI 1640 buffered with bicarbonate and 20 mM Hepes + 5% FCS, 2 mM glutamine and 50 μM 2-mercaptoethanol. IL-6 (10–100 U/ml) is added to this basal medium to stimulate cell growth.

(c) Culture conditions: grow the cells in 5–10 ml of medium in 25 cm^2 flasks. Sub-culture every 3–4 days by suspending the cells using a Pasteur pipette and diluting this suspension 1:5–1:10 in fresh medium.

Protocol 3. Proliferation assays of cytokine bioactivity—IL-1, IL-2, and IL-6

Equipment required

- humidified 37°C CO_2 (5%) incubator
- flat-bottomed tissue-culture microtitre plates
- 12-tipped micropipette (capable of delivering 20–100 μl) and boxed sterile tips

A. *General method*

1. Make eight serial dilutions (between two- and four-fold) of the analyte in flat-welled microtitre plates leaving a final volume of 50 μl. Use the basal medium for the individual cell-lines (*Protocol 2*) as diluent. At least duplicate dilution series should be made for each sample. The specificity of the response may be assessed by adding a suitable neutralizing antibody to the dilutions of the sample.
2. Harvest the appropriate sensitive cells on the third day following sub-culture and wash once in basal medium. Re-suspend at a concentration of 1×10^5 cells/ml. The medium for the IL-1 assay (D10(N4)M cells) should be supplemented with 60 U/ml rhIL-2.
3. Add 50 μl of the cell suspension to each well and incubate at 37 °C for 3 days (1–2 days for the CTLL cells).
4. Determine the index of viable cell numbers as per *Protocol 1*.

B. *Special recommendations for assays using serum or plasma*

1. Blood samples for bioassay should be taken into low-endotoxin heparinized tubes (Kabi Diagnostica). Clear the plasma fraction of platelets prior to freezing by high-speed centrifugation in a bench-top microfuge. Serum samples can also be assayed, though the clotting process will induce cytokine release from leukocytes.
2. IL-1 bioassay: this assay is inhibited by plasma/serum components that can be removed by precipitation by polyethylene glycol (PEG) (6). The procedure is as follows:
   (a) In a microfuge tube, dilute the sample 1 + 1 with sterile solution of PEG (mol. wt. 8000) 24% (w/v) in saline. Mix well and keep at 4°C for 30 min. After centrifugation for 5 min in a bench-top microfuge, remove the supernatant for bioassay.
   (b) Dilute this sample 1 + 1 with assay medium and conduct the bioassay as described above but incorporating PEG 8000 in the assay diluent to give a final concentration of 3% (w/v).
3. IL-6 bioassay: many plasma/serum samples kill the B9 cell-line by a complement-mediated mechanism. Heat the sample to 56°C for 30 min before assaying to prevent this.

3. Cytotoxicity bioassays

Tumour necrosis factor (TNF) (and lymphotoxin (LT)) can be determined by bioassays based on cytokine-induced cytotoxicity of appropriately sensitive cell-lines. A description of the assay using the WEHI 164 clone 13 fibrosarcoma cell-line (7) is given in *Protocol 4*.

Protocol 4. Bioassay of TNF/LT

A. *Maintenance of cell-line*

1. Cell-line: WEHI 164 clone 13, a murine fibrosarcoma cell line. Sources:
   (a) Dr T. Espevik, Institute of Cancer Research, University of Trondheim, N-7006, Trondheim, Norway.
   (b) Dr A. Meager, National Institute for Biological Standards and Control, South Mimms, Potters Bar, Hertfordshire EN6 3QG, UK.
2. Culture medium: RPMI 1640 buffered with bicarbonate and 20 mM Hepes + 5% FCS and 2 mM glutamine.
3. Culture conditions: grow the cells in 75 cm^2 tissue-culture flasks using 10–20 ml of culture medium. The cells are sub-cultured every 3 days by splitting 1:10. To detach the cells from the culture flask, remove the culture medium, wash the cell monolayer with PBS (calcium- and magnesium-free), and cover the monolayer with 1 ml sterile 0.005% (w/v) EDTA–PBS. Stand at room temperature for 3–5 minutes and then assist the detachment of the cells by firmly striking the wall of the flask on a rubber mat, or the palm or thigh (whichever is least painful!). The detached cells are quickly suspended in 10 ml of culture medium and washed once prior to sub-culture or use in the assay.

B. *Other reagents*

This assay incorporates actinomycin D, an RNA polymerase inhibitor, to increase the sensitivity of the cell-line to TNF/LT cytotoxicity. Actinomycin D–mannitol (Sigma No. A 5156) is readily water-soluble and a stock solution can be prepared in RPMI 1640 medium for use in this assay.

C. *Assay procedure*

1. Make eight serial dilutions (between two- and four-fold) of the analyte in flat-welled microtitre plates leaving a final volume of 50 μl. Use the basal medium as diluent. At least duplicate dilution series should be made for each sample. The specificity of the response may be assessed by adding a suitable neutralizing antibody to the dilutions of the sample.
2. Harvest the cells on the third day after sub-culture and suspend the washed cells at a concentration of (5–6) $\times$ 10^5 cells/ml in medium to which actinomycin D (1 μg/ml) has been added. Add 50 μl to each well.
3. Incubate at 37°C for 18–24 h and determine the index of viable cell numbers using the procedure described in *Protocol 1*.

4. Enzyme release bioassays

Interleukin-8 induces degranulation by granulocytes. Cytochalasin B pre-treatment of the granulocytes ensures that the contents of the lysosomes are released into the extracellular medium, rather than into phagocytic vesicles. The assay described here (*Protocol 5*) measures peroxidase activity as an indicator of myeloperoxidase release (8). Other enzyme markers, such as elastase, could also be used. This assay is not sensitive enough to be recommended for use with clinical samples of serum/plasma and the clinician should make use of suitable immunoassays.

Protocol 5. Interleukin-8 bioassay

This assay is based on the ability of IL-8 to stimulate lysosomal enzyme release from cytochalasin B-treated granulocytes.

- V-well and flat-well microtitre plates and pipettes as described in *Protocol 3*
- microtitre plate reader with 486 nm (or 490 nm) filter

A. *Isolation of human granulocytes and cytochalasin B treatment*

1. Leukocyte buffy coats from citrate-anticoagulated blood can be obtained from blood banks and provide a good source for the large numbers of human granulocytes needed for this assay.
   (a) Dilute the buffy coat 1:2 with PBS.
   (b) Remove the mononuclear cells by centrifugation (400*g* for 30 min) on Ficoll–Hypaque cushions (Pharmacia).
   (c) Gently remove the white cell layer resting on the red cell pellet and lyse the contaminating red cells in 0.85% (w/v) ammonium chloride solution. Wash the granulocytes twice in PBS and finally re-suspend at a concentration of 1×10^7 cells/ml in PBS containing 0.9 mM $CaCl_2$, 0.5 mM $MgCl_2$, and 0.1% (w/v) bovine serum albumin (PBS–BSA).

2. A stock solution of cytochalasin B (1–5 mg/ml) is prepared in dimethylsulphoxide (DMSO) and stored in small aliquots at −20°C. Just prior to the assay add cytochalasin B to the granulocyte suspension to give a final concentration of 5 µg/ml. Incubate the cells at 37°C for 5 min and use immediately in the assay.

B. *Assay procedure*

1. Make eight serial dilutions (between two- and four-fold) of the analyte in V-welled microtitre plates leaving a final volume of 100 µl. Use PBS–BSA as diluent. At least duplicate dilution series should be made for each sample. The specificity of the response may be assessed by adding a suitable neutralizing antibody to the dilutions of the sample. The maximal

Protocol 5. *Continued*

response can be mimicked by lysing the cells in wells containing 100 μl of PBS–BSA containing 0.01% (w/w) Triton X-100.

2. Add 100 μl of cytochalasin B-treated granulocytes to each well and incubate for 30 min at 37°C.
3. Pellet the cells by centrifugation (150*g* for 5 min) and transfer 100 μl volumes of the supernatant from each well to the corresponding wells of a flat-bottomed microtitre plate.
4. Determine the myeloperoxidase activity released into the supernatant by adding 100 μl of OPD reagent (10 mM *o*-phenylenediamine dihydrochloride (OPD) in 0.1 M citrate/phosphate buffer (pH 5) containing 0.001% (v/v) hydrogen peroxide). After 10 min at room temperature the reaction is stopped by adding 50 μl of 2 M sulphuric acid. Measure the optical density at 486 nm.

5. Data analysis

In all the bioassays described here a semi-logarithmic plot of the dose–response relationship is sigmoid. A 'hook' effect may occasionally be seen with high analyte concentrations. The analysis of the dose–response curves can proceed at many levels of sophistication, and the choice of method depends on the purpose of the assay, the quality and completeness of the data, and the rigour with which the researcher wishes to pursue the analysis. Three approaches will be outlined using a typical data set for a cell proliferation bioassay.

5.1 Raw data

The simplest procedure is to sketch a plot of the average response (optical density) against the logarithm of the dose or dilution (*Figure 1* A). Using logarithms to the base of the dilution factor facilitates this stage. The plot demonstrates that although the dose–response curves appear to be parallel, only sample C provides complete information on the full dose–response curve. Sample A inhibits the assay at maximal concentration, but this inhibition is diluted out by the second serial dilution. The data for this curve are edited to remove the aberrant point from further calculations. Sample B is not sufficiently potent to achieve maximal stimulation of the cell-line. The apparent parallelism of the dose–response curves strongly suggests that the same growth factor is being assayed in each of the three samples. This plot enables a rough estimate to be made of the dose of sample C that gives half-maximal response (ED_{50}). This is at approximately the fifth three-fold dilution, 1:243 (i.e. 0.004), and so the sample could be described as having approximately 243 U/ml.

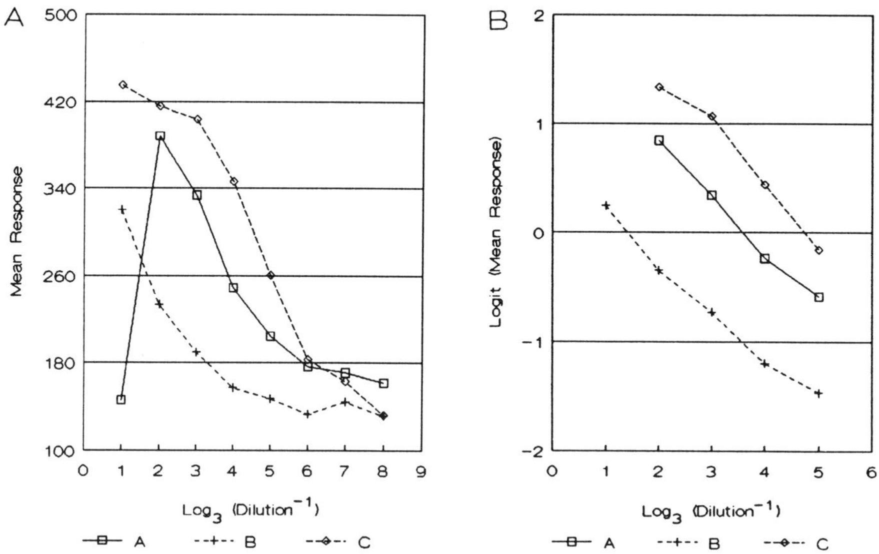

Figure 1. A, semi-logarithmic plot of three typical bioassay data sets. B, Logit–log plots of portions of the same data.

5.2 Straightening the curve

The logit transformation provides a quick method for linearizing sigmoid curves. A plot of logit(response) versus log(dose) is generally substantially more linear than the semilogarithmic plot of the raw response data. The logit has a range from approximately −3 to +3, covering the region of the dose–response curve from 5% to 95% of the maximal response. A logit value of zero is equivalent to 50% of the maximal response. Consequently, the intersection of the logit–log plot with the *x*-axis gives the ED_{50}. This can be determined graphically, or by interpolation after linear regression analysis of the largest linear portion of the plot. The data points for the most linear portion of the logit–log plots are graphed in *Figure 1* B. Estimated ED_{50} values for the three samples are given in *Table 1*.

Table 1. Estimates of ED_{50} (U/ml) for the example data

Method	Sample A	Sample B	Sample C
Raw data plot	—	—	0.0041 (243)
Logit–log plot	0.018 (54)	0.202 (5)	0.0055 (181)
Four-parameter logistic (ALLFIT)	0.024 (42)	0.219 (5)	0.0055 (181)
Logistic spline fit (FLEXIFIT)	0.024 (42)	0.221 (4)	0.0053 (189)

Relative potency (R) is a ratio of equipotent doses from two preparations. Since the ED_{50} values are, by definition, equipotent, the ratio enables the investigator to express the potency of a test sample in terms of a multiple of the potency of a standard preparation. Therefore, for the example data, sample B is approximately one eleventh (5:54) of the potency of sample A, which, in turn, is approximately 30% (54:181) of the potency of sample C.

To perform logit transformation of bioassay data:

(a) Calculate the proportion of maximal response (p) for each dose level

$$p = \frac{\text{response at dose } x - \text{minimum response}}{\text{maximum response} - \text{minimum response}}.$$

(b) Calculate the logit of this proportion

$$\text{logit}\,(p) = \log_e \left(\frac{p}{1-p}\right).$$

The validity of the bioassay requires that the dose–response curves be parallel with equivalent asymptotes. Analysis of variance procedures using single degree of freedom contrasts provide means for analysing pairs of dose–response curves to confirm that there are no deviations from parallelism, and that the transformed dose–response data have a linear relationship. Confidence intervals for estimates of R can be made using Fieller's theorem. These procedures are explained in detail by Finney (9), but shorter accounts of the procedures, together with numerical examples, are given by Colquhoun (10) and Wardlaw (11).

5.3 Non-linear fitting of raw response data

In order to use the logit transformation on continuous data, such as cytokine bioassay data, it is necessary to estimate the maximum and minimum responses. This can introduce complications over which values to use, since the available data may not include the 'true' maximum and minimum values. A simpler, but computationally more complex, procedure is to fit the raw data directly to a mathematical function that describes a sigmoid curve and to estimate the ED_{50} and asymptote values directly. Rodbard and colleagues have made extensive use of the four-parameter logistic function to describe dose–response data from a wide range of bio- and immunoassays. This function has parameters for the upper and lower asymptotes, a symmetrical point of inflection of the sigmoid (ED_{50}), and a slope parameter. This procedure is implemented in the computer program ALLFIT (12) and can be used to estimate these parameters for individual dose–response curves. By simultaneously fitting several dose–response curves from one assay, and by comparing the parameters obtained with and without constraining parameters, such as slope and asymptote parameters, to equivalence, the analyst can construct F statistics to test the similarity of the curves.

An extension of the idea of fitting data to an expression that describes the underlying dose–response relationship is to extract that relationship from the data under investigation. This approach has been described by Guardabasso and implemented in the computer program FLEXIFIT (13). Raw bioassay data can be related to the log(dose) by a set of knotted splines— a mathematical 'joint-the-dots'—and the underlying sigmoid curve can be determined by removing the lateral displacement of each dose–response curve that is due to differences in potency of the test samples. As with the four-parameter logistic, the analyst can determine the goodness-of-fit of each dose–response curve to the underlying, essential dose–response curve. Testing for parallelism is done by fitting the data twice, once with and once without constraining the slope parameters to unity, and constructing F-statistics to compare the residuals from the two fits. Parameter constraint is also useful in situations where some of the dose–response curves are incomplete, but there is good reason to believe that the same analyte is being compared in all the curves.

The estimates of ED_{50} values obtained by the ALLFIT and FLEXIFIT routines for the three example data sets are given in *Table 1*. The results were obtained by constraining the data to have equivalent upper asymptotes and F statistics confirmed that the resulting curves had similar, parallel slopes.

The use of vertical scaling parameters also enables the analyst to confirm that dose–response curves taken from separate assays conform to the same underlying shape.

ALLFIT and FLEXIFIT are available from Dr P. J. Munson, Laboratory of Theoretical and Physical Biology, NICHHD, NIH, Bethesda, MD 20892, USA, in IBM and Macintosh formats.

6. Standards and quality control

Bioassays should use two types of standard:

(a) 'in-house' standards which may be either commercially available recombinant proteins, or conditioned medium from stimulated cytokine-secreting cells (e.g. silica-stimulated macrophages)
(b) international standards or interim reference reagents

The international standards are in limited supply and the sole use of these materials is for the calibration of the 'in-house' standards. Details of the current international standards for cytokines are available from the National Institute for Biological Standards and Control, South Mimms, Potters Bar, Hertfordshire EN6 3QG, UK, and also from Biological Response Modifiers Program, NCI, PO Box B, Frederick, MD 21701, USA. Quality-control procedures for bioassay are similar to those for other assay types. Samples with high, medium, and low activities should be stored in small aliquots at −70°C and only thawed once. These samples should be matched with the other samples under assay with respect to the matrix, e.g. plasma or tissue-culture medium. Control charts can be established on the basis of the variation observed with 20 consecutive assays. The ED_{50} and potency of the quality-control samples with respect to the assay standard should be monitored, and aberrant assays can be easily flagged. The slope parameter obtained from the non-linear curve-fitting routine will give a further indication of the sensitivity of the cell line. A comparison of the dose–response curves of the standard preparation from several assays can be made using FLEXIFIT. This will enable the analyst to make frequent between-assay checks on the responsiveness of the cell-line.

Acknowledgements

F. P. Winstanley is supported by the Scottish Hospitals Endowment Research Trust and the Cunningham Trust.

References

1. Mosmann, T. (1983). *J. Immunol. Methods,* **65,** 55.
2. Hansen, M. B., Nielsen, S. E., and Berg, K. (1989). *J. Immunol. Methods,* **119,** 203.
3. Hopkins, S. J. and Humphries, M. (1989). *J. Immunol. Methods,* **120,** 271.
4. Gillis, S., Ferm, M. M., Ou, W., and Smith, K. A. (1978). *J. Immunol.,* **120,** 2027.
5. Aarden, L. A., De Groot, E. R., Schaap, O. L., and Lansdorp, P. M. (1987). *Eur. J. Immunol.,* **17,** 1411.
6. Hopkins, S. J. and Humphries, M. (1990). *J. Immunol. Methods,* **133,** 127.
7. Espevik, T. and Nissen-Meyer, J. (1986). *J. Immunol. Methods,* **95,** 99.
8. Schroder, J-M., Sticherling, M., Henneicke, H. H., Preissner, W. C., and Christophers, E. (1990). *J. Immunol.,* **144,** 2223.
9. Finney, D. J. (1971). *Statistical Method in Biological Assay.* Griffin, London.
10. Colquhoun, D. (1971). *Lectures in Biostatistics.* Clarendon, Oxford.
11. Wardlaw, A. C. (1985). *Practical Statistics for Experimental Biologists.* Wiley, Chichester.
12. DeLean, A., Munson, P. J., and Rodbard, D. (1978). *Am. J. Physiol.,* **235,** E97.
13. Guardabasso, V., Rodbard, D., and Munson, P. J. (1987). *Am. J. Physiol.,* **252,** E357.

12

Strategies for the production of human monoclonal antibodies

M. KURPÌSZ and G. WILSON

1. Introduction

Monoclonal antibodies are now routinely used to identify and localize a wide variety of biological materials, providing an essential tool for structural and functional analysis. Among the different research topics in medicine, perhaps the most urgent is the need to analyse tumour growth and metabolism and then successfully treat and/or manage these tumours in the clinic. For this purpose the majority of monoclonal antibodies in current use were derived by immunization of rodents with human tumour cell preparations. This technique, however, has the major disadvantage that many of the resulting antibodies reflect the differences between murine and human cells in general, rather than the malignant nature of the human cell. Thus, in most cases, the anti-tumour monoclonal antibodies which were obtained were found to identify common epitopes on a variety of cell types, mostly containing carbohydrate structures (1).

In a clinical situation, monoclonal antibodies derived from rodents present high immunogenicity to humans. An elicited 'anti-mouse' immune response eliminates the possibility of repeated administration of the particular antibody and a short half-life of such antibody in a patient's serum.

Therefore, for both fundamental investigations or medical practice, the ability to generate human monoclonal antibodies against human tumour antigens would be of enormous importance. Due to the large number of problems associated with the present methodology used for the production of human monoclonal antibodies, the number of antibodies with potential clinical value which are currently available is relatively small.

Although there has been a substantial amount of work dedicated to the production of human monoclonal antibodies directly, many others have used genetic manipulation or antibody re-engineering in order to 'humanize' a valuable rodent antibody (to escape the destructive immunological response of the recipient against xenoantibodies). Two main approaches to human monoclonal antibody production still dominate the scene:

(a) classical fusion of human B cells to a suitable partner cell-line (either in normal or heterohybridoma combination)

(b) Epstein–Barr virus (EBV) transformation alone or with subsequent fusion (the latter one is called the EBV–hybridoma method)

Many attempts have been made to fuse human B lymphocytes to fusion partners from a variety of sources, but a suitable human fusion partner has yet to be found. Two common strategies were practised by a number of researchers. One, previously mentioned as the heterohybridoma combination, used human B cells and mouse cell partners (2, 3) thus taking advantage of better fusion frequency when fusing with mouse myelomas (4). The second approach involved human B cells and a human cell for human–human hybrids and explored quite a range of available partner cell-lines (5). However, these were not able to combine the two most highly desired features, i.e. a good growth potential and high antibody secretion. The majority of human lymphoblastoid cell-lines developed for fusion do proliferate vigorously but have low antibody production, while human myelomas produced quite the opposite effect.

Heterohybridomas, which grow better and secrete more antibody were often found to be genetically unstable, which resulted in the loss of antibody production (6). Thus, frequent recloning was necessary to minimize karyotype drift (7) and to maintain antibody secretion. Another theoretical disadvantage to this system is the possibility of post-transcriptional modifications to the human monoclonal antibody made by an interspecies hybrid. The heteromyelomas instability can be overcome by using recently established interspecies (tetra- or sextaploid) hybrids as fusion partners (8). As a matter of fact, such cell-lines were very much in favour at the recently organized Workshop for Human Monoclonal Antibody (9).

Epstein–Barr virus has been successfully used by many researchers to produce human monoclonal antibodies to a range of antigens, including tumour antigens (10–14). Although EBV transformation may be potentially the simplest way of obtaining human monoclonals there are several disadvantageous points which have to be emphasized here:

(a) the low stability of EBV-transformed antibody-producing cell-lines

(b) the low level of immunoglobulin production

(c) the rapid decrease of antibody production with time (especially for IgG)

(d) difficulties in cloning

As we have mentioned before, the combination of EBV infection with the subsequent cell fusion could be proposed as a method of choice. This technique was successfully developed by Kozbor and co-workers (15) in 1982, generating antibody-secreting hybridomas against tetanus toxoid. EBV infection pre-selects antibody-producing cells prior to fusion, while EBV-infected cells provide higher fusion frequencies than non-transformed lymphocytes (1×10^{-5} versus 4×10^{-7} (16)). The EBV–hybridoma technique can be therefore suggested as a satisfying alternative to EBV transformation alone.

EBV infects human B lymphocytes through binding of a viral protein to the C3d receptor, the CD21 molecule (17–19), which is present on the surface of mature resting B lymphocytes and this results in the polyclonal activation of the cells in a T-cell-independent manner.

The infection of B lymphocytes with EBV has been shown to lead to two forms of response (20), short-term and long-term:

(a) The short-term response lasts for only a few days and involves proliferation of the B lymphocytes and differentiation of the cells into antibody secreting cells.

(b) The long-term response involves those cells which have become 'immortalized' by EBV infection and transformed into permanent lymphoblastoid cells. This response is associated with a change in the morphology of the infected cell, acid production, and rapid proliferation, although the cells maintain the phenotypic properties of the cell surface and the secreted immunoglobulins. This response is found in only a fraction of the cells, possibly only 4% (of B cells); however, if the researcher has an efficient selection procedure then it is from this group that the establishment of a monoclonal antibody producing cell-line will come.

There is no reliable cell marker available in order to estimate an EBV genome integration into the host genome, but EBV-infected lymphocytes express at least one new antigen, called the EBV nuclear antigen (EBNA) (21). EBV stimulates DNA synthesis in infected cells about 20 h after EBNA synthesis begins, i.e. approximately 24–36 h after exposure to virus (22).

2. EBV infection of human B lymphocytes: a practical approach

2.1 Source and preparation of B lymphocytes

A variety of sources may be used to provide the B lymphocytes for EBV transformation. These include peripheral blood lymphocytes as well as, with particular reference to tumour immunobiology, tumour-infiltrating lymphocytes and lymphocytes isolated from involved lymph nodes, spleen, and ascitic fluid.

Before attempting to transform B lymphocytes with EBV it is advisable to obtain a relatively pure population of cells. Although it is possible to proceed straight to the EBV transformation step, it is advantageous to remove any cells which may have an adverse effect on the efficiency of transformation or the production of lymphoblastoid cells, such as anti-EBV cytotoxic T lymphocytes.

If the source of the lymphocytes is a piece of solid tissue then it must first be dissociated. This is a relatively straightforward procedure which can simply involve mechanical dissociation of the tissue and suspension of the dissociated cells in a suitable solution (for example a balanced salt solution), although frequently enzymic digestion may be required (see Chapter 1). The next step is to collect the mononuclear cells present in the sample. These include lymphocytes, monocytes, neutrophil precursors, and platelets. The procedure for the isolation of mononuclear cells is shown in *Protocol 1*.

Protocol 1. Isolation of mononuclear cells

1. Dilute the sample in phosphate-buffered saline (PBS).
2. Place a Ficoll–Hypaque separating solution in a centrifuge tube.
3. Overlay with 10 ml of the sample (5:3 proportion of sample to gradient solution).
4. Centrifuge at 400*g* for 20 min at room temperature.
5. Remove the mononuclear cell interface.
6. Transfer the cells to complete medium.
7. Centrifuge at 150*g* for 10 min at room temperature (washing).
8. Re-suspend the cells in complete medium.

If the lymphocytes are being isolated from a tumour specimen then tumour cells may also be present in the mononuclear cell population. To remove any tumour cells present it is necessary to include a further stage. The procedure for the removal of tumour cells is shown in *Protocol 2*.

Protocol 2. Removal of tumour cells for a mononuclear cell suspension (23)

1. Place 5 ml of Ficoll–Hypaque (100% solution) in a centrifuge tube.
2. Overlay with 5 ml of a 75% Ficoll–Hypaque solution.
3. Overlay with the sample.
4. Centrifuge at 400*g* for 20 min at room temperature.
5. Remove the cells from the interface of the 75%/100% Ficoll–Hypaque layers (the less-dense tumour cells band at the 75%/medium interface).
6. Transfer the cells to complete medium.
7. Centrifuge the cells at 150*g* for 10 min at room temperature.
8. Re-suspend the cells in complete medium.

The next step is to remove the adherent cells present in the sample. These consist mainly of monocytes and macrophages and may be removed by the procedure in *Protocol 3*.

Protocol 3. Removal of adherent cells

1. Place the sample in a tissue-culture flask.
2. Incubate the flask horizontally for 3 h at 37°C.
3. Gently remove the culture medium and non-adherent cells from the flask.

The final step is the removal of the T lymphocytes. This may be achieved by spontaneous T-cell rosetting with sheep red blood cells (SRBC) (24). The affinity of SRBC binding can be enhanced by addition of foetal calf serum (FCS) previously absorbed with SRBC. The sample is incubated with other solutions in proportion 1:1:1 v/v (lymphocyte sample:SRBC:absorbed FCS). Another way to increase SRBC binding is to pre-treat them with neuraminidase or 2 amino-ethylisothioronium bromide hydrobromide (25). Using T-cell rosetting, it is possible to remove over 90% of T lymphocytes present in the sample. *Protocol 4* shows the procedure involved.

Protocol 4. Removal of T lymphocytes by sheep red blood cell (SRBC) rosetting

1. Add equal volumes of sample and neuraminidase-treated sheep red blood cells to a centrifuge tube and mix.
2. Incubate for 10 min at 37°C.
3. Centrifuge at 150*g* for 5 min at 4°C.
4. Incubate on ice for 1 h.
5. Gently re-suspend the cell pellet.
6. Underlay with an equal volume of Ficoll–Hypaque.
7. Centrifuge at 400*g* for 20 min at room temperature.
8. Transfer the cells from the interface to complete medium.
9. Repeat steps **1–8**.
10. Centrifuge cells at 150*g* for 10 min at room temperature.
11. Re-suspend in complete medium.

At this stage, the cell suspension should contain a relatively pure population of B lymphocytes. As you will appreciate, it is necessary to start with as large a sample as possible in order to have a workable number of cells remaining at this point. It is now possible to proceed to the EBV transformation stage or to select for minority groups of B lymphocytes, for example surface-IgG positive cells. These can be selected using a method similar to that used for T-cell rosetting. Steinitz and Klein (26) used rabbit anti-human immunoglobulins coupled to ox erythrocytes to select for surface-IgG positive B lymphocytes. Similar selections can be made by incubating sensitized B cells on dishes previously coated with antigen of interest (this method has been described as 'panning' in the literature). Alternatively, lymphocyte selection can also be carried out using magnetic beads and a magnetic column. The different lymphocyte sub-sets may therefore be isolated according to their function (especially for the purpose of an *in vitro* re-immunization scheme) and magnetic beads can be attached to the appropriate anti-CD antibodies or anti-human immunoglobulin classes. Thompson *et al.* (27) reported that the secretion of IgG by EBV-transformed B lymphocytes was restricted to the ecto-5′nucleotidase-positive subset, and this could form yet another means of selection.

2.2 Source of EBV

Although EBV may be obtained from a number of sources, the most widely used is the B95-8 marmoset cell-line. The B95-8 cell-line grows in culture as a loosely adherent monolayer and spontaneously releases the virus into the surrounding culture medium.

In order to obtain the virus at a usable concentration the cell-line should be grown to confluence and then left undisturbed for around 10–14 days. As the medium becomes yellow it is recommended that the cells are 'cold-stressed' (incubated overnight at 4°C) in order to increase the rate of virus release from the cells. After this time the medium should be removed from the flask, centrifuged to remove the cells and then filtered through a 0.45 μm filter to remove any cell debris. The virus-containing medium should be aliquoted and stored at −70°C until use. The virus remains stable for at least a year at −70°C, or even longer if stored in liquid nitrogen.

The B95-8 cell-line should be kept completely free of mycoplasma since the cloning efficiency of B cells infected with EBV is drastically reduced in its presence.

This cell-line, as with all sources of EBV, should be handled in a class-II hood to ensure both sample and operator protection. The hood should be fitted with a UV light for decontamination, since EBV is extremely susceptible to UV light.

To test the potency of the virus-containing medium, titrate it against its ability to induce DNA synthesis in B lymphocytes as measured by the uptake of $[H^3]$thymidine 3 days after infection with the virus (2).

2.3 *In vitro* culture systems to improve efficiency of EBV transformation

As we previously mentioned, the proportion of successfully and stably transformed cells which arise from the total B-lymphocyte populations is rather low. This is even more striking when we have to take into account the small percentage of cells in peripheral blood which are actually sensitized to the antigen of interest. These two points, when combined, do not encourage one to enter the EBV transformation technique when one has to consider the rather random success of immortalization of a clone, while at the same time preserving its ability to produce antibodies. To increase the chances of successful EBV infection (of antibody-producing cells) several variations of *in vitro* culture systems have been proposed for use, prior to viral transformation.

2.3.1 *In vitro* secondary antigen stimulation

This type of *in vitro* culture is performed when the lymphocytes from poorly sensitized human individuals are subjected to further *in vitro* manipulations. The target antigen is added to B lymphocytes together with a variety of other factors (5).

Protocol 5. Principles of secondary *in vitro* antigenic stimulation prior to EBV transformation

1. Immunodeplete the T suppressor/cytotoxic lymphocytes by:
   - SRBC rosetting
   - separation on nylon wool columns (adjustment of adherent:non-adherent cells into 1:1 proportion)
   - lysis of T cells with complement + monoclonal antibody
   - Sephadex G-10 column
   - panning procedures
2. Add the antigen in optimal proportion (this has to be tested for each antigen: a proposed range varies between 40 ng and 10 μg of protein per ml of culture).
3. Add the exogenous growth factors (IL-2, IL-4; conditioned media after PHA or PWM stimulation, etc.).
4. Stimulate the production of endogenous growth factors by mitogens: PHA, LPS, MDP, SAC-I, PWM.
5. Supplement the culture medium with human AB serum.
6. Culture the cells for 3–5 days with a concentration of $(3–5) \times 10^6$ cells/ml of culture.
7. Transform the cells with EBV.

Abbreviations: SAC I—*Staphylococcus aureus* Cowan I; Con A—concanavalin A; LPS—lipopolysaccharide; MDP—muramyl dipeptide; PHA—phytohaemagglutinin; PWM—pokeweed mitogen.

The main problem with *in vitro* secondary stimulation is that one is uncertain of the stage of lymphocyte sensitization *in vivo*. Therefore, one successful re-stimulation procedure cannot be automatically translated onto another system (or even individual), which may present a different status of sensitization, B-cell clonal expansion, etc. In most situations, therefore, each attempt will be a random trial. In our hands we found a simple mitogen stimulation (PWM) or antigenic stimulation alone (prior to EBV infection) more favourable than all other attempts of synergistic action by mitogen, antigen, and exogenous factors altogether (29).

2.3.2 *In vitro* primary antigenic stimulation

As we pointed out earlier, there can be some problems with *in vitro* secondary antigenic stimulation. In this context, it may seem easier to start with naive cells and conduct a primary *in vitro* sensitization. As a matter of fact, a majority of recent spectacular successes in generation of human monoclonal antibodies by the EBV–hybridoma method were mainly due to primary antigenic immunization prior to EBV infection (30, 31). The principles of this technique are listed in *Protocol 6*.

Protocol 6. Primary antigenic stimulation *in vitro* prior to EBV infection

1. Immunodeplete the T suppressor/cytotoxic cells by:
   - column with magnetic beads (anti-CD-8 antibodies)
   - cell lysis with anti-CD-8 monoclonal antibody and complement
   - adherent:non-adherent cell methodology (plastic dish adherence or nylon wool column)
   - use methyl esters (leucyl-leucine methyl ester 150–250 μM in serum-free medium for 15 min at room temperature)
2. Add the antigen (optimal concentrations have to be determined)
3. Add the exogenous growth factors:
   - 10–25% v/v of PWM conditioned medium
   - IL-2—range of 5–20 U/ml of medium
   - interferon gamma—range of 10–400 U/ml of medium
4. Supplement medium with AB serum.
5. Culture the cells for 7 days at lymphocyte concentration of 3×10^6 to 10^7/ml of culture.
6. Transform the cells with EBV.

It has to be pointed out that in our hands (M. Kurpìsz, unpublished data) the action of methyl esters remains unclear and its selective effect on T suppressor/cytotoxic cells doubtful. However, the change in proportion of lymphocyte cell subsets for *in vitro* antigenic challenge seems to be absolutely necessary (32). Monocytes and T helper cells must be saved in such manipulations in order to provide sufficient antigenic presentation. Simultaneous addition of conditioned media with IL-2 is recommended, although some doubts remain about the necessity of supplementing with interferon gamma. AB serum works really well in this type of system, but its influence on screening procedures (testing human antibody activity from supernatant against human antigens) must be seriously considered.

2.3.3 The Banchereau system

Recently, another system for initiating and supporting B-cell proliferation was described (33), which is more efficient (up to 40% of B cells activated) for B-cell stimulation than EBV infection. B cells activated by this protocol, however, can be maintained only up to 10 weeks *in vitro*. The components of the system are listed in *Protocol 7*.

Protocol 7. The components of the Banchereau system for B-cell activation

1. Add anti-CD40 cross-linking monoclonal antibody (approximately 30 ng/ml of medium).
2. Add a 'cross-linking amplification factor'—the fibroblastic mouse cell-line expressing FcγRII/CDw32, treated thus before addition:
   (a) Irradiate the cells with 7500 rads.
   (b) Wash the cells three times at 250*g* for 10 min at room temperature.
   (c) Re-suspend the cells in concentration—2.5×10^3 per microwell.
3. Add IL-4 at 100 U/ml of medium.

This system may create very good conditions for the initial stages of both secondary and primary antigenic stimulation (optional addition of antigen). Also, the complementary influence of IL-10 can be considered. After several weeks of B-cell activation, an EBV infection or fusion with a suitable partner cell will inevitably become necessary.

2.3.4 SCID-hu mice technology

The use of severe combined immunodeficiency (SCID) mice for human monoclonal antibodies seems to be quite a promising prospect. SCID mice are unable to mount an effective cellular or humoral response (34) and therefore they can be reconstituted with human tissues or different cell types. There are several options which can be considered when beginning to use SCID mice for EBV infection. These mice can propagate EBV-infected cell-lines and/or enhance their antibody secretion. They can also be used for the initial stages of both *in vitro* primary or secondary antigenic stimulation; recent reports are quite encouraging in this respect (35, 36). The present degree of knowledge with the SCID mouse is very much in favour of intraperitoneal administration of relatively large numbers of human lymphocytes (e.g. 50×10^6) from EBV-negative donors. EBV-infected cells transferred in this number will rapidly develop a highly invasive tumour in such mice, although antibody production can be maintained for up to 20 weeks after transfer of EBV-transformed cells (37). For non-infected lymphocytes, cell transfer with subsequent antigen challenge *in vivo* can be recommended. The antigen dose should be tested in each case, although 100 μg per mouse in intraperitoneal injection should be a good starting point.

2.4 EBV transformation of B lymphocytes

A standard protocol for the transformation of B lymphocytes by EBV is set out in *Protocol 8*.

Protocol 8. Standard EBV transformation protocol (38)

1. After preparation of the B lymphocytes (see *Protocols 1–4*) for transformation the cells should be washed twice and re-suspended in 20 ml of complete medium.
2. Determine the number of viable cells.
3. Centrifuge the cells (150*g* for 10 min) and discard the supernatant.
4. To the cell pellet, add 100 μl FCS per 10^6 cells and 1–2 ml of EBV-containing medium.
5. Incubate the virus–cell mixture at 37 °C for 1–1.5 h.
6. Centrifuge at 150*g* for 10 min at room temperature and re-suspend in complete medium containing 20% FCS.
7. Dispense the cells at a concentration of $(2–4) \times 10^6$ cells into the wells of a 24-well tissue-culture plate. Add complete medium, to 2 ml.

The plates should be incubated at 37 °C in a humidified atmosphere containing 5% CO_2. An alternative to the lengthy preparation of peripheral B cells is to use the whole leukocyte suspension and cyclosporin A to prevent the induction of an anti-EBV cytotoxic T-cell response.

Protocol 9. EBV transformation with the use of cyclosporin A [a]

1. Dissolve 1 mg of cyclosporin A in absolute ethanol.
2. Add 0.2 ml of Tween 80, and mix well.
3. Top up with serum-free RPMI 1640 to give a final cyclosporin concentration of 100 μg/ml.

4. Filter and store at −20°C.
5. Prepare a mononuclear leukocyte suspension—approximately 5×10^6 cells per ml.
6. Spin the cells down and re-suspend in 1 ml EBV filtrate (*Protocol 8*).
7. Incubate at 37°C for at least 1 h.
8. Add 0.2 ml of cyclosporin A (from the stock solution) and 8 ml of RPMI with 10% FCS.
9. Incubate at 37°C for 7 days.
10. Tip off supernatant (the cells will stay packed) and add 10 ml of complete RPMI medium.
11. At the end of 10 days, transfer the cells to a bigger flask and treat as a normal EBV-transformed cell-line.

[a] Instead of cyclosporin A, phytohaemagglutinin may be added to the medium in which the cells are initially re-suspended. PHA agglutinates T cells (among them T suppressor/cytotoxic cell sub-set).

Transformed cells established in 24-well plates should be fed weekly by removing 1 ml of medium from each well and replacing it with 1 ml of fresh medium. The wells should be checked at regular intervals for the appearance of clumps of viable cells, although any clumps which appear during the first week should be disregarded. Any clumps of viable cells should be carefully transferred to a fresh culture well and then on to a 25 cm^2 tissue-culture flask.

As with the B95-8 cell-line, all procedures involving EBV should be carried out in a class-II hood, although EBV-transformed B cells do not secrete virus and are not infective.

2.5 Screening for immunoglobulin production

After two to three weeks of culture, the supernatant from each well which contains viable EBV-transformed cells should be assayed for the production of immunoglobulin. If a negative result is obtained then it is not worth proceeding with the culture of that well. Human monoclonal antibodies may be assayed by ELISA, according to the method of Vollmers *et al.* (39).

Once it has been established that immunoglobulin is being produced the specificity of that antibody should be tested. This may be done using a live-cell ELISA procedure (40) or by screening against frozen tissue sections (41). Again, if a negative result is obtained then it is not worth proceeding. If a positive result is obtained then it may be worthwhile isotyping the immunoglobulin of interest.

Cells secreting antibody of the IgM type can be examined for a spontaneous immunoglobulin class-switch (into IgG). This procedure can be less laborious when using a FACS sorter but for less well-equipped laboratories, this can be addressed by extensive ELISA screening (see *Figure 1*).

2.6 Maintenance of EBV-transformed cell-lines

EBV-transformed cell-lines may be maintained in the same manner as other antibody-producing cell-lines, although the researcher should always attempt to establish the optimum growth conditions for their particular cell-line.

There are several factors which have to be considered as worth trying. These include feeder layers, antibody cross-linking, conditioned media, and cytokines.

2.6.1 Feeder cells

When proceeding with human culture systems it is a matter of choice as to whether to use human feeder cells. All types of allogeneic cells can be considered, i.e. lymphocytes, lymphoblastoid cells, fibroblasts, etc. Cord blood lymphocytes, which have been reported to be superior to the other sources, in fact need much laborious preparation prior to use (42). Human allogeneic feeder cells have to be irradiated with a dose of 2000–3000 rads. Their concentration does not need to exceed 10^4 cells per microwell. Among the xenogeneic feeder cells, splenocytes have to be irradiated, thymocytes can be used straight; xenogeneic feeders (usually taken from mice) have to be present in larger numbers than the human ones—from 10^5 to 10^6 per microwell. From our observations, we have concluded that EBV infection of purified B-cell populations do require feeder layers (43). In cases where irradiation is not available, a pre-treatment with mytomycin-C can be applied (*Protocol 10*).

Protocol 10. Mitomycin C pre-treatment of cells for feeder layers

1. Add 2 ml RPMI (serum-free) to a 2 mg vial of mitomycin C. (**Attention**: avoid the need to weigh out the mitomycin powder. It is extremely toxic. Once dissolved, the solution can be stored for up to 2 weeks at 4°C.)
2. Make cells up to 5×10^7/ml in serum-free medium.
3. Add 25 μg mitomycin C per ml of cells.
4. Incubate at 37°C for 20 min.
5. Fill up the tube with wash medium and spin for 10 min at 250*g* at room temperature.
6. Re-suspend the cells in culture medium at the desired density.

2.6.2 Enhanced stimulation of B-cell populations by cross-linking B-cell surface antigens

When working with the Banchereau system, it is advisable to try to cross-link surface antigenic structures which are stable and present on EBV-

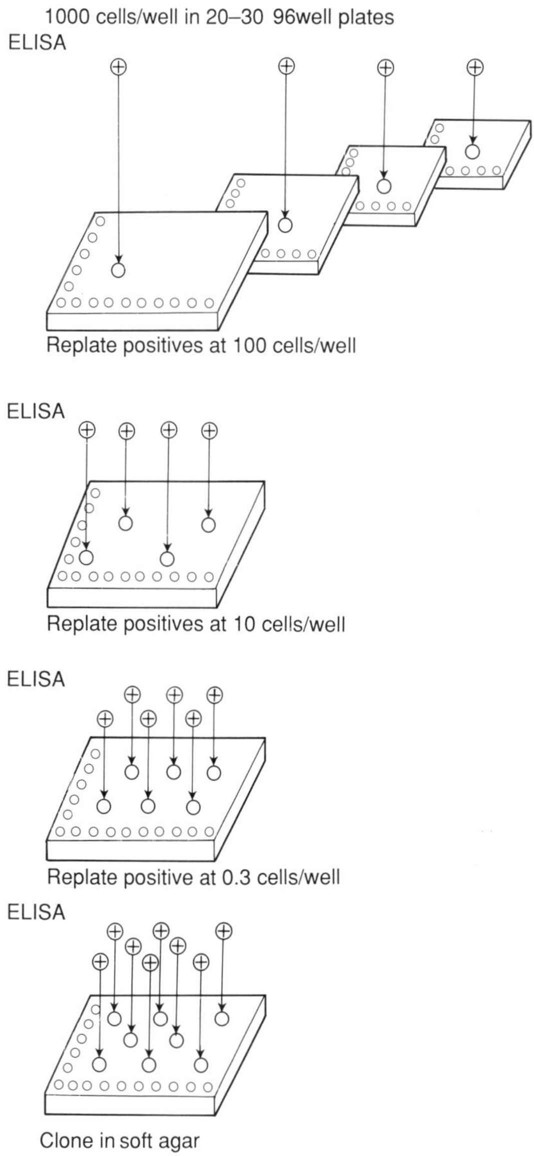

Figure 1. Switch immunoglobulin selection.

transformed cell-lines (with preserved antibody production). It is known from other observations that at least two clusters could be particularly promising, i.e. CD 38 (plasma cells) and CD 71 (receptor for transferrin (44)). On the other hand, a simple anti-immunoglobulin M cross-linking can also have a good effect (45).

2.6.3 Conditioned media

There are a variety of these, as mentioned earlier. Pokeweed mitogen supernatant can be particularly recommended (31), when harvested after 24 h from irradiated T cells. Alternatively, rat mixed thymocyte or mixed splenocyte (two-way MLC) culture supernatants taken after 48 h of incubation (46) can be used. After termination of cultures, cells are pelleted and supernatants aseptically filtered and stored in aliquots at −70°C.

2.6.4 Cytokines

The role of various growth factors in cell growth and antibody production by EBV-transformed cell-lines has recently been extensively investigated. It has been shown by several groups that various T lymphocyte and monocyte-derived cytokines (including IL-1, IL-2, IL-4, and IL-6 and interferon-gamma) have an influence both on the immunoglobulin production and proliferation of EBV-transformed cell-lines (47–50). Of the listed cytokines, the beneficial effect of IL-2 (in high doses) was confirmed (29, 45). The hopes for IL-6 were not realized either in our hands (M. Kurpìsz, unpublished data) or those of others (51). IL-4, although promoting the IgG isotype preference, was only documented to be helpful in the Banchereau system (33) and had a tendency to inhibit the cell growth of established EBV-infected lines (29, 45). It has also been shown that EBV cell-lines have the ability to produce at least some of these factors (52, 53). A recent report by Jochems *et al.* (54) has demonstrated a heterogeneity in the amount and type of cytokines produced by different EBV-transformed cell-lines which (it is claimed) may account for the range of responses exhibited by EBV-transformed cell-lines to various exogenously added lymphokines. Again, it is up to individual researchers to examine this on their own cell-lines.

2.7 Limiting cell dilution

Limiting cell dilution has been difficult to achieve in EBV-transformed cell-lines (55) due to the importance of cell-to-cell contact in the growth of these cells. Several attempts have been made to overcome this problem, including the use of human foreskin fibroblast feeder cells (56) and cloning in soft agar (57).

Tiebout *et al.* (58) reported an increased efficiency in the growth of EBV transformants at low cell numbers by growth in conditions which favour close cell-to-cell contact. These include the use of V-bottomed tissue-culture plates as well as the addition of irradiated autologous EBV transformants as feeder cells. Further growth enhancement could be achieved by the addition of the tumour promoter phorbol-myristate acetate to the culture medium.

Other groups reported success with methods of doubling dilutions when sub-cloning them beginning from a concentration of 1000 cells per well and then halving the numbers (in every round) up to the point of 10 cells per well

(59). This suggests that a gradual adjustment of cells may acclimatize them for growth (see also *Figure 1*).

2.8 Fusion of EBV-transformed cell-lines

Once a cell-line with the appropriate specificity has been established it may be possible to fuse it to a suitable fusion partner. This allows the advantages of both fusion and EBV transformation to be coupled. The specificity of the EBV-transformed cell-line can be combined with the higher cloning efficiency and increased immunoglobulin production levels of a myeloma cell-line. Any standard fusion protocol may be used (60, 61) although the addition of dimethylsulphoxide content in 30–45% solution of polyethylene glycol seems to increase the fusogenic properties.

A way of selecting for human cells which have fused is to use a fusion partner with resistance to ouabain. After fusion, the addition of ouabain to each culture well at a final concentration of 2 μM will prevent the growth of unfused cells and HAT selection removes unfused myeloma cells. It is advisable to pre-incubate fused hybrids for 24 h in complete medium or HT medium before the full range of selecting compounds is added (HAT + ouabain).

3. Clinical use of antibody from EBV-transformed cell-lines

The clinical administration of antibodies derived from an EBV-transformed cell-line carries a theoretical risk of passing infectious virus to the patient. However, supernatants from EBV-transformed cell-lines apparently contain no infectious agents. This appears to be due to the behaviour of the cell-lines which restrict viral replication despite the fact that in all cases the viral genome may be detected within the nuclear DNA (62). Even though no infectious agents may be detected in the culture supernatant further study is required before it may be considered absolutely safe to use these antibodies clinically.

The decisions as to whether or not antibodies derived from heterohybridomas are safe for clinical use is far more difficult. This relies heavily on extensive testing, biochemical analysis, and excluding the possibility of cytopathogenic effects of any viruses present, especially retroviruses.

4. Conclusions

There are many available methodologies for the production of human monoclonal antibodies. This reflects the fact that there is not one which is comparable to the production of mouse monoclonals and so there is still no 'standard'.

EBV transformation can result in the production of human anti-tumour antibodies (63, 64) but care has to be taken in maintaining the lines and screening them. Good luck!

References

1. Magnani, J. L., Spitalnik, S. L., and Ginsburg, V. (1987). *Meth. Enzymol.*, **138,** 195.
2. Gigliotti, F., Smith, L., and Insel, R. A. (1984). *J. Clin. Infect. Dis.*, **149,** 43.
3. Hirata, Y, and Sugawara, I. (1987). *Microbiol. Immunol.*, **31,** 231.
4. Smith, L. H. and Teng, N. N. H. (1987). In *Human Hybridomas; Diagnostic and Therapeutic Applications*, (ed. A. J. Strelkauskaus), pp. 121–58. Marcel Dekker, New York.
5. James, K. and Bell, G. T. (1987). *J. Immunol. Methods,* **100,** 5.
6. Koropatnick, J., Pearson, J., and Harris, J. F. (1988). *Mol. Biol. Med.*, **5,** 69.
7. Lane, H. C. and Fauci, A. S. (1983). In *Monoclonal Antibodies. Probes for the Study of Autoimmunity and Immunodeficiency*, (ed. B. F. Hayes and G. S. Eisenbarth). Academic, New York.
8. Kurpìsz, M. (1990). In *Gamete Interaction: Prospects for Immunocontraception*, (ed. N. J. Alexander, D. Griffin, J. M. Spieler and G. M. H. Waites), pp. 377–400. Wiley-Liss, New York.
9. 11th Eur. Fed. Immunol. Soc., Helsinki. (1991), *Book of Abstracts*, Ch. 14.
10. Al-Azzawi, F., Stimson, W. H., and Govan, A. D. T. (1987). *J. Clin. Lab. Immunol.,* **22,** 71.
11. Boylston, A. W., Gardner, B., Anderson, R. L., and Hughes-Jones, N. C. (1980). *Scand. J. Immunol.,* **12,** 355.
12. Kirkwood, J. M. and Robinson, J. E. (1990). *Cancer Immunol. Immunother.,* **32,** 228.
13. Kozbor, D., Steinitz, M., Klein, G., Koskimies, S., and Makela, O. (1979). *Scand. J. Immunol.,* **10,** 187.
14. Steinitz, M., Klein, G., Koskimies, S., and Makela, O. (1977). *Nature,* **269,** 420.
15. Kozbor, D., Lagarde, A. E., and Roder, J. C. (1982). *Proc. Natl Acad. Sci. USA,* **79,** 6651.
16. Roder, J. C., Kozbor, D., Cole, S. P. C., Atlaw, T., Campling, B. C., and McGarry, R. C. (1985). In *Human Hybridomas and Monoclonal Antibodies*, (ed. E. G. Engleman, S. K. H. Foung, J. Larrick, and A. A. Raubitschek). Plenum, New York.
17. Arman, P., Henriksson, E. B., and Klein, G. (1984). *J. Exp. Med.,* **159,** 208.
18. Boyd, A. W. and Fecondo, J. (1988). *Immunol. Cell. Biol.,* **66,** 159.
19. Fingeroth, J. D., Weis, J. J., Tedder, T. F., Strominger, J. L., Biro, P. A., and Fearon, D. T. (1984). *Proc. Natl Acad. Sci. USA,* **81,** 4510.
20. Tosato, G., Blaese, R. M., and Yarchuan, R. (1985). *J. Immunol.,* **135,** 959.
21. Pope, J. H., Scott, W., Reedman, B. M., and Water, M. K. (1971). In *Recent Advances in Human Tumor Virology and Immunology,* (ed. W. Nakahara, K. Nishioka, T. Hirayama, and Y. Ito), pp. 177–88. University of Tokyo Press.
22. Einhorn, L. and Ernberg, I. (1978). *Int. J. Cancer,* **21,** 157.
23. Whiteside, T. S., Miescher, S., MacDonald, H. R., and van Fliedner, V. (1986). *J. Immunol. Methods,* **90,** 221.
24. Minden, M. D., Buick, R. N., and McCulloch, E. A. (1979). *Blood,* **54,** 186.

25. Winger, L., Winger, C., Shastry, P., Russell, A., and Longenecker, M. (1983). *Proc. Natl Acad. Sci. USA,* **80,** 4484.
26. Steinitz, M. and Klein, G. (1980). *J. Immunol.,* **125,** 194.
27. Thompson, L. F., Rvedi, J. M., Low, M. G., and Clement, L. T. (1988). *J. Clin. Invest.,* **82,** 902.
28. Robinson, J. and Miller, G. (1975). *J. Virol.,* **15,** 1065.
29. Fiszer, D., Niedbała, W., Fernandez, N., and Kurpìsz, M. (1992). *Arch. Immunol. Therap. Exp.* (In press.)
30. Borrebaeck, C. A. K. (1989). *J. Immunol. Methods,* **123,** 157.
31. Borrebaeck, C. A. K., Danielsson, L., and Moller, S. A. (1988). *Proc. Natl Acad. Sci. USA,* **85,** 3995.
32. Boyd, J. E. and James, K. (1989). *Monoclonal Antibodies: Production and Application,* pp. 1–43. Liss, New York.
33. Banchereau, J., DePaoli, P., Valle, A., Garcia, E., and Rousset, F. (1991). *Science,* **251,** 70.
34. McCune, J. M., Namikawa, R., Kaneshima, H., Shultz, L. D., Lieberman, M., and Weisman, I. L. (1988). *Science,* **241,** 1632.
35. Carlsson, R., Martesson, C., Ohlin, M., and Borrebaeck, C. A. K. (1991). *Book of Abstracts, 11th Eur. Fed. Immunol. Soc., Helsinki,* Abstract 14–2.
36. Matoso-Ferreira, A., Laari, T., and Kaartinen, M. (1991). *Book of Abstracts, 11th Eur. Fed. Immunol. Soc., Helsinki,* Abstract 14–20.
37. Mosier, D. E., Gulizia, R. J., Baird, S. M., and Wilson, D. B. (1988). *Nature,* **335,** 257.
38. Hudson, L. and Hay, F. C. (ed.) (1980). *Practical Immunology* (2nd edn), pp. 458–9. Blackwell Scientific, London.
39. Vollmers, H. P., O'Connor, R., Muller, J., Kirchner, T., and Muller-Hermelink, H. K. (1989). *Cancer Res.,* **49,** 2471.
40. Posner, M. R., Antoniou, D., Groffin, J., Schlossman, S. F., and Lazarus, H. (1982). *J. Immunol. Methods,* **48,** 23.
41. Bannerjee, D., Karim, R., Hearn, S. A., and Geddes, D. (1990). *Hum. Antibod. Hybridomas,* **1,** 55.
42. Clement, L. T., Vink, P. E., and Bradley, G. E. (1990). *J. Immunol.,* **145,** 102.
43. Kurpìsz, M., Simon, L. L., and Alexander, N. A. (1987). *Am. J. Reprod. Immunol. Microbiol.,* **15,** 61.
44. James, K., Gardner, J., Skibinski, G., McCann, M., and Thorpe, R. (1991). *Hum. Antibod. Hybridomas.* (In press.)
45. Skibinski, G. and James, K. (1989). *Arch. Immunol. Therap. Exp.,* **37,** 295.
46. Micklem, L. R., McCann, M. C., and James, K. (1987). *J. Immunol. Methods,* **104,** 81.
47. Falkoff, R. J. M., Butler, J. S., Dinarello, C. A., and Fauci, A. S. (1984). *J. Immunol.,* **133,** 692.
48. Gallagher, G., Taylor, N., and Willdridge, J. (1987). *Scand. J. Immunol.,* **26,** 295.
49. Richter, W., Eirmann, T. H., and Scherbaum, W. A. (1990). *Hybridoma,* **9,** 1.
50. Tosato, G., Gerrard, T. L., Goldman, N. G., and Pike, S. E. (1988). *J. Immunol.,* **140,** 4329.
51. Jochems, G., Klein, M., Brakenhoff, J., Aarden, L., Zeijlemaker, W., and Van Lier, R. (1991). *Book of Abstracts, 11th Eur. Fed. Immunol. Soc., Helsinki,* Abstract 14–15.

52. Acres, R. R., Larsen, A., Gillis, B., and Conlon, P. J. (1987). *Mol. Immunol.*, **24,** 479.
53. Lotz, M., Tsoukas, C. D., Fong, S., Dinarello, C. A., Carson, D. A., and Vaughan, J. H. (1986). *J. Immunol.*, **136,** 3537.
54. Jochems, G. J., Klein, M. R., Jordens, R., Pascual-Salado, D., Van Boxtel-Oosterhof, F., Van Lier, R. A. W., *et al.* (1991). *Hum. Antibod. Hybridomas,* **2,** 57.
55. Tiebout, R. F., Stricker, E. A. M., Hagenaars, R., and Zeijlemaker, M. P. (1984). *Eur. J. Immunol.,* **14,** 399.
56. Zurawski, J. R., Haber, E., and Black, P. H. (1987). *Science,* **199,** 1439.
57. Sasaki, T., Endo, F., Mikami, M., Sekiguchi, Y., Tada, K., Ono, Y., *et al.* (1984). *J. Immunol. Methods,* **72,** 157.
58. Tiebout, R. F., Sauerwein, R. W., Van der Meer, W. G. J., Van Boxtel-Oosterhof, F., and Zeijlemaker, M. P. (1987). *Immunology,* **60,** 187.
59. Górny, M. K., Giaanakakos, V., Sharpe, S., and Zolla-Pazner, S. (1989). *Proc. Natl Acad. Sci. USA,* **86,** 1624.
60. Posner, M. R., Elboim, H., and Santos, D. S. (1987). *Hybridoma,* **6,** 611.
61. Schoenfeld, Y., Hsu-Lin, S. C., and Gabriels, J. E. (1982). *J. Clin. Invest.,* **70,** 205.
62. Gerber, P. and Lucas, S. J. (1972). *Cellular Immunol.,* **5,** 318.
63. Gallagher, G., Al-Azzawi, F., Walsh, L. P., Wilson, G., and Handley, J. (1991). *Br. J. Cancer.*, **64,** 35.
64. Al-Azzawi, F., Smith, J., and Stimson, W. H. (1987). *Br. Med. J.*, **294,** 545.

13

Radiolabelling antibodies for imaging and targeting

M. V. PIMM and S. J. GRIBBEN

1. Introduction

The generation of monoclonal antibodies against tumour-associated antigens over the last ten or so years had led to there being a need for techniques for studying their interaction with target antigen on the surface of malignant cells not only *in vitro*, but also *in vivo*. The use of radioactive tracers for following the *in vivo* fate of biologically important substances such as antibodies has proved to be one of the most powerful and sensitive methods available.

Although it is possible to label antibodies, particularly monoclonal antibodies, endogenously with radioisotopes (i.e. to incorporate the tracer into the antibody molecule during its biosynthesis) it is the ability to label exogenously by introducing a gamma-emitting isotope on to the antibody after its purification which makes this such a powerful technique.

It is possible, by relatively simple chemical manipulations, to introduce on to antibody molecules radioactive elements not intrinsically present in antibodies. Of greatest importance here have been radioactive iodines such as ^{125}I and ^{131}I. The ready availability of these, their ease of attachment to antibodies and their high counting efficiencies in gamma spectrometers, with virtually no necessity for sample preparation, explains their widespread use in numerous radioimmunoassays.

In addition to *in vitro* use, it is possible to follow *in vivo* the biodistribution and fate of radioidine-labelled antibodies by determining the amount of radiolabel (and thus of antibody) in blood and other tissue. 'Amount' here is usually determined as the count rate of the radioactive decay of the radioiodine under set conditions of the gamma spectrometer. By relating this to the count rate of known amounts of the original material (e.g. counts/min/mg of antibody) the concentration of the labelled material can be calculated. (It is not usual to even attempt to determine the absolute amount of the radiotracer itself, which is quantified only by the rate of its radioactive decay.)

1.1 Choice of radioisotopes for antibody labelling

Starting in the early 1980s, the use of monoclonal antibodies against tumour-associated antigens for detection, in patients, of primary and metastatic disease by localization of antibody in these tumour deposits required the development of appropriately labelled antibodies and detection systems. For the visualization (usually termed 'imaging' or 'scanning') of the biodistribution of radiopharmaceuticals, gamma cameras had been available for many years for routine clinical investigations, but there was now the need to label antibodies with gamma emitters suitable for detection with these cameras and which also gave minimal radiation doses to the patients. Of the two radioiodines readily available (^{125}I and ^{131}I) only ^{131}I was suitable. Even with ^{131}I, its long half-life of about eight days, and beta as well as gamma emissions, and its poor detection on gamma cameras due to the high energy of its gamma emission (at 364 keV) meant that it was far from ideal.

Although another radioisotope of iodine, ^{123}I, is available and has more acceptable characteristics than ^{131}I, it is not as readily obtainable as other radioiodines, and its short half-life of 12 h meant that shipping from manufacturer to user exactly when it was required to label antibody for a clinical investigation was often technically difficult. These problems were circumvented by the introduction of methods for labelling antibodies with two other radioisotopes which had a long history of use in labelling conventional radiopharmaceuticals. These were isotopes of the metals indium, ^{111}In, and technetium, ^{99m}Tc. At first sight these seem bizarre isotopes for labelling antibodies, since they not only do not occur naturally in the body (unlike iodine which does occur in thyroxine and therefore has some biological role) but they have no natural biological function. Indeed, technetium does not even occur in nature being a 'synthetic' element generated by the decay of radioactive molybdenum. The choice of these isotopes has been governed by the fact that they are two of the very few isotopes with suitable energies of gamma emission for detection by gamma camera, and with suitable half-lives and radiation doses to patients following clinical administration (1, 2).

In this chapter we describe the most widely used methods of labelling antibodies with radioactive iodine, indium, and technetium. Although iodine is the most universally used for *in vitro* tests and for experimental investigations *in vivo*, the use of the radiometals is of growing importance as antibodies against tumour-associated antigens are being developed for clinical imaging trials. *Table 1* summarizes the characteristics and general uses of the radioisotopes most commonly used for antibody labelling. The use of such labelled antibodies for *in vivo* pharmacokinetic studies in animals and imaging in patients is outside the scope of this chapter and is dealt with elsewhere (1, 2).

Throughout, we have assumed that antibody is available already in purified form, awaiting labelling. Such purified antibody will be in buffer solution, and phosphate-buffered saline (PBS) at pH 7.2 is widely used. Although through-

Table 1. Radioisotopes used for labelling antibodies

Isotope	Physical half-life	Principal gamma energy (keV)	Uses and advantages	
			In vitro	*In vivo*
^{125}I	60 days	35	Ideal for *in vitro* assays	Ideal for *in vivo* studies not requiring gamma camera imaging
^{131}I	8 days	365	Can be used for *in vitro* assays but ^{125}I preferred. Ideal for labelling control immunoglobulin	Ideal for *in vivo* studies to label control immunoglobulin. Can be used for gamma camera imaging. Used for clinical imaging, but its use is declining
^{123}I	13 h	159	Expense and short half-life precludes *in vitro* use	Suitable for gamma camera imaging. Used clinically, but not widely
^{111}In	2.8 days	171 and 245	Expense and short half-life precludes *in vitro* use	Good for gamma camera imaging. Widely used for clinical imaging
^{99m}Tc	6 h	140	Short half-life precludes *in vitro* use	Ideal for gamma camera imaging. Becoming used clinically

out we refer to 'antibody' the techniques are equally applicable to antibody fragments, heterospecific antibody constructs, etc., and to antibody–drug conjugates where the antibody moiety can be labelled.

2. Handling and measurement of radioisotopes

2.1 Legal responsibilities and safety in handling radioactive materials

It should be recognized that radioactive materials are potentially dangerous. In almost every country legislation will exist to control acquisition, use and disposal of radioactive materials. In the UK this is governed particularly by the Radioactive Substances Act (1960) and Ionising Radiations Regulations (1986). Each establishment using radioactive materials must have a Radiation Protection Adviser, and in addition each department or area in which they are used should have a Departmental Radiation Supervisor whose responsibility it is to oversee safe storage, use, and disposal of radioactive materials. Generally, the use of radioactive materials will only be permitted following registration of individual workers with the Radiation Protection Adviser, and after appropriate training and guidance from the Departmental Radiation Supervisor. Other countries will have their own legislation.

2.2 Detection and measurement of gamma-emitting isotopes

Radioactivity is measured in terms of the rate at which nuclear transformations or disintegrations occur. The older unit, the curie, and its sub-unit the millicurie (mCi) are still sometimes encountered. This is a cumbersome unit since its basis is the number of disintegrations per second from 1 g of radium. The newer SI unit, the becquerel, has a more immediate practical appeal. A becquerel is one transformation (or disintegration) per second. Larger units are the kilobecquerel (kBq), being 10^3 disintegrations per second, the megabecquerel (MBq), being 10^6 disintegrations per second, and the gigabecquerel (GBq), which is 10^9 disintegrations per second.

Measurement or 'counting' of gamma-emitting isotope is usually carried out in a crystal-well scintillation counter, which measures as 'counts' the number of gamma rays detected as scintillations in the crystal. Count rates are usually expressed in counts per minute (c.p.m.).

By setting the discrimination of the counter to the appropriate energy of gamma emission (measured in keV), optimum detection of a particular isotope is achieved. Some machines have two or more channels, each of which can be set to different energies, enabling two isotopes to be counted separately but simultaneously. This can be particularly useful in dual-label studies in which an antibody can be labelled with, say, ^{125}I and a control immunoglobulin with ^{131}I, and their fate, either *in vivo* or *in vitro*, can be followed simultaneously.

The efficiency with which counters detect radiation will depend on the quality and thickness of the detector crystal, because the thicker the crystal the more gamma rays will be detected. However, counting efficiency will also depend on the energy of gamma emission, since the higher the energy the more will pass through the crystal without producing scintillation. Thus although the becquerel, at one disintegration per second, gives some indication of the likely count rate, the higher the energy the lower the efficiency of counting. ^{125}I (35 keV) will often be detected with 80% efficiency, but ^{131}I (365 keV) with only 20%.

2.3 Specific activity of radiolabelled preparations

The specific activity of a radiolabelled preparation is the amount of radioactivity per unit weight of material, for example MBq/mg of antibody. Knowledge of specific activity allows an estimate of the amount of material to give any desired count rate, bearing in mind counting efficiency for the particular isotope. Obviously, for short-lived isotopes there will be a significant decline in specific activity over a few days, and this needs to be borne in mind.

Although it is possible to label some proteins (such as hormones used in hormone radioimmunoassays) to specific activities of several hundred MBq/mg, it is usual to label antibodies to only a few MBq/mg. Antibodies can be damaged by high direct incorporation of radioactive iodine or attachment of chelators for labelling with radiometals. The immune function of antibodies should always be confirmed after labelling.

3. Labelling with radioiodine

^{125}I and ^{131}I are available from many suppliers. For example, Amersham International supply both, specifically formulated for protein iodination. They are as sodium iodide, in sodium hydroxide solution at pH 7–11, free from reducing agent (see below). They are at concentrations of 1.5 GBq/ml (^{131}I) and 3.7 GBq/ml (^{125}I). ^{125}I is carrier free, in that no non-radioactive iodide has been added, although by virtue of its manufacture ^{131}I is only 20% ^{131}I at the time of preparation, the rest being stable iodine. The eight day half-life of ^{131}I means that if several weeks elapse between its manufacture and delivery or use, then the vast majority of iodide present will be stable iodide and not radioactive iodide. Labelling to high specific activity may be introducing on to the antibody more iodine than is appreciated at first sight, and this could damage antibody function.

^{123}I is less readily available, and is not supplied in a radiochemical form specifically designed for protein iodination. This isotope has been little used in the USA for labelling monoclonal antibodies. In Europe it is produced in the UK by the Atomic Energy Research Establishment at Harwell, in Switzerland by the Swiss Federal Institute for Reactor Research, and in Belgium by the National Institue for Radioelements, from whom it is available commercially from IRE-Medgenix, Fleurus, Belgium.

3.1 Oxidative methods of radioiodination

In the most widely used methods for iodination of antibody, the radioiodine is treated with a mild oxidizing agent in the presence of the antibody. Cationic iodine (I^+) is presumed to be formed under these oxidizing conditions and there is an electrophilic aromatic substitution into mainly the tyrosine amino acids of the protein, although histidine can also be labelled. Oxidizing agents can have deleterious effects on the function of some antibodies, because of oxidation of various amino acid residues, and with each antibody the chosen method of labelling must be shown not to compromise the reactivity of the antibody.

It is unlikely that there will be 100% incorporation of the radioiodine into antibody, and so it is necessary to remove unreacted radioiodide before the labelled antibody is ready for use. The most widely used and simple technique here is gel filtration, and Sephadex G25 or G50 (Pharmacia) is most commonly used. Because the reaction volume from the labelling reaction is small (usually no more than 1 ml), only small columns of Sephadex are needed for efficient separation of proteins from free radioiodide. Small pre-packed columns of Sephadex G25 (PD-10 Columns, Pharmacia) are available and are ideal for this purpose. The mixture from the labelling reaction is added to the top of the column and eluted by addition of buffer such as PBS. These pre-packed columns have a surface tension net at the top of the gel so that the liquid can only drop to the top of the gel bed (the column cannot run dry). Addition of, say, 0.5 ml of buffer to the top is followed by simultaneous elution of the same volume from the bottom. Thus, small fractions can be eluted from the column and the count rate in each determined. The labelled antibody elutes first from the column, and the free radioiodine comes off later. Efficiencies of labelling can be calculated from the input count rate of radioiodine and that recovered in the labelled antibody fractions.

3.1.1 The Iodogen method

In 1978 Fraker and Speck (3) introduced 1,3,4,6-tetrachloro-3α,6α-diphenylglycoluril as an oxidizing agent giving minimal exposure of proteins to oxidation during radioiodination. This is now probably the most widely used agent for radioiodination of antibodies. The material is available commercially as Iodogen (Pierce Chemical Company).

Iodogen is virtually insoluble in water, and for protein iodination it is coated on the inner surface of the reaction vessel by evaporating, under a stream of nitrogen, a solution of the material in chloroform or methylene chloride (carry this out in a fume cupboard!). Small glass or solvent-resistant plastic (e.g. polypropylene) tubes capable of holding up to 1 or 2 ml should be used, and conical 'microfuge' tubes with screw caps are ideal. They can be prepared in large numbers and be stored refrigerated for many months. The amount of Iodogen coated on to the surface of the reaction tube varies in published reports but it is generally up to about 100 μg. This amount will produce a visible film of material on the surface of the tube. Smooth coating is virtually impossible to achieve, but tubes with a somewhat 'lumpy' appearance usually work quite satisfactorily.

Iodination reactions are carried out by adding the appropriate volume of antibody solution and radioiodine to the coated tube, mixing, and leaving, usually at room temperature, for a few minutes. The reaction is stopped by removing the reactants from the presence of the iodogen simply by transferring the solution into a fresh container. *Protocol 1* outlines the procedure.

Protocol 1. Antibody labelling by the Iodogen method

Reagents required

- Iodogen
- Analar-grade methylene chloride
- polypropylene conical microfuge tubes, 1.5 ml volume
- antibody in phosphate-buffered saline at 1 mg/ml[a]

- PD-10 column of Sephadex G25
- radioiodine, ^{125}I or ^{131}I, protein-labelling grade
- phosphate-buffered saline, pH 7.2 (PBS)

Method

1. Dissolve the Iodogen in methylene chloride to 400 μg/ml.
2. Dispense 0.3 ml of solution into the tubes.
3. Evaporate the contents of each tube to dryness under a stream of nitrogen. Rotate the tube slowly as methylene chloride evaporates to leave a film of Iodogen. This procedure should be carried out in a fume cupboard. Cap the tubes and store them in a desiccator in a refrigerator.
4. Wash the PD-10 column through with 10 ml of PBS.
5. Add 0.5 ml of antibody[b] solution to a tube with dried Iodogen, followed by 15 MBq of radioiodine. Mix with a Pasteur pipette and leave the reaction at room temperature for 10 min. This, and step **6**, must be carried out in a fume cupboard to prevent inhalation of volatile radioiodine during the labelling procedure.
6. Position a collection tube beneath the PD-10 column. Transfer the antibody/radioiodine mixture to the top of the PD-10 column, collecting the 0.5 ml of eluant which will flow out of the bottom. Add 19 × 0.5 ml aliquots of PBS to the top of the column, collecting 0.5 ml from the bottom after each addition.
7. Determine the radioiodine count rate in fractions. The count rate will be too high for counting of the samples themselves, and so aliquots of 10 μl should be withdrawn from each for the counting. Under these conditions, labelled protein will be eluted in fractions 7–10, and free radioiodide around fraction 15 onwards. Pool the two or three fractions of the first peak of radioactivity as the labelled antibody preparation.

[a] Antibody at higher or lower concentrations can be used, and the volume to be labelled and the amount of radioiodine can be varied. This protocol should yield a final labelled antibody at about 200 μg/ml with a specific activity of about 20 MBq/mg.

[b] If a large volume of solution is used, most will be above the level of dried Iodogen, and labelling efficiency may be reduced. If small volumes are used, it is difficult to mix without significant loss of solution into the mixing pipette.

3.1.2 Other oxidative methods

Other agents can be used for oxidative iodination of antibodies. One widely used before the introduction of Iodogen was Chloramine-T (4). This is the sodium salt of *N*-chloro-*p*-toluene sulphonamide. Because it slowly produces hypochlorous acid in aqueous solution, it is a mild oxidizing agent. For this method of labelling, antibody is mixed with the radioiodine, and an aqueous solution of freshly prepared Chloramine-T added. This can be prepared at such concentration that only microlitre amounts need to be added to the reaction vessel. Reaction times and conditions which have been used vary widely, but generally 10 to 20 μg of Chloramine-T are used for each 37 MBq of radioiodine. The amount of Chloramine-T is dictated by the amount of radioiodide, not by the amount of antibody, since it is the iodide which is being oxidized. Reaction times also vary, but are usually in the range of 2–5 min, usually at room temperature. The shorter the time the less likely is oxidative damage to the antibody. The oxidizing action of the Chloramine-T is then usually stopped by the addition of an appropriate amount of a reducing agent, usually sodium metabisulphite.

As an alternative to the use of Chloramine-T as a solution, non-porous polystyrene beads coated with an immobilized form of the chemical are commercially available (IODO-BEADS, Pierce Chemical Company). These beads are about one-eighth of an inch in diameter. Beads are added to the radioiodine solution about 5 min before the addition of antibody solution. The reaction can be stopped simply by removing the beads from the solution, and there is no need for the addition of reducing agent. Reaction conditions can be varied by the use of different numbers of the beads.

Other methods of oxidative iodination include the enzyme lactoperoxidase, which in the presence of hydrogen peroxide catalyses the incorporation of radioiodine into tyrosine amino acids of proteins (5). An alternative oxidizing agent recently introduced is *N*-bromosuccinimide (6). This is water soluble, and is added in solution directly to the antibody/radioiodine mixture.

3.2 Non-oxidative labelling

An alternative to oxidative labelling is the use of ^{125}I-labelled Bolton and Hunter reagent (7). This is *N*-succinimidyl 3-(4-hydroxy 5-[^{125}I]iodophenyl) propionate and is available commercially (e.g. Amersham International). This reacts directly with antibody, amide bonds being formed with the lysine groups of the antibody molecule. This material is destroyed by hydrolysis if it comes into contact with water and is supplied dissolved in benzene. The required amount of solution should be evaporated to dryness under nitrogen, and antibody in solution added. Unreacted, hydrolysed, material can be removed by small-scale gel filtration.

3.3 Causes of poor labelling

Labelling efficiency will be at its highest, often approaching 100%, with small volumes of reactants (less than 1 ml) and antibody at concentrations of several mg/ml. Sometimes it is found that a particular preparation of antibody labels poorly, and there are a number of possible reasons for this. With the oxidative methods of labelling such as Iodogen, any reducing agent present will interfere with the reaction. Radioiodines available commercially for protein labelling are specifically free of reducing agents, but other reactants, or the antibody itself, may have become contaminated. We have often found that with an antibody preparation that 'won't label', dialysis against fresh buffer, such as phosphate-buffered saline, will clean it up, possibly by removal of reducing agents, so that it can now be labelled.

Poor labelling with Chloramine-T can be due to deterioration of this chemical on long storage, and fresh material should be obtained periodically.

Good labelling efficiency with oxidative methods, but with poor immunological reactivity of the final product, suggests that the antibody in question is intrinsically sensitive to oxidation. As an alternative the use of Bolton and Hunter reagent should be examined.

3.4 Detection of free radioiodine in labelled preparations

If preparations are purified efficiently after labelling the amount of free radioiodine will be only a few per cent. However, on storage, some radioiodide may become detached. Consequently it is advisable to check the amount of free radioiodide in preparations, particularly those stored for more than a week or so. The simplest way to do this is by TCA (trichloracetic acid) precipitation which depends on the rapid denaturation and precipitation of proteins in highly acidic conditions which will leave free radioiodide in solution.

A trace of the labelled preparation can be diluted into a convenient volume, say 0.5 ml. containing approximately 10% bovine serum albumin and an equal volume of a 20% solution of trichloracetic acid (TCA) in water added to make the solution 10% with respect to TCA. The carrier albumin and the monoclonal antibody will be rapidly precipitated. Centrifugation can be used to separate the precipitate from supernatant, and radioiodine measured in the pelleted precipitate and in the supernatant. (TCA is highly corrosive—handle with care.)

A refinement of this procedure, which does not require the addition of carrier protein, is to spot the labelled material 1 cm from the bottom edge of a small strip (1 × 15 cm) of filter paper, and then to stand the paper with its bottom in a 10% solution of TCA to produce a simple ascending chromatogram. This is best carried out in a closed vessel, such as a gas jar, with the atmosphere pre-saturated to prevent drying of the strip. The paper strip can then be cut, and radioiodine count rates determined of the origin (where acid precipitation of antibody-bound material will occur), and the rest of the strip including the ascending solvent front with which any free radioiodide will have moved.

4. Labelling with radioindium

Indium cannot be introduced directly into proteins in the way that iodine can, and radiolabelling with ^{111}In is carried out by pre-conjugation to the antibody of a chelating agent. The most widely used chelating agent now is diethylenetriaminepentacetic acid (DTPA) (8). The bicyclic anhydride of DTPA (DTPA anhydride, or DTPAA) will react with epsilon amino groups of lysine residues in proteins with the formation of amide bonds. Remaining negatively charged carboxyl groups on the DTPA will subsequently bind by ionic interaction to the positively charged indium ions (In^{3+}). DTPAA is commercially available (e.g. Sigma Chemical Company).

To prevent hydrolysis of DTPAA it has to be kept dry. Following its addition to antibody solution, part will be hydrolysed to DTPA and part will react with the antibody. It is usual to add DTPAA to antibody at a molar ratio about 2:1 to achieve about one conjugated DTPA group per antibody molecule. DTPAA is a solid, but weighing the very small amounts needed to react with milligram quantities of antibody is impractical. The most convenient way is to dissolve the DTPAA in anhydrous dimethylsulphoxide, and then to add the required volume of this to antibody. Dimethylsulphoxide is miscible with aqueous solutions and addition of a series of small aliquots to the antibody solution with continual stirring allows sufficient reaction with antibody before hydrolysis. Optimum pH conditions for the reaction of DTPAA with antibody are within the range of 7 to 9. In our experience, antibody in PBS at pH 7.2 can be used quite successfully. Unreacted DTPA can be removed from the reaction mixture either by gel filtration, using for example Sephadex G25, or dialysis, and the antibody–DTPA conjugate may be returned to phosphate-buffered saline. Aliquots of antibody–DTPA can be stored in the same way as antibody, awaiting ^{111}In labelling.

Subsequent radiolabelling of antibody–DTPA conjugates is carried out by the addition of ^{111}In. This is available as a solution of indium chloride (e.g. Amersham International). Chelation of the radioindium takes place most efficiently at pHs below 5, and to prevent the formation of colloidal forms of the indium it is necessary to add acetate or citrate to the reaction mixture. It is advisable to add an equal volume of 1 M sodium acetate or citrate to the solution of indium chloride before its addition to the antibody. A convenient alternative which we have found quite satisfactory with many antibodies is to transfer the antibody–DTPA conjugate into 0.3 M citrate buffer at pH 6 during gel filtration or dialysis following reaction with DTPA anhydride. Under these conditions radioindium as chloride can be directly added to the antibody–DTPA conjugate without any pre-treatment. *Protocol 2* outlines the overall procedure. Unreacted ^{111}In can be removed by small-scale gel filtration as outlined above for the purification of radioiodine labelled preparations.

Protocol 2. Labelling of antibody with ^{111}In by DTPA chelation

Reagents required

- DTPA anhydride. This must be kept dry, and should be stored in a desiccator

- anhydrous dimethylsulphoxide, Analar grade
- antibody in PBS at 1 mg/ml
- magnetic stirrer
- dialysis tubing
- citrate phosphate buffer, 0.3 M, pH 6.0
- PD-10 column of Sephadex G25
- ^{111}In as indium chloride
- phosphate-buffered saline (PBS), pH 7.2

Method

1. Weigh out 470 μg of DTPA anhydride into a dry vessel. To ensure dryness, a glass bijou bottle should be used which has been dried in an oven and allowed to cool in a desiccator. Dissolve the DTPA anhydride in 1 ml of dimethylsulphoxide. (Do this in a fume cupboard.)
2. Add 100 μl of DTPA anhydride solution to 10 ml of the antibody as 10 × 10 μl aliquots stirring continuously with the magnetic stirrer. This is a 2:1 molar ratio of DTPA to antibody.[a]
3. Transfer the solution to dialysis tubing and dialyse against 200 times its own volume of citrate buffer at pH 6.0, changing the medium twice over a 24 h period. Carry out this dialysis in a closed vessel to prevent dimethylsulphoxide vapour entering the atmosphere. It is best to carry this out in a refrigerated room (~6°C).
4. Determine the protein concentration spectrophotometrically, given that $O.D._{280}$ of immunoglobulin at 1 mg/ml is 1.43.
5. Dispense antibody–DTPA conjugate into suitable aliquots, of say 1 mg, and store frozen at −20°C.
6. For ^{111}In labelling add 37 MBq of indium chloride to a thawed aliquot[b] of antibody–DTPA, incubating at room temperature for 5 min.
7. Wash PD-10 column through with 10 ml of PBS.
8. Transfer the solution to the PD-10 column and proceed as for steps **6** and **7** of *Protocol 1*.

[a] A different volume of antibody, at higher or lower concentrations can be used, with a corresponding correction to the concentration of DTPAA (the molecular weight of DTPAA is 357 Da).

[b] The amount of antibody–DTPA to be labelled and the amount of indium can be varied. This protocol should yield a final labelled antibody at about 500 μg/ml with a specific activity of about 30 MBq/mg.

4.1 Causes of poor labelling

Because DTPA anhydride will be hydrolysed to unreactive DTPA on contact with water, it must be kept dry, preferably in a desiccator. The DMSO used must also be anhydrous. This can be produced by distillation of the commercial material, the fraction boiling at 189°C being collected. Alternatively, or in addition, the material should have desiccant material such as Molecular Sieve added to absorb water (the 3Å pore size potassium aluminosilicate Molecular Sieve is suitable).

Because the final ^{111}In uptake is by chelation, contamination with or bi- or trivalent cations can compete with the In^{3+} for reaction with DTPA on the antibody. Although in our hands solutions prepared with conventionally distilled or deionized water are perfectly satisfactory, some reports using this method advocate additional treatment with ion exchangers.

4.2 Detection of free radioindium in preparations

The amount of free ^{111}In in preparations is most easily measured by silica gel thin layer chromatography. Here the preparation is spotted 1 cm from the bottom of a 1 × 10 cm strip of silica-gel-coated instant thin-layer chromatography medium, and eluted by ascending solvent consisting of 0.1 M sodium acetate with 10 mM EDTA (ethylenediaminetetraaceticacid, disodium salt). Antibody-bound ^{111}In remains at the origin, while unbound ^{111}In migrates with the solvent front. Assay of the radioactivity of each portion will give the proportion of the total ^{111}In bound to antibody.

5. Labelling with technetium

^{99m}Tc is widely used in hospital radiopharmacies for preparation of radiopharmaceuticals (1). It is produced by the decay of radioactive ^{99}Mo in ^{99m}Tc generators. These contain ^{99}Mo adsorbed to alumina. ^{99m}Tc produced by decay of the molybdenum, but not the molybdenum itself, can be eluted with saline. Such generators are available commercially, and virtually all hospital radiopharmacies can be expected to have them.

Many techniques have been described for labelling antibodies with ^{99m}Tc (9), but they are often cumbersome to perform. One of the simplest was described by Schwarz and Steinstrasser (10) and is often referred to as the 'Schwarz method'. Essentially this involves treatment of antibody with a reducing agent such as mercaptoethanol to cleave some of the intrachain disulphide bonds to give free –SH (sulphydryl or thiol) groups. Ionization of –SH to $-S^-$ allows reaction with positively charged Tc^{4+}.

^{99m}Tc eluted from generators is as pertechnetate (TcO_4^-). Before it will react with reduced antibody the pertechnetate itself has to be reduced to Tc^{4+}. This is usually carried out with Sn(II) as stannous chloride as the reducing agent. The method of Schwarz, expanded and described by Mather and Ellison (11), takes advantage of conventional methylene diphosphonate (MDP) pharmaceutical kits used to prepare ^{99m}Tc-labelled MDP for bone scanning. These kits contain stannous chloride, which will reduce the pertechnetate, and MDP to which the Tc^{4+} will chelate before transchelation to the reduced antibody. The labelled antibody can be purified from these reactants by passage through Sephadex G25. *Protocol 3* outlines the practical aspects of this method.

Protocol 3. Reduction-mediated labelling of antibody with ^{99m}Tc [a]

Reagents required

- antibody at 10 mg/ml in phosphate-buffered saline (PBS)
- 2-mercaptoethanol
- PD-10 columns of Sephadex G25
- methylene diphosphonate (MDP) bone-scanning kit (e.g. Amerscan, Amersham International)
- sodium [^{99m}Tc]pertechnetate eluted from ^{99m}Tc generator

Method

1. Add 4.7 µl of 2-mercaptoethanol to each ml of antibody solution, with stirring. This is a 1000:1 molar ratio of mercaptoethanol to antibody. (The molecular weight of 2-mercaptoethanol is 78 Da, and it is a liquid of density 1.114 g/ml.) Incubate at room temperature for 30 min. (Mercaptoethanol is noxious and should be handled in a fume cupboard.)
2. Purify the reduced antibody by passage through Sephadex G25 using PBS for elution. With less than 2 ml of solution this can be with a PD-10 column. Identify fractions with antibody, by determination of $O.D._{280}$, pool and store reduced antibody at −20°C in 1 mg aliquots.
3. Reconstitute MDP kit with 5 ml of 0.9% saline.
4. Add 0.1 ml of MDP solution to 1 mg of antibody.
5. Add the required amount of [^{99m}Tc]pertechnetate[b] to the antibody/MDP mixture, and leave at room temperature for 10 min.
6. Purify labelled antibody through a PD-10 column, eluting in PBS, as in steps **6** and **7** of *Protocol 1*.

[a] Based on the protocol of Mather and Ellison (11).
[b] Because ^{99m}Tc has a half-life of 6 h, antibody should be labelled to a specific activity of several tens of MBq/mg.

5.1 Causes of poor labelling

This method depends on adequate reduction of antibody to yield –SH gropus. Re-oxidation will prevent subsequent labelling with ^{99m}Tc. There is a suggestion that some residual mercaptoethanol in the reduced antibody is advantageous in this respect. Simple gel filtration after mercaptoethanol treatment, which may leave some residual mercaptoethanol, is probably better than extensive purification. It is possible that some antibodies might be fragmented by mercaptoethanol by cleavage of interchain disulphide bonds, yielding an unreactive product. Other reducing agents can be used, such as ascorbic acid (11), but we have no experience of their use.

5.2 Detection of free ^{99m}Tc in preparations

The purity of the ^{99m}Tc-labelled antibody can be assessed by chromatography on silica gel, using 0.9% saline, free ^{99m}Tc moving with the solvent front. The strip should be cut and ^{99m}Tc count rates determined as for assessment of purity of radioiodine-labelled preparations.

6. Materials and suppliers

Material	Supplier
Iodogen	Pierce Chemical Company UK: Pierce and Warriner, 44 Upper Northgate Street, Chester CH1 4EF
Iodobeads	Pierce Chemical Company
^{125}I-labelled Bolton and Hunter reagent	Amersham International UK: Amersham, Buckinghamshire HP7 9NA USA: 2636, South Clearbrook Drive, Arlington Heights, IL 60005
DTPA anhydride (diethylenetriaminepentaacetic acid anhydride)	Sigma Chemical Company UK: Fancy Road, Poole, Dorset BH17 7TG USA: PO Box 14508, St Louis, MO 63178
PD-10 columns (small disposable columns pre-packed with Sephadex G25)	Pharmacia LKB Biotechnology UK: Davey Avenue, Knowlhill, Central Milton Keynes MKN5 8PH USA: 800 Centenniel Avenue, PO Box 1327, Piscataway, NJ 08855-1327

Acknowledgement

The authors' work is supported by the Cancer Research Campaign, London, UK.

References

1. Sampson, C. B. (ed.) (1990). *Textbook of Radiopharmacy*. Gordon and Breach, New York.
2. Perkins, A. C. and Pimm, M. V. (1991). *Immunoscintigraphy—Practical Aspects and Clinical Applications*. Wiley-Liss, New York.
3. Fraker, P. J. and Speck, J. C. (1978). *Biochem. Biophys. Res. Commun.*, **80,** 849.
4. Greenwood, F. C., Hunter, W. M., and Glover, J. S. (1963). *Biochem. J.,* **89,** 114.
5. Marchanolis, J. J. (1969). *Biochem. J.,* **113,** 299.
6. Mather, S. J. and Ward, B. C. (1987). *J. Nucl. Med.,* **28,** 1034.
7. Bolton, A. E. and Hunter, W. M. (1973). *Biochem. J.,* **133,** 529,
8. Hnatowich, D. J., Layne, W. W., Childs, R. L., Lanteigne, D., Davis, M. A., Griffen, T. W., *et al.* (1983). *Science,* **220,** 613.
9. Verbruggen, A. M. (1990). *Eur. J. Nucl. Med.,* **17,** 346.
10. Schwarz, A. and Steinstrasser, A. (1987). *J. Nucl. Med.,* **28,** 721.
11. Mather, S. J. and Ellison, D. (1990). *J. Nucl. Med.,* **31,** 692.
12. Thakur, M. L. and DeFulvio, J. D. (1991). *J. Immunol. Methods,* **137,** 217.

14

Preparation of multispecific $F(ab)_2$ and $F(ab)_3$ antibody derivatives

MARTIN J. GLENNIE, ALISON L. TUTT, and JOHN GREENMAN

1. Introduction

IgG antibody, as produced by normal B cells, is a symmetrical four-chain molecule capable of recognizing two matching antigenic determinants through its Fab arms. Over the last few years a range of techniques has developed to generate asymmetric antibodies that engage two different antigenic sites. These bispecific reagents have potential as highly versatile protein cross-linkers in a number of diagnostic and therapeutic situations. For example, they have been used in immunohistochemistry to tether an indicator molecule (such as peroxidase) to a tissue marker, and as possible therapeutic reagents where the bispecific antibody (BsAb) targets pharmacological substances (e.g. drugs or toxins), or cellular effectors (e.g. T cells, monocytes, or NK cells), against unwanted cells. In each of these applications the BsAb provides a cross-linking function between two different antigenic moieties.

Three different types of BsAb are currently available: IgG-heterodimers, in which two IgG antibodies are disulphide bonded together using a lysyl-reactive cross-linker such as *N*-succinimidyl-3-(2-pyridyldithio)-propionate (SPDP) (1); $F(ab)_2$ fragments, where two antibody Fab arms are disulphide (2) or thioether (3) linked together via hinge-region SH-groups; and bispecific IgG, secreted from a 'hybrid-hybridoma' or 'quadroma' produced when two antibody-producing hybridoma cells are fused together (4). In this chapter we shall concentrate on techniques developed in this laboratory for the generation of BsAb, and more recently trispecific antibodies (TsAb), through chemical linkage of two or three antibody Fab fragments (5–7).

The first bispecific $F(ab)_2$ derivatives were constructed in the early 1960s by Nisonoff and Mandy (2). Reduced Fab fragments from two selected rabbit IgG antibodies were allowed to reoxidize, via their hinge-region SH groups, and produce a mixture of $F(ab)_2$ products. Unfortunately, because the conjugation was random, these products contained both hetero- and homo-Fab dimers which could only be separated by sequential adsorption and elution from two immunoadsorbents, each containing one of the two antigens. Brennan *et al.* (3) modified this approach and proposed a scheme in which the SH-groups of one of the Fab species are protected by dithio-bis(2-nitrobenzoic acid) (DTNB; Ellman's reagent), thus allowing directed disulphide exchange with the second, reduced, Fab species and hence minimizing the formation of homodimers. This procedure is highly efficient and results in a good yield of intact $F(ab)_2$ heterodimers with the same number of inter-H chain disulphide bonds as the parent antibodies (most mouse IgG isotypes contain three).

Over the past few years BsAb have been prepared in this laboratory using the chemical cross-linker, *o*-phenylenedimaleimide (*o*-PDM) (5). Using this reagent Fab fragments from the desired antibodies have been thioether linked, primarily through their hinge region SH groups, to produce bispecific $F(ab)_2$ and $F(ab)_3$ and trispecific $F(ab)_3$. These derivatives are produced in good yield, are of known composition, and are stable to reduction by thiol. The bispecific $F(ab)_2$ and $F(ab)_3$ have been used to deliver toxins (saporin and ricin) to target cells to inhibit protein synthesis *in vitro* and *in vivo*, and also to redirect the lytic activity of cellular effectors such as monocytes, NK cells, and T cells. We are investigating various trispecific $F(ab)_3$ antibodies, with one Fab binding site for a target cell and two different binding sites for cytotoxic T cells, for their abilities to recruit and activate T cells for cytotoxicity; the interest in having two arms attached to the effector cell stems from the extra activation thereby induced during the lytic process (6, 7).

In this chapter we outline the methodology for preparing these multivalent antibodies.

2. Buffers used in the preparation of multispecific derivatives

i. 2M 'Tris base' containing EDTA, pH 8.0, (2 M TE8)

- Tris[hydroxymethyl]aminomethane (Sigma catalogue No. T1503), 242 g
- ethylenediaminetetraaceticacid (BDH catalogue No. 10093), 37.2 g
- hydrochloric acid (BDH catalogue No. 19066), 200 ml

Make up to 1 litre with distilled water.

Prepare 0.2 M and 0.02 M Tris base containing EDTA pH 8.0 (0.2 M TE8 and 20 mM TE8) using 2 M TE8 diluted 1:10 and 1:100 with distilled water respectively.

ii. 0.05 M Tris containing EDTA, pH 7.0, (50 mM TE7)

- Tris[hydroxymethyl]aminomethane, 6.06 g
- ethylenediaminetetraaceticacid, 0.75 g

Dissolve in distilled water, pH to 7.0 with HCl and make up to 1 litre with water.

iii. 1 M Tris base, pH 9.2

- Tris[hydroxymethyl]aminomethane, 121.1 g

Make up to 1 litre with distilled water.

iv. 1 M sodium chloride containing Tris base and EDTA, pH 8.0 (1 M NTE8)

- Sodium chloride (BDH catalogue No. 10241), 58.4 g
- Tris[hydroxymethyl]aminomethane, 24.2 g
- ethylenediaminetetraaceticacid, 3.72 g
- hydrochloric acid, 20 ml

Make up to 1 litre with distilled water.

v. Prepare 0.5 M and 0.2 M sodium chloride containing Tris base and EDTA, pH 8.0 (0.5 M NTE8 and 0.2 M NTE8) using 1 M NTE8 diluted 1:2 and 1:5 with distilled water respectively.

vi. Ammonia thiocyanate for immunosorbent elution

- Ammonia solution (about 35% NH_3) (BDH catalogue No. 10012), 40 ml
- potassium thiocyanate, 97.18 g

Make up to 1 litre with distilled water.

vii. 0.1 M glycine containing EDTA, pH 3.0 (0.1 M GE3)

- Glycine (BDH catalogue No. 10119), 7.51 g
- ethylenediaminetetraaceticacid, 0.74 g

Dissolve in distilled water, pH to 3.0 with HCl and make up to 1 litre with water.

viii. 0.05 M acetate buffer containing EDTA, pH 5.2 (0.05 M AE)

- Anhydrous sodium acetate (BDH catalogue No. 10236), 3.35 g
- ethylenediaminetetraaceticacid, 0.186 g
- acetic acid glacial (BDH catalogue No. 10001), 0.526 ml

Make up to 1 litre with distilled water.

ix. Bicarbonate buffer, pH 9.6, for coating ELISA plates

- Na_2CO_3, 1.59 g
- $NaHCO_3$, 2.93 g

Make up to 1 litre with distilled water.

x. Substrate for ELISA

- Citric acid (19.2 g/litre), 24.3 ml
- Na_2HPO_4 (28.4 g/litre), 25.7 ml

- *o*-phenylenediamine tablet (Sigma catalogue No. P-5412), 1 (200 μmol)
- hydrogen peroxide solution (60%) (BDH catalogue No. 10399), 20 μl
- distilled water, 50 ml

Important: dissolve *o*-phenylenediamine tablet in citrate solution (in dark) before adding other constituents and make up immediately prior to use in ELISA.

xi. F(ab)$_2$ reducing solution (220 mM 2-mercaptoethanol)
- 2-mercaptoethanol (2-ME; BDH catalogue No. 44143), 1.54 ml
- ethylenediaminetetraacetic acid, 37.2 mg

Make up to 100 ml with distilled water.

3. Chromatography equipment

The following list of equipment is suitable for synthesizing multispecific derivatives:

(a) Columns: Two columns packed with Sephadex G25 medium (Pharmacia catalogue No. 17-0033-02) are required for small-scale preparation (2–30 mg) of F(ab)$_2$ or F(ab)$_3$ derivatives. These must be fitted with two end-flow adaptors and water jackets to allow chilling throughout the preparation. Pharmacia K series columns are ideal:

- column 1 (XK 16/40, catalogue No. 18-8774-01) 1.6 cm in diameter, packed with 25 cm of gel and pumped at approximately 60 ml/h
- column 2 (XK 26/40, catalogue No. 18-8786-01) 2.6 cm in diameter, packed with 20 cm of gel and pumped at approximately 200 ml/h

Two larger columns packed with polyacrylamide agarose gel (Ultrogel AcA44; IBF Biotechnics, France; catalogue No. 230161) are used for the size-exclusion chromatography of bi- and trispecific antibody products. The columns are joined in series using Teflon (PTFE) capillary tubing (Pharmacia catalogue No. 18-4370-01). Chilling through water jackets is not required at this stage in the preparation, and fractionation can be run at room temperature. Two Pharmacia columns are suitable:

- column 3 (XK 26/100, catalogue No. 18-8770-01) 2.6 cm in diameter, packed with approximately 80 cm of gel and pumped at 30 ml/h

(b) Chromatography pumps: Two pumps are required capable of delivering buffer to the various columns at between 15 and 200 ml/h. We use a single-channel peristaltic pump P-1 (Pharmacia catalogue No. 19-4610-01) and a Gilson Minipuls 2 single-channel pump (Anachem, Luton, UK; catalogue No. E17340).

(c) Chromatography monitoring and collecting equipment: A suitable UV monitor, chart recorder, and fraction collector are required. We use a Uvicord SII monitor fitted with flowcell and 280 nm interference filter (Pharmacia), a two-channel chart recorder (Pharmacia), and a SuperFrac fraction collector (Pharmacia).

(d) Chiller/water circulator: A suitable means of chilling chromatography columns is required. This can be achieved with a chiller/circulator (e.g. Conair Churchill chiller thermocirculator 0.2 series, Uxbridge, Middlesex, UK) or a simple water bath (0–4°C) with an appropriate pumping system to supply the water jackets of columns 1 and 2. For example, a large polystyrene box containing water and crushed ice and a submersible garden pond pump delivering approximately 10 litre/min will suffice.

(e) High-pressure liquid chromatography (HPLC) system: At each stage of construction, antibody fragments and multispecific derivatives are checked for yield and purity by rapid size fractionation. For this purpose one of the many HPLC systems is required. We use a system supplied by Waters Associates Ltd, UK, consisting of a U6K universal injector, 6000A solvent delivery system, 440 absorbance detector, and 680 gradient controller. The fractionation is performed at 0.5 ml/min on a Zorbax^R bio series GF250 column (Du Pont Company, Wilmington, USA) equilibrated in 0.2 M phosphate, pH 7.0, containing 10 mM sodium azide. Each assessment requires approximately 20 min.

(f) Immunosorbent columns:

- A 5 ml sheep IgG anti-mouse Fcγ immunosorbent was prepared. Preparation of immunosorbent columns is described in detail in other volumes in this series (8). Briefly, sheep were first hyperimmunized with mouse IgG (mixture of IgG1 and IgG2a monoclonal antibodies; see below). Serum was prepared and IgG affinity purified by elution from a column of mouse IgG. 7S IgG was then isolated by size-exclusion chromatography on polyacrylamide agarose gel (Ultrogel AcA34; IBF Biotechnics). Finally all detectable anti-mouse Fab activity was removed from this 7S pure IgG by exhaustive absorption against a 25 ml immunosorbent column of mouse $F(ab)_2$ fragments. The remaining IgG antibody (anti-mouse Fcγ) was coupled to cyanogen-bromide-activated Sepharose CL-4B beads (Pharmacia catalogue No. 17-0430-02) according to the manufacturer's instructions and stored at 4°C in 0.1 M NTE8.

- An immunosorbent of recombinant Protein A was made again using cyanogen-bromide-activated Sepharose CL-4B beads. The Protein A was supplied by Porton Products Ltd, Maidenhead, Berks, UK and coupled at 10 mg/ml of swollen gel. The capacity was approximately 40 mg of human IgG/ml at pH 8 and 20°C. Storage as for the anti-Fcγ column above.

4. Preparation of mouse IgG and its $F(ab)_2$ fragments

4.1 Preparation of mouse IgG

The isolation of mouse IgG from ascites fluid and culture supernatant has been detailed in a previous volume in this series (9). Throughout the current work mouse IgG1 and IgG2a antibodies were isolated from ascitic fluid taken from hybridoma-bearing mice using a Protein A column. Preparations normally start when 50–300 ml of ascites has been collected. Prior to preparation, electrophoresis (EP) of a small sample of fluid allows a monoclonal band to be identified and its concentration estimated. *Figure 1* shows EP strips for eight ascitic fluids, each with monoclonal bands which migrate within the gamma or beta region. Ascites fluid without a detectable monoclonal antibody band is not processed. IgG and its fragments are stored in phosphate (e.g. PBS) or a Tris base buffer, pH 8.0. To avoid significant losses, purified Ig are stored at high concentration (1–10 mg/ml). The concentration of all pure antibodies and Fab derivatives are estimated by measuring UV absorbance at 280 nm, taking the $A^{1\%}/1$ cm to equal 1.35.

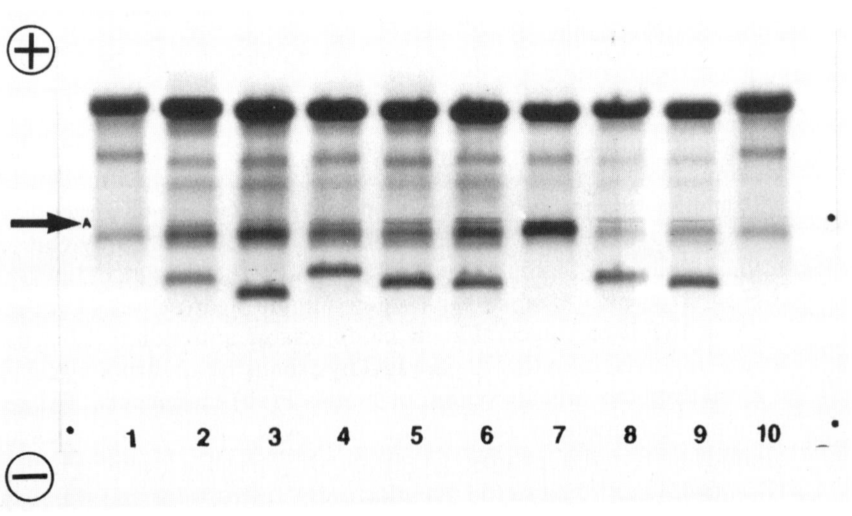

Figure 1. Detection of monoclonal antibody in mouse ascitic fluid by electrophoresis. Samples of eight different ascitic fluids (tracks 2–9) and mouse normal serum (tracks 1 and 10) were separated according to the manufacturer's instructions using a Paragon Electrophoresis System (Beckman Instruments Ltd, High Wycombe, UK). Each ascitic fluid, with the exception of that in track 7, shows a clear monoclonal band in the gamma region of the electrophoretic strip. The sample in track 7 has a band migrating in the beta region of the strip close to the sample-application point (arrow). Anode and cathode are indicated by + and −.

Protocol 1. Preparation of mouse IgG1 and IgG2a

1. Filter the ascites fluid through a 24 cm Whatman 113 filter paper (Whatman International Ltd, Maidstone, UK catalogue No. 1113 240).
2. Add an equal volume of 0.2 M NTE8 buffer.
3. Equilibrate the Protein A immunosorbent in 0.2 M NTE8 and load the diluted ascites at approximately 2 ml/min. The IgG-binding capacity of the column will vary depending on the coupling efficiency of Protein A to Sepharose. Routinely, we use a column of 2.6 cm diameter by 7 cm length and load approximately 300 mg of IgG. This amount corresponds to about 50 ml of ascites. Always save the IgG-depleted effluent from the column and check for monoclonal band by EP.
4. Wash the column thoroughly with 0.2 M NTE8 until no further protein is eluted, as judged by a stable baseline on the UV (280 nm) recorder.
5. Elute the bound IgG by flushing the column through with 0.1 M GE3 buffer. Re-equilibrate the Protein A column in 0.2 M NTE8 and store at 4°C.
6. Rapidly dialyse the IgG solution using the appropriate sized visking tubing (Medicell International Ltd, London, UK) into cold 0.2 M NTE8 and then into 20 mM TE8, ready for $F(ab)_2$ preparation. The purity of IgG can be checked by EP and by chromatography on HPLC (*Protocol 7*).

4.2 Preparation of $F(ab)_2$

The production of $F(ab)_2$ by limited proteolysis of mouse IgG has been described by many groups (10, 11). All the mouse IgG isotypes, with the exception of IgG2b, can generally be cleaved to a $F(ab)_2$ product. Until recently, the enzyme of choice for this preparation from mouse IgG1, IgG2a, and IgG3 would have been pepsin, but today a number of other enzymes, in particular bromelain and ficin, are proving more useful at least for some mouse IgG1 antibodies (12, 13). For example, Mariani *et al.* (13) found that, in contrast to pepsin (which was highly pH-dependent and gave variable levels of digestion) ficin consistently gave high yields of $F(ab)_2$ from a panel of monoclonal IgG1 antibodies. In our own work ((7) and A. Tutt, unpublished data), two mouse IgG1 monoclonal antibodies (C4/120 and R73) which are consistently sensitive to pepsin, give good yields of $F(ab)_2$ when treated with the pineapple enzyme, bromelain. The other advantage of ficin and bromelain is that the digestion can be maintained at neutral pH and the antibody avoids the acid environment necessary for proteolysis with pepsin. Unfortunately, ficin, bromelain, and various other proteolytic enzymes have failed to replace pepsin for the production of $F(ab')_2$ from mouse IgG2a and IgG3 antibodies. In addition, none of these enzymes produces a $F(ab)_2$ from mouse IgG2b antibodies.

It should be noted that a prime in antibody fragments, such as $F(ab')_2$ or Fab′, indicates that they have been produced by digestion with pepsin.

A standard-size $F(ab)_2$ preparation would normally start with 50–200 mg of pure mouse IgG. However, with newly acquired antibodies we normally perform a 'pilot' digestion on 5–10 mg of IgG.

Protocol 2. Preparation of $F(ab')_2$

1. Concentrate the pure mouse IgG1 or IgG2a antibody (we have no experience with IgG3 antibodies) to approximately 10 mg/ml by suitable means. We use an Amicon ultrafiltration stirred cell (Amicon Ltd, Stonehouse, UK) with PM10 filtration membrane and nitrogen pressure at 25 lb/in^2.
2. Stir the antibody in a suitable container and adjust the pH to 4.1 to 4.2 by adding 2 M sodium acetate.
3. Dissolve pepsin (Sigma catalogue No. P6887) to 10 mg/ml in 0.07 M sodium acetate containing 0.05 M NaCl, pH 4.0. Add this dissolved pepsin to the antibody solution at a 3% ratio (w/w) to give the final digest mixture.
4. Incubate the reaction at 37°C in a water bath. At 1 h intervals remove 10 μl samples and fractionate them on Zorbax GF250 bio series HPLC column (*Figure 2*). When less than 10% remains as IgG or when the $F(ab')_2$ peak is no longer increasing, stop the digestion by adjusting the pH back to 8 with 1 M Tris base, pH 9.2. Under these conditions, most IgG1 antibody digestions will require 4–8 h to achieve completion. However, due to the extreme sensitivity of pepsin to pH, the period of digestion can be extended or reduced very significantly by adjusting the pH by just 0.1 of a unit. Digestions which are not completed in a working day can be left overnight at 4°C and then continued the following day.
5. Fractionate the digest mixture on two columns (connected in series) of Ultrogel AcA44 (see 'column 3' in chromatography equipment above) which have been equilibrated in 0.2 M TE8 and harvest the $F(ab')_2$ species.

Protocol 3. Preparation of $F(ab)_2$ from mouse IgG1 using bromelain

1. Concentrate IgG1 as described in *Protocol 1*, then dialyse into 50 mM TE7.
2. Dissolve 10 mg of bromelain (Sigma catalogue No. B 5144) in 1 ml of 50 mM TE7 and activate it by adding 2-ME to a final concentration of 0.5 μM. Incubate for 15 min at 37°C. Add bromelain to the IgG1 solution to give a final concentration of 4% (w/w) and then incubate at 37°C.

3. At 1 h intervals, remove 10 μl samples and fractionate on Zorbax GF250 bio series HPLC column as described for the pepsin digestion in *Protocol 1* (see *Figure 2*). Stop the digestion by adding iodoacetamide (BDH catalogue No. 44181) to a final concentration of 0.5 mM when intact IgG represents less than 10% of digest mixture.
4. Fractionate $F(ab')_2$ on Ultrogel AcA44 as described for the pepsin digestion.

5. $F(ab)_2$ and $F(ab)_3$ multispecific antibody derivatives

5.1 Background

The directed formation of thioether bonds joining two or more Fab fragments through a bifunctional maleimide cross-linker is the key to the synthesis of all

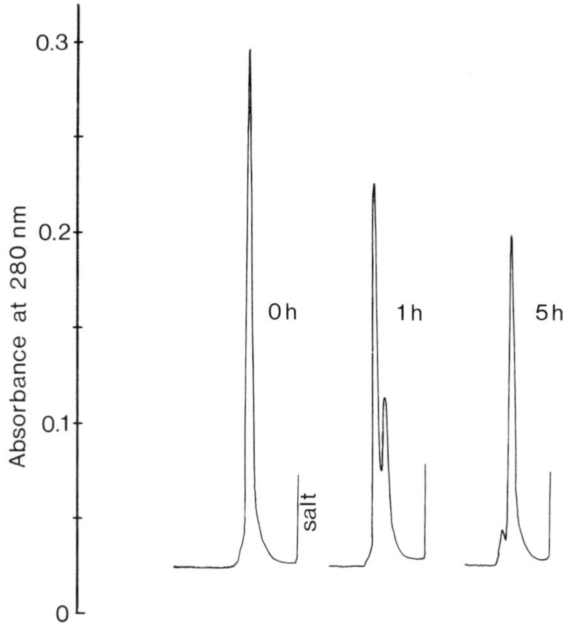

Figure 2. Three HPLC profiles (see Section 4.2) obtained with samples taken at times 0, 1, and 5 h during digestion of a mouse IgG1 monoclonal antibody (8 mg/ml) with 3% pepsin at pH 4.2. At time 0 h the digest mixture shows a single peak of IgG. By 1 h this has been partially converted to $F(ab')_2$ and the trace shows a doublet with the IgG still representing the major species. After 5 h the bulk (>95%) of the IgG (very small leading peak) has been converted to $F(ab')_2$ (single major peak) together with smaller fragments and peptides. This latter material elutes with the 'salt' peak (only the leading edge is shown in each trace).

the multispecific Fab derivatives described in the following sections. The first step in this procedure is the production of $F(ab)_2$ fragments from the required parent antibodies (see above). These fragments, when exposed to low levels of thiol, release univalent FabSH containing free sulphydryl groups which can be employed in chemical cross-linking.

Mouse IgG1 and IgG2a each possess two H–L chain and three inter-H chain S–S bonds. It follows, therefore, that Fab(SH) from such molecules possess five SH groups ($Fab(SH)_5$): two from a H–L chain bond and three from inter-H chain bonds. In the current procedure, these SH groups on one parent antibody (antibody A) are alkylated with a large molar excess of the cross-linker *o*-PDM to yield univalent Fab(mal). Immunochemical studies have shown a strong tendency for *o*-PDM in this reaction to cross-link adjacent SH-groups intramolecularly (14). Thus the SH-group on the C-terminal end of the light chain and its adjacent partner on the H chain, and two SH-groups in the hinge region probably become linked together through *o*-PDM, leaving a solitary SH in the hinge region to react with just one end of the linker ((14) and *Figure 3*). The Fab(mal) is thus left with a single reactive maleimide group ($Fab(mal)_1$) to react with Fab(SH) from a selected partner (antibody B). It should be noted that, under the conditions employed to reduce the $F(ab)_2$, while all hinge-region S–S bonds are broken, only about 50% of those between the H and L chain become reduced. However, this incomplete reduction is not important to the preparation, since, as discussed above, only certain maleimide groups introduced into the hinge-region remain reactive for subsequent conjugation.

The $Fab(mal)_1$ from antibody A is now mixed with $Fab(SH)_5$ from antibody B under conditions which favour cross-linking of maleimide and SH groups and avoid reoxidation of SH groups. When $Fab(mal)_1$ and $Fab(SH)_5$ are mixed in equal amounts the major product is $F(ab)_2$ heterodimer. It is likely that in most cases maleimide will react with SH groups in the hinge region of $Fab(SH)_5$, since they will be more exposed than SH buried between the H and L chain. However, we cannot exclude the possibility that in any Fab(SH) molecules where H–L disulphide bonds have been reduced this latter reaction sometimes occurs (5).

Recently we have found that by increasing the proportion of $Fab(mal)_1$ in the reaction mixture, a significant amount of $F(ab)_3$ derivative is produced in which two molecules of $Fab(mal)_1$ react with one molecule of $Fab(SH)_5$. We do not see large amounts of $F(ab)_4$ or higher polymers from this reaction and we believe that the reaction of more than two Fab(mal) with the SH-containing hinge is sterically difficult. As two of the Fab arms in the bispecific $F(ab)_3$ derivative arise from the maleimidated partner it is possible to control the configuration of antibody specificities in the final product. Thus for use in cellular re-targeting we are able to construct $F(ab)_3$ molecules with either two Fab arms reacting with the effector cell and one Fab arm binding to the target or vice versa (6).

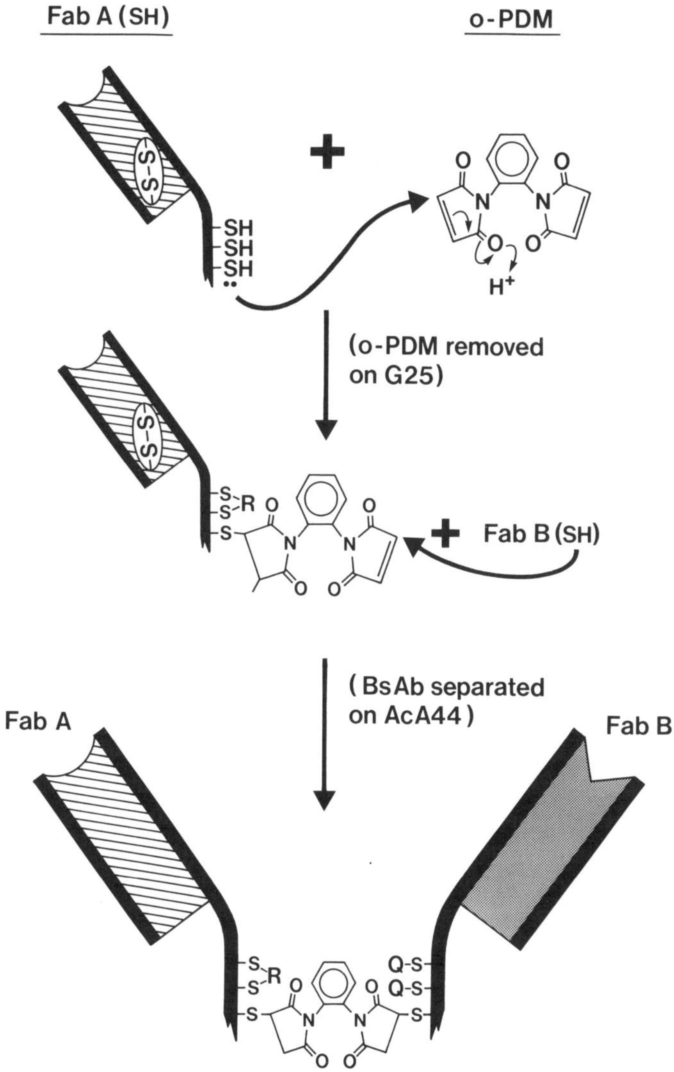

Figure 3. Flow diagram to show conjugation of two antibody Fab fragments using maleimide cross-linker. The various stages in BsAb production are discussed in Section 5 and *Protocol 4*. The proposed typical structure of bispecific $F(ab)_2$ antibody is constructed from Fab fragments derived from mouse IgG1 or IgG2a antibody. Alternative but functionally equivalent structures are discussed in the text. Using a higher ratio of Fab A(mal):Fab B(SH) during conjugation will favour production of bispecific $F(ab)_3$ in which two molecules of Fab(mal) are linked to one molecule of Fab(SH) (*Figure 5A*). Groups joined to cysteinyl sulphur: Q, carboxyamidomethyl; R, *o*-phenyenedisuccimimidyl (as shown linking the two H chains).

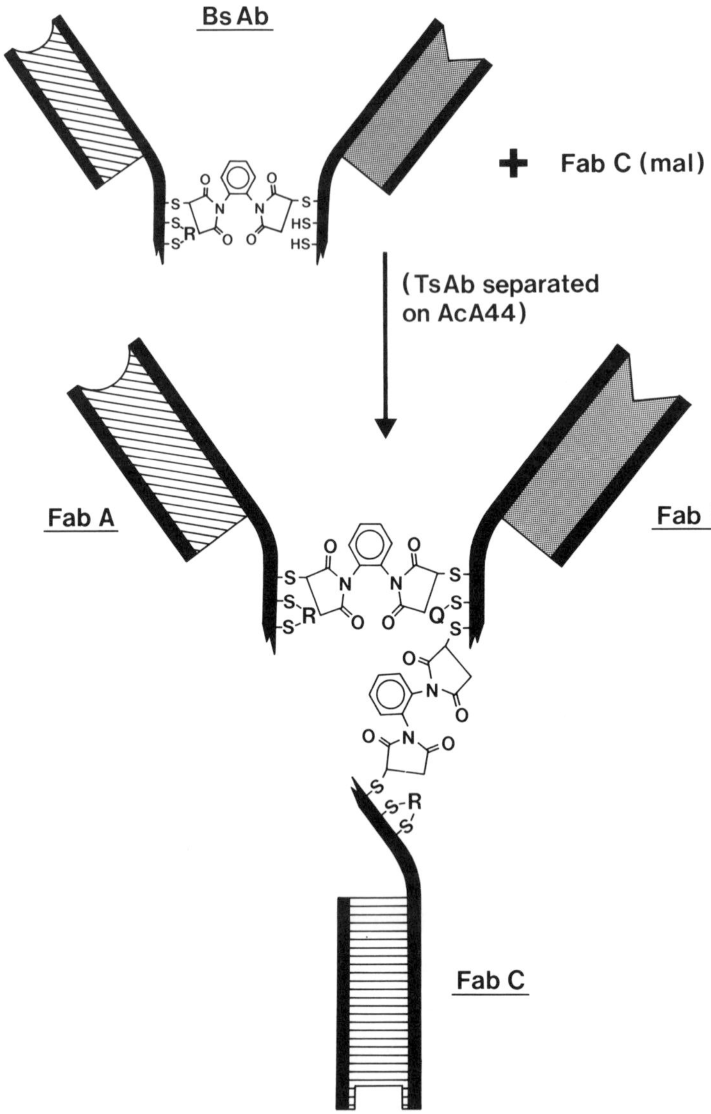

Figure 4. Production of trispecific $F(ab)_3$. BsAb ([Fab A × Fab B](SH)) is conjugated to Fab C(mal) as described in *Protocol 6* to give the proposed $F(ab)_3$ structure. Groups joined to cysteinyl sulphur are as given in *Figure 3*. Note that before the final product was alkylated with iodoacetamide, one hinge-region sulphydryl group remained, offering the potential for linking at least one more Fab′(mal) fragment to yield $F(ab')_4$ (see *Figure 5*).

Because this methodology relies on a single remaining SH after intramolecular cross-linking by *o*-PDM, the species of Fab chosen to bear the maleimide group must be derived from IgG with an odd number of hinge disulphide bonds: among the mouse IgG subclasses IgG1, IgG2a (both with three bonds), and IgG3 (one bond) qualify, while IgG2b (four bonds) does not. The same restriction does not apply to the Fab(SH) partner, and in this case the number of hinge-region SH groups controls the size of Fab derivatives produced. Thus, while it is possible to construct $F(ab)_3$ and $F(ab)_4$ derivatives using mouse Fab(SH), when this species is substituted by rabbit Fab(SH), which contains only one hinge-region SH group, the major product is always bispecific $F(ab)_2$ with little $F(ab)_3$ or $F(ab)_4$ (5). Failure to produce significant amounts of $F(ab)_3$ and $F(ab)_4$ with rabbit Fab(SH) (5) indicates that the hinge-region SH group is the primary site of conjugation and that, under the conditions adopted, relatively little use is made of SH groups arising from the reduction of the H–L chain disulphide bond.

The protocol for preparing a trispecific $F(ab)_3$ is to first prepare bispecific $F(ab)_2(SH)$ containing antibody A and antibody B Fab fragments, and, having isolated this reagent, to link it to Fab from antibody C (*Figure 4*). Bispecific $F(ab)_2$ is prepared and isolated as usual, but SH groups are left in a reduced state and not alkylated at the end of the preparation (*Protocol 4*). This $F(ab)_2(SH)$ is then used in a second conjugation with an excess of $Fab(mal)_1$ from the third antibody. From this second conjugation we obtain $F(ab)_3$ and small amounts of putative $F(ab)_4$ (see *Figure 5* B) which would have arisen if two $Fab(mal)_1$ fragments from antibody C had combined with one $F(ab)_2(SH)_{>2}$ molecule. The same restrictions apply to the selection of the third Fab fragment, Fab C, regarding SH groups and maleimidation, as they did to Fab A (above).

Once isolated, multispecific antibody preparations are dialysed into PBS, filter sterilized and stored in aliquots at −20°C.

5.2 Preparation of multispecific derivatives

Protocol 4. Preparation of bispecific $F(ab)_2$

Conditions given are for small-scale preparation (1–5 mg) of BsAb. Larger quantities will require appropriate scaling up of the two G25 columns.

1. $F(ab)_2$ fragments from the two selected antibodies are concentrated to between 5 and 12 mg/ml by ultrafiltration in an Amicon unit and, if necessary, dialysed into 0.2 M TE8. For these small (1–5 mg) sized preparations we process 1 ml samples of each fragment.
2. Reduce both $F(ab)_2$ preparations by addition of 1/10 volume of 220 mM 2-ME (final concentration 20 mM; see Section 2). Samples are incubated at 30°C for 30 min and then chilled in an ice-bath. It is important that temperature is maintained below 4°C for the rest of the preparation.

Protocol 4. *Continued*

3. Select the Fab (Fab A) sample to be maleimidated, and remove all reducing agent by chromatography on column 1 (G25) equilibrated in 0.05 M AE buffer and maintained at 4°C (see Section 3 (a)). Collect protein in minimum volume (8–10 ml) in a plastic universal placed in an ice-bath. Avoid any contamination by the 2-ME peak at all costs. Leave the column flowing to remove all 2-ME (this column is required again in preparation).
4. Check condition of Fab A(SH) from G25 samples by chromatography on HPLC (see *Protocol 7*).
5. While the Fab A(SH) is on the G25 column, dissolve 16.1 mg *o*-phenylenedimaleimide (*o*-PDM; Sigma catalogue No. P 7518) in 5 ml dimethylformamide (DMF; BDH catalogue No. 10322) which gives a 12 mM solution and immediately chill in a methanol ice-bath.
6. Transfer the Fab A(SH) sample, complete with ice-bath, to a magnetic stirrer, add a small magnetic flea, and stir rapidly. Add one half-volume (normally about 4 ml) of cold 12 mM *o*-PDM quickly; allow the two liquids to mix before turning off the stirrer. Leave the reaction mixture in an ice-bath for 30 min.
7. When all 2-ME is washed from column 1 (G25), load the second reduced F(ab)$_2$ preparation (Fab B(SH)) and separate as for Fab A(SH).
8. Collect 8–10 ml of Fab B(SH) from the column in a suitable container suspended in an ice-bath and check its size on HPLC (*Protocol 7*).
9. Load Fab A(mal) (maleimidated) via the peristaltic pump on to column 2 (G25; Section 3 (a)). Deliver Fab A(mal) directly into a container holding Fab B(SH) while it stands in an ice-bath. It is always a useful precaution at this stage to take a small sample of Fab A(mal) as it emerges from column 2 and again check its size on HPLC.
10. Rapidly concentrate the Fab A(mal) and Fab B(SH) mixture to approximately 5 mg/ml (normally back to starting volume of F(ab)$_2$ fragments) by ultrafiltration in an Amicon chamber at below 5°C. Carefully remove the reaction mixture from the Amicon into a suitable container (such as a plastic universal) and leave at approximately 4°C overnight. Always slightly over-concentrate sample in the Amicon and wash all residue from chamber with a little fresh chilled buffer.
11. Add 1/10 volume 1 M NTE8 followed by 1/10 volume 220 mM 2-ME (see Section 2). Incubate at 30°C for 30 min and alkylate by adding 1/10 volume 250 mM iodoacetamide in 0.2 M TE8. Any precipitate which may have formed during concentration (step **10**) should have now cleared. However, it may be advisable to centrifuge the sample (1500*g*) for 20 min to remove any slight aggregates before final chromatography.

12. Load the reaction mixture via the peristaltic pump on to two AcA44 columns connected in series (Section 3 (a)) and collect 7.5 ml fractions (see *Figures 3* and *5A*). These columns are equilibrated and stored in 0.2 M TE8. Characteristically three main protein peaks are eluted with the larger central peak, which represents more than 50% of the eluted material, being bispecific $F(ab)_2$. The position of this peak is approximately the same as that of the $F(ab)_2$ fragments isolated after proteolysis of mouse IgG. Other species eluted include an IgG-sized derivative, which we believe is $F(ab)_3$ (see below), and any unconjugated Fab. For unexplained reasons Fab(SH) and Fab(mal) in this latter peak sometimes partially resolve to give a double peak or a main peak with shoulder. Much later in the fractionation run a 'salt' peak will appear containing reducing and alkylating agents.

13. Harvest and pool required material taking only the central two-thirds of any peak to avoid contamination from neighbouring material. It is always a good idea to run the final product on HPLC to check its homogeneity.

14. Concentrate in an Amicon chamber and dialyse into PBS.

The derivative is now ready to be checked for contamination by mouse Fcγ (*Protocol 9*).

Protocol 5. Preparation of bispecific $F(ab)_3$

Conduct steps **1–14** as for *Protocol 4* except that the ratio of Fab A(mal):Fab B(SH) should be increased from 1:1 to at least 2:1. The UV trace in *Figure 5A* shows a typical elution profile for $F(ab)_3$ preparation.

Protocol 6. Preparation of trispecific $F(ab)_3$

1. Perform steps **1–13** of *Protocol 4* with the following modifications

(a) Ideally start BsAb preparation with 10–20 mg each of Fab A and Fab B in 3 ml or less of 0.2 M TE8. Three millilitres of protein is the maximum volume which can be 'desalted' safely on column 1 in steps **3** and **9** of *Protocol 4*. Smaller starting quantities can be used but difficulties may be experienced later in the preparation, especially if a low yield of BsAb is obtained during this first conjugation.

(b) It is **essential to omit** the alkylation step with iodoacetamide in step **11**. This leaves SH groups in the [Fab A × Fab B] ([Fab A × Fab B](SH)) BsAb on which to couple a third Fab.

2. Concentrate [Fab A × Fab B](SH) to between 2 and 5 mg/ml in an Amicon.

Protocol 6. *Continued*

3. $F(ab)_2$ from Fab C is concentrated to 5–10 mg/ml and if necessary dialysed into 0.2 M TE8. Each 1 mg of [Fab A × Fab B](SH) BsAb will need 2 mg of Fab C for this second conjugation.
4. Incubate Fab C and [Fab A × Fab B](SH) with 1/10 volume of 220 mM 2-ME (final concentration 20 mM) at 30°C for 30 min and then chill in an ice-bath. Throughout the remainder of the conjugation maintain temperature below 4°C.
5. Perform steps **3–6** of *Protocol 4* with Fab C.
6. Perform steps **7** and **8** of *Protocol 4* with [Fab A × Fab B](SH).
7. Load Fab C(mal) via peristaltic pump on to column 2 (G25; see Section 3(a)). Deliver Fab C(mal) directly into a container with [Fab A × Fab B](SH] while it stands in ice-bath. Ensure to take a small sample of Fab C(mal) as it emerges from column 2 and check its size on HPLC (*Protocol 7*).
8. Rapidly concentrate the Fab C(mal) and [Fab A × Fab B](SH) mixture to approximately 5 mg/ml (i.e. approximately starting volume) by ultrafiltration in an Amicon chamber at below 5°C.
9. Remove sample from Amicon and perform steps **11–14** of *Protocol 4*. A typical UV trace obtained by chromatography of the final reaction mixture on AcA44 is shown in *Figure 5B*. It shows that the major products of the conjugation are trispecific $F(ab)_3$ and $F(ab)_4$.

5.3 Analysis of antibody fragments on HPLC

For rapid analysis of antibody fragmentation during proteolysis and conjugation during multispecific antibody preparation, an HPLC system fitted with a Zorbax^R bio series GF250 column is used (see Section 3(e)). This will resolve IgG-, $F(ab)_2$-, and Fab-sized molecules in approximately 20 min and can be performed while the IgG digestion or the multispecific antibody preparation is in progress. For most purposes a small sample of antibody or antibody derivative (10–100 μg) is simply loaded directly on to the column and the eluted product monitored at 280 nm. However, we have found that when monitoring multispecific antibody preparations, reduced Fab fragments (Fab(SH)) rapidly reoxidize to form $F(ab)_2$ while on the Zorbax column. The following protocol overcomes this problem.

Protocol 7. Alkylation of small antibody samples for HPLC

1. Dissolve 9.3 mg of iodoacetamide in 1 M NTE8 (50 mM).
2. Add 5 μl of iodoacetamide solution to 45 μl of Fab(SH) and leave at room temperature for 2 min. The Fab(SH) is sampled as it elutes from the G25

column (column 1), at the very top of the protein peak to maintain sufficient concentration for the HPLC run. By dissolving the iodoacetamide in a strong buffer (1 M NTE8) the pH of the Fab(SH) sample (pH 5.2 when it emerges from G25 column) will be raised close to 8.0, a level at which alkylation proceeds very rapidly.

3. Load approximately 10 μl on the HPLC and fractionate. By monitoring the column effluent at two UV wavelengths (254 nm and 280 nm) it is possible to distinguish protein from salt peaks. Proteins absorb more strongly than salts at 280 nm, while at 254 nm the reverse is the case.

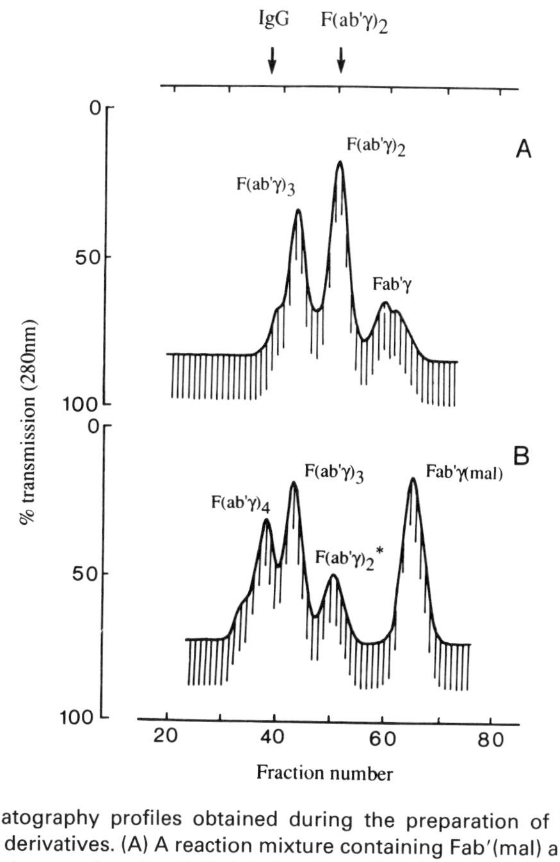

Figure 5. Chromatography profiles obtained during the preparation of bispecific and trispecific $F(ab')_3$ derivatives. (A) A reaction mixture containing Fab'(mal) and Fab'(SH) at a weight ratio 1.5:1 was reduced and alkylated and then fractionated on Ultrogel AcA44 in 0.2 M TE8. The unreacted Fab' fragments and the putative bispecific $F(ab')_2$ and $F(ab')_3$ are indicated. (B) A reaction mixture containing bispecific $F(ab')_2$(SH) and Fab'(mal) at a weight ratio of 4:1 was reduced and alkylated and then fractionated as for A. Putative trispecific $F(ab')_3$ is indicated. The arrows indicate the elution position of protein standards from the same columns. (From reference (5).)

5.4 Checking and removing contaminating Fcγ

Our experience has shown that, despite considerable care when preparing multispecific Fab antibodies according to the above methods, they are almost always contaminated with trace amounts of intact IgG antibody and/or Fcγ fragments. This material remains after the initial proteolysis of mouse IgG with pepsin or bromelain and is harvested first with the $F(ab)_2$ fragments and then with the multispecific derivatives. In a number of biological assays even a small amount of intact IgG may invalidate any results. For example, it has been a particular problem when using $F(ab)_2$ BsAb to redirect the cytotoxicity in human T cells without inadvertently recruiting NK cells via their Fcγ receptors (CD16). Also, when examining the separate roles of CD2 and CD16 in activating lymphocytes, we have found contaminating IgG a major problem ((6) and A. Tutt, unpublished data).

To overcome this problem all multispecific Fab preparations can be checked for the presence of mouse Fcγ by immunoassay and, if necessary, absorbed by immunoaffinity chromatography. Typically, contaminating Fcγ (and/or IgG), which might be present at 2–4 ng/μg of derivative, is undetectable by ELISA after one passage through the anti-Fcγ immunosorbent.

Protocol 8. Enzyme-linked immunosorbent assay (ELISA) for mouse Fcγ

1. Dispense 100 μl aliquots of affinity pure sheep anti-mouse IgG (see Section 3(f)) at 5 μg/ml in bicarbonate buffer (see Section 2) into Nunc 96-well Immuno plates (Gibco catalogue No. 4-42404) and leave overnight at 4°C. Individual batches of anti-IgG should be pre-titrated to determine optimal working concentration and avoid high background 'signals'.
2. Discard contents of plate by 'flicking out' into a sink and add 150 μl of PBS containing 1% BSA. Incubate at 37°C for 60–90 min.
3. Wash the plate three times in PBS containing 0.05% Tween 20 (Sigma catalogue No. P 1754) and discard the contents.
4. To each well add 100 μl of test samples (antibody derivative at 20–1 μg/ml) or mouse IgG standard (40–1 ng/ml) diluted in PBS containing 1% BSA. Incubate at 37°C for 90 min. A seven-point standard curve is set up in duplicate on each plate using the parent mouse monoclonal IgG antibodies.
5. Wash the plates five times with PBS containing 0.05% Tween 20 and discard the contents.
6. Add 100 μl aliquots of peroxidase-labelled sheep anti-mouse Fcγ (Serotec, Kidlington, Oxford, UK catalogue No. AAC 01P) diluted 1/1000 in PBS containing 1% BSA and incubate for 90 min at 37°C. Individual batches of peroxidase-labelled antibody should be titrated for optimal working dilution.

7. Wash the plates five times with PBS/0.05% Tween 20 and discard.
8. Add 100 μl of *fresh* substrate (see Section 2) to each well and allow the colour to develop in the dark for 30 min at room temperature.
9. Stop the reaction by adding 50 μl of 2.5 M sulphuric acid to each well.
10. Read the absorbance on an automatic plate reader at 490 nm. The standard curve can be plotted (O.D. against IgG concentration) and the line of best fit drawn. The concentration of IgG in test samples can then be taken from standard curve and expressed as ng of IgG/μg of derivative.

Protocol 9. Removal of mouse Fcγ and IgG from multispecific derivatives

1. Connect anti-Fcγ immunosorbent to a suitable UV monitor and pen recorder with capillary tubing and wash thoroughly with PBS at room temperature. Since multispecific Fab preparations contain only trace amounts of Fcγ or IgG the capacity of the anti-Fcγ column is not critical. For all preparations we use 4 ml of immunosorbent gel packed in a 5 ml Gillette syringe barrel. The gel is retained in the barrel with a thin pad of quartz wool and buffer is introduced via a 19-gauge syringe needle passed through an appropriately sized silicon bung.
2. Allow excess PBS to drain from the top of immunosorbent. Load and wash sample through the column with fresh PBS.
3. Collect the eluted protein in a suitable container.
4. Test Fcγ content of derivative by ELISA (*Protocol 8*).
5. Equilibrate the immunosorbent column in 0.5 M NTE8 and clean with half the column volume of ammonia thiocyanate (see Section 2). Ensure ammonium thiocyanate remains on the column for the minimum time possible and re-equilibrate in 0.5 M NTE8. Finally store the column in 0.2 M NTE8 at 4°C.
6. Filter sterilize multispecific antibody through a 0.2 μm filter and store in suitable aliquots (100–1000 μg) at −20°C. Once an aliquot has been thawed it should be kept sterile at 4°C and not re-frozen, to avoid precipitation.

References

1. Karpovsky, B., Titus, J. A., Stephany, D. A., and Segal, D. M. (1984). *J. Exp. Med.,* **160,** 1686.
2. Nisonoff, A. and Mandy, W. J. (1962). *Nature,* **194,** 355.

3. Brennan, M., Davison, P. F., and Paulus, H. (1985). *Science,* **229,** 81.
4. Milstein, C. and Cuello, A. C. (1983). *Nature,* **305,** 537.
5. Glennie, M. J., McBride, H. M., Worth, A. T., and Stevenson, G. T. (1987). *J. Immunol.,* **139,** 2367.
6. Tutt, A., Greenman, J., Stevenson, G. T., and Glennie, M. J. (1991). *Eur. J. Immunol.,* **21,** 1351.
7. Tutt, A., Stevenson, G. T., and Glennie, M. J. (1991). *J. Immunol.,* **147,** 60.
8. Arvieux, J. and Williams, A. F. (1988). In *Antibodies,* Vol. 1, (ed. D. Catty), pp. 113–36. IRL Press, Oxford.
9. Catty, D. and Raykundalia, C. (1988). In *Antibodies,* Vol. 1, (ed. D. Catty), pp. 75–6. IRL Press, Oxford.
10. Lamoyi, E. and Nisonoff, A. (1983). *J. Immunol. Methods,* **56,** 235.
11. Parham, P. (1983). *J. Immunol.,* **131,** 2895.
12. Milenic, D. E., Estaban, J. M., and Colcher, D. (1989). *J. Immunol. Methods,* **120,** 71.
13. Mariani, M., Camagna, M., Tarditi, L., and Seccamani, E. (1991). *Mol. Immunol.,* **28,** 69.
14. Stevenson, G. T., Pindar, A., and Slade, C. J. (1989). *Anti-Cancer Drug Design,* **3,** 219.

15

Construction and expression of Ig fusion proteins

MARTHA S. HAYDEN, H. PERRY FELL, and NICHOLAS F. LANDOLFI*

1. Introduction

The techniques of molecular biology have made the production of modified and/or novel proteins commonplace. The immunoglobulin (Ig) molecule has been a popular target for modification with the intent of improving the therapeutic potential of a given antibody (reviewed in reference (1)). Prominent examples include 'chimeric' and 'humanized' antibodies intended to minimize human anti-mouse Ig responses and to optimize effector functions mediated by the Fc portion of the molecule in patients. Further manipulations have sought to combine the specificity of an Ig molecule with the functional attributes of another molecule. The majority of this 'antibody engineering' has focused on maintaining the antigen specificity of the original immunoglobulin molecule. These forms of Ig fusion proteins will be referred to here as 'antibody fusions' and are discussed further in Section 5.

More recently, some effort has been directed to combining the effector functions of the Ig constant region, such as Fc receptor binding or complement fixation, with a non-Ig moiety. In this case, the variable region of the Ig molecule is replaced with a non-Ig moiety that confers the binding specificity. Such molecules are referred to as 'immunoligands' (the term immunoadhesion has also been used for Ig/adhesion molecule fusion proteins). In addition to these engineered molecules, antibody structure may be modified to produce single-chain forms of immunoglobulin molecules which either maintain only the binding specificity, or include effector functions as well. 'Single-chain antibodies' which incorporate effector functions are a type of Ig fusion protein. Because the antigen binding specificity of an antibody serves as a substitute, or artificial ligand for a specific receptor, these molecules are functionally equivalent to an 'immunoligand'. Future references will therefore include single-chain antibodies under the designation 'immuno-

* Author to whom correspondence should be addressed.

Table 1. Examples of immunoligands (ligand domains fused to Ig constant regions) that have been constructed and expressed

Ligand	**Ig constant region**	**Expression system**	**Reference**
Human IL-2	Human IgG1	Murine myeloma	2
Human CD4	Human IgG1	Human embryonic kidney	3
Human CD4	Murine IgG2a, IgM	Murine myeloma	4
Human CD8	Human IgG1	COS	5
Human CD44	Human IgG1	COS	5
Murine homing receptor	Human IgG1	Human embryonic kidney	6
Human ELAM-1	Human IgG1	COS	7
Human Leu 8	Human IgG1	COS	7
Human GMP 140	Human IgG1	COS	8
Human CD22	Human IgG1	COS	9
Human VCAM	Human IgG1	COS	10
Human CD7	Human IgG1	COS	10
Human ICAM 1 and 2	Human IgG1	COS	11
Human CD31	Human IgG1	COS	11
Human B7	Human IgG1	COS cells, CHO cells	12
Human CTLA4	Human IgG1	COS cells, CHO cells	13
Anti-tumour L6	Human IgG1 (NO CH1)	COS cells	Hayden *et al.* (in preparation)

ligand'. Examples of some of the immunoligands that have been constructed are presented in *Table 1*. A schematic representation of these types of molecules are shown in *Figure 1*.

The utility of creating such molecules ranges from their value as experimental reagents to their potential usefulness as therapeutic agents. The addition of an Ig constant region can turn a particular ligand into a versatile probe. For example, the presence of an Ig constant region can greatly simplify the purification of the reagent (e.g. Protein A affinity chromatography), and can serve as a valuable molecular tag for detection by ELISA, fluorescent, or autoradiographic assays. The potential value of an immunoligand as a therapeutic agent is much more speculative. The addition of an immunoglobulin constant region to a ligand imparts to that ligand the antibody effector functions attributed to the constant region. These include Fc receptor binding (and thus the potential to mediate antibody-dependent cellular cytotoxicity), long serum half-life, complement fixation, and placental transfer. Thus, if the ligand has specificity for a cell type that is characteristic of a disease state (e.g. neoplasia) the immunoligand may be an effective form of passive immunotherapy.

While many of the immunoligands that have been constructed have replaced the variable domain with another member of the Ig superfamily, the use of ligand domains that are not members of this superfamily has also been successful. Thus, one should be able to construct an immunoligand using any

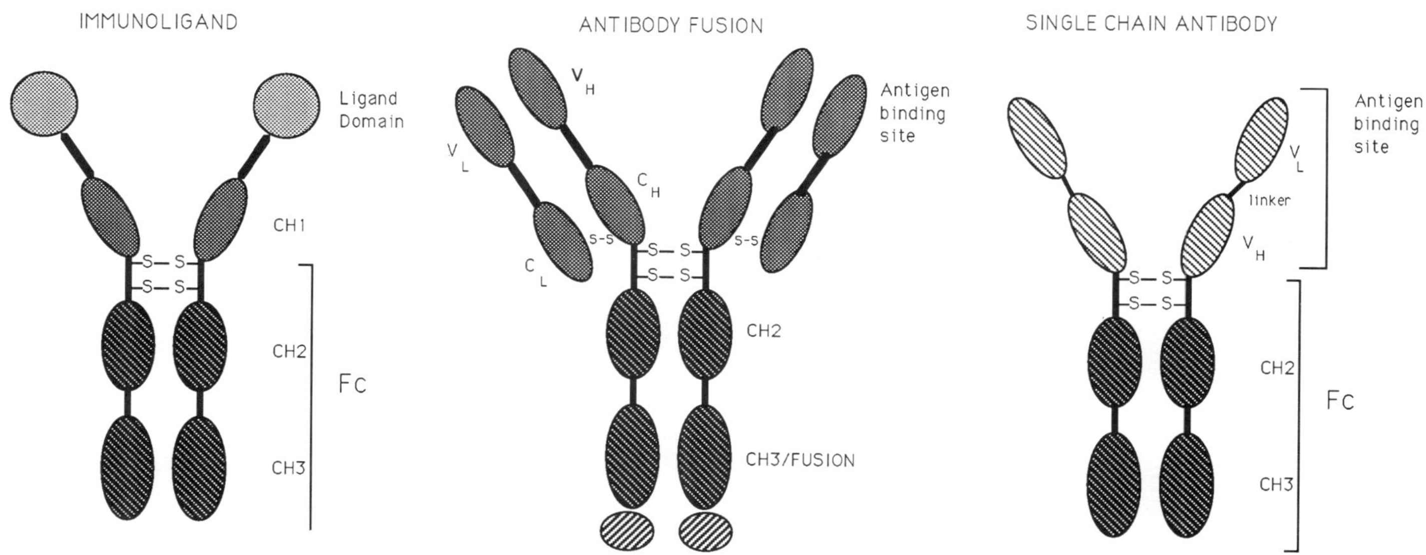

Figure 1. Schematic representation of various Ig fusion proteins. Three basic structures are presented. The 'immunoligand' maintains an Ig Fc region, but has the variable region replaced with a ligand domain from another molecule. The 'antibody fusion' retains its original specificity for antigen by virtue of its variable-region domains, but incorporates novel activity in conjunction with the Fc portion of the molecule. Finally, 'single-chain antibodies' possess both antigen binding and Fc sequences on a single protein chain which can form homodimers, thus providing Ig effector functions. CH, constant region of the Ig heavy chain; CL, constant region of the Ig light chain; VH and VL, variable region of the Ig heavy and light chain, respectively.

binding moieties (e.g. hormone, receptor, lectin, peptide, etc.), and subsequent characterization of the molecule will reveal to what level it retains the functional activity of the ligand and Ig domains. This characterization should include analysis of the binding activity of the ligand domain, as well as any other assayable activity of the ligand. In addition, the status of the Ig effector function should be assayed.

2. Design and construction of an immunoligand

As *Table 1* indicates, a variety of non-Ig domains have been successfully substituted for the variable region of the Ig heavy chain (or light chain). The resulting chimeric molecules all exhibit the original binding specificity of the ligand, and those that contain the Ig Fc region that have been assayed for Ig effector function possess these capacities. This implies that a variety of ligands can be successfully utilized in the construction of an immunoligand, with the only limitation being one's creativity.

The assembly and construction of an immunoligand expression vector involves basic molecular biology techniques and the reader is directed to technique manuals that describe these methods in detail. The choice of the expression system used will dictate the appropriate elements of the vector (a variety of expression systems have been successfully used to produce these chimeric molecules: see *Table 1*).

3. Expression

3.1 Transient mammalian expression of fusion proteins

Initial characterization of the functional properties of Ig Fc-bearing fusion proteins can be simply and rapidly performed using a transient expression system. We have adapted an existing system (14) for transient mammalian expression of cDNA to express constructs encoding such proteins in COS cells. The expression vector pCDM8 was modified to contain a portion of cDNA encoding the human IgG1 heavy-chain hinge, CH_2, and CH_3 domains (*Figure 2*). Various truncations of the heavy-chain constant regions may be used depending on the effector functions desired. Constructs which incorporate all of the heavy chain from CH1 to CH3 or which delete the CH1 domain have been successfully expressed and characterized. In the example shown in the figure, the leader segment from the anti-tumour antibody L6 (15) light-chain gene was cloned just upstream to direct secretion of the eventual fusion protein. Other secretory signal peptides might be substituted depending on the sequences available. Unique restriction sites should be located at the fusion junctions between the leader sequence and the Fc tail to facilitate the cloning of ligand domains in the intervening region. The desired domains may be amplified by PCR using primers which terminate with these restriction sites. The design of these oligonucleotides must maintain the reading frame

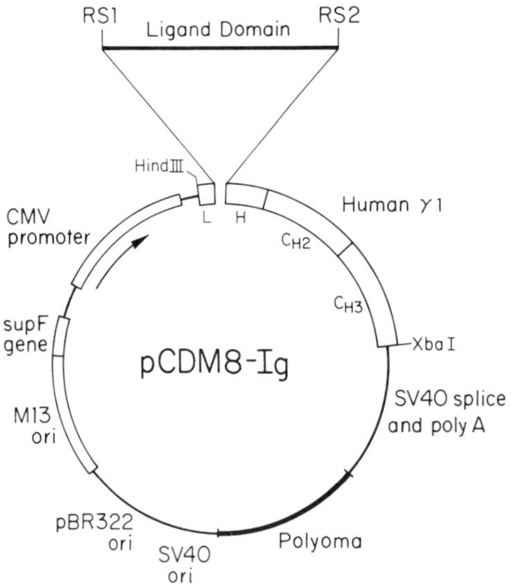

Figure 2. Modification of pCDM8. The expression vector pCDM8 can be modified by removal of the stuffer fragment and replacement with adaptor sequences for expression of single-chain antibody molecules, immunoligands, or antibody fusions. A *Hind*III-*RS1* (restriction site No. 1) fragment encoding the leader peptide from the variable region of the αL6 light chain is inserted to achieve secretion of the expressed molecules. The Fc domain of human IgG1 is included downstream as a *RS2-Xba*I segment to facilitate detection, purification, and characterization of fusion constructs. Between these two sequences, a fusion cassette may be inserted that encodes antibody variable regions separated by an amino acid linker such as $(Gly_4Ser)_3$ or the ligand domain of interest.

introduced by the leader segment, often requiring the addition or deletion of a few amino acids at the junction between domains. It is particularly important that maintenance of the reading frame be verified when constructing molecules which combine several specificities. Insertion of several domains and associated linker segments between the leader and the Fc region increases the potential for frameshifts resulting in failure to express the desired protein. After the PCR fragment is ligated into the expression vector, the construct is transformed into bacteria for propagation and screening. It is recommended that individual clones be sequenced to verify the integrity of the construct. Plasmids with the correct sequence are expressed by transient transfection of COS cells using the DEAE–dextran procedure (see *Protocol 1*).

Protocol 1. Transient transfection of COS cells with DEAE–dextran

1. On the day before transfection, plate COS cells as follows in DMEM (GIBCO-BRL) containing 10% FBS:
   - 3×10^5 cells/60 mm dish (3 ml at 1×10^5/ml)

Protocol 1. *Continued*

- 2×10^6 cells/150 mm dish (15 ml at 1.35×10^5/ml)

Tissue-culture petri dishes may be 60 mm—Corning 25010, 100 mm—Corning 25020, or 150 mm—Falcon 3025.

2. Make the transfection medium on the day of the experiment:
   - 50 ml serum-free DMEM
   - 20 µl 0.25 M chloroquine in PBS (0.2 µm filtered, keep frozen until use) or some multiple of the proportions above.
3. Make a DNA cocktail by mixing with PBS and DEAE–dextran 50 mg/ml in PBS (0.2 µm filter, keep frozen until ready to use) **in the order below** (or DNA will precipitate out of solution):

	Per 60 mm dish	Per ten 150 mm dishes
DNA	3–10 µg pure plasmid or 12–15 µl of 30 µl miniprep DNA (*x* µl)	350–400 µg DNA *x* ml (100–400 µl)
PBS	68 µl (80-*x* µl)	(6.25-*x*) ml
DEAE–dextran	20 µl	1.25 ml
Total volume	100 µl	7.5 ml

4. Add the DNA cocktail to 1.7 ml transfection medium/60 mm dish for small plate transfections. For large 150 mm plates, add 7.5 ml of DNA cocktail to 110–120 ml transfection medium.
5. Aspirate the culture medium from COS cells and add the DNA mix. (1.8 ml/plate—60 mm, or 11–12 ml/plate—150 mm.)
6. Incubate 2.5–3.5 h at 37°C.
7. Aspirate the DNA-containing medium.
8. Add 10% DMSO in PBS (0.2 µm filtered) (2–3 ml—60 mm, or 10 ml—150 mm). Incubate for 1–2 min and no more. Timing is not critical—but do not overshock the cells or they will fail to adhere to the plate.
9. Aspirate and wash once with serum-free DMEM.
10. Add 3–3.5 ml DMEM/10% FBS per 60 mm dish or 12–15 DMEM/10% FBS per 150 mm dish. Incubate at 37°C.
11. If serum-free medium is desired, aspirate DMEM/10% FBS after 24 h following transfection. Wash once with serum-free DMEM and add 3–3.5 ml/60 mm or 12–15 ml/150 mm dish serum-free DMEM. Incubate at 37°C.
12. Collect medium for assay at 72–96 h post-transfection. Cells can also be harvested at this time if desired. For small plate transfections, cells and supernatants may be harvested at 48 h instead of 72–96. Fresh serum-free DMEM may be added (1–2 ×) for an additional 72 h prior to harvesting.

A total of two to three harvests of cell supernatants is usually performed for large plate transfections.

13. Spin out cells from culture supernatants in a table-top or other centrifuge at 1000*g* Transfer the liquid to a new tube. If desired, 10% sodium azide may be added to a final concentration of 0.1% to prevent microbial contamination.
14. Analyse the culture supernatants as described in later sections of this chapter.

The DEAE–dextran transient transfection technique is particularly suitable for constructs which express a desired sub-set of specificities or activities and for discriminating between molecules containing engineered variations in structure, because the time elapsed between construction and expression of protein in active form is only three days. Refolding or other manipulations are unnecessary, eliminating tedious and often fruitless attempts to recover correctly folded, active protein from the host cells.

3.2 Transfection for stable expression

Transfection for stable expression will result in a cell-line that constitutively produces the immunoligand. Several cell-lines have been successfully employed for the stable production of recombinant products. We have successfully used electroporation to introduce the vector, together with a drug-resistance encoding plasmid into the non-secreting murine myeloma cell-lines Sp2/0 or Ag8.653.

Protocol 2. Transfection of Sp2/0 cells by electroporation

1. Wash the Sp2/0 cells once in cold 0.05 M PBS. Re-suspend the cells at a concentration of 10^7/ml in cold PBS. Keep the cells on ice until electroporation.
2. Place 1 ml of the cell suspension in the electroporation cuvette.
3. Add 10–50 μl of vector DNA (at a 1 mg/ml concentration).
4. Electroporate the cells at 300–400 V (BioRad Gene Pulser or equivalent).
5. Place the cells on ice for 10 min.
6. Add 9 ml of DMEM + 10% FCS to the cells and plate 100 μl per well into a 96-well tissue-culture plate.
7. Incubate the cells for 24 h before placing them under drug selection.
8. Monitor the wells for the appearance of resistant colonies.

The concentration of the drug used for selection should be empirically determined beforehand as the lowest concentration that will cause 100%

death of the recipient cell-line. The supernatant from wells containing drug-resistant transfectants can be assayed for the production of the immunoligand by ELISA (*Protocol 3*) once the transfectants cover an area equal to or greater than 25% of the well.

Transfectants that are positive in the ELISA assay should be ranked in terms of their relative level of production. This can be done by assaying various dilutions of the supernatants from positive transfectants. The transfectant that gives the strongest signal in the ELISA assay at a given dilution is the best producer and should be selected for cloning and subsequent analysis of the clones. Absolute levels of expression can be determined by two or three rounds of cloning; subsequent selection of the highest producer should result in a stable transfectant.

4. Detection and characterization of immunoligands

Since the molecules described in this section bear immunoglobulin Fc regions, detection and purification can be carried out as for monoclonal antibodies.

4.1 ELISA

Protocol 3. Detection of immunoligand by ELISA

1. Pre-coat a 96-well ELISA plate (e.g. Immulon 1, Dynatech Laboratories) by adding 100 μl of a 1:500–1:1000 dilution in PBS of a commercially prepared heavy-chain-specific goat anti-human IgG (GαHIgG) to each well and incubate overnight at 4°C.
2. Add 200 μl of ELISA blocking buffer (0.05 M PBS pH = 7.4, 1% (w/v) BSA, 0.5% (v/v) Tween 20) to each well and incubate for 1 h at room temperature to block all unoccupied protein binding sites in the well.
3. Wash wells three times with 200 μl of ELISA wash buffer (0.05 M PBS pH = 7.4, 0.5% Tween 20) to remove excess GαHIgG and BSA. (Wells may be washed using an ELISA plate washer, or by simply filling wells and flicking the wash solution into a sink.)
4. Add 100 μl of sample to be tested for presence of immunoligand (may be neat supernatant or a dilution). Also add 100 μl of 100 ng–10 μg/ml of human IgG1 to a well(s) to serve as the positive control, and 100 μl of fresh tissue-culture medium to a well(s) to serve as the negative control.
5. Incubate for 1 h at room temperature.
6. Wash wells three times as above.
7. Add 100 μl of a 1:500–1:1000 dilution of a commercially prepared horseradish peroxidase-conjugated GαHIgG in ELISA blocking buffer.

8. Incubate 1 h at room temperature.
9. Wash wells three times as above.
10. Add the substrate. Prepare substrate solution just prior to use by adding 4 ml of *o*-phenylenediamine dihydrochloride (OPD) stock solution (10 mg/ml in H_2O, aliquots can be stored at −20°C) to 10 ml of phosphate/citrate buffer (0.0486 M citric acid, 0.103 M Na_2HPO_4 pH = 5.0). Add 4 µl of 30% H_2O_2. Add 100 µl substrate solution per well. (**Caution**, OPD is a potential carcinogen.)
11. Stop the reaction after colour development in the positive control (5–15 min) by adding 50 µl of 2.5 M H_2SO_4 per well. The appearance of a yellow colour indicates the presence of human IgG determinants in the tested supernatants. The plate may be read at 492 nm on an ELISA reader to quantify the results.

4.2 Biochemical characterization by immunoprecipitation

Immunoprecipitation analysis from the supernatant of biosynthetically labelled transfectant cells will confirm the chimeric nature of the ligand/Ig fusion protein by verifying the predicted molecular weight of the product. In addition, such analysis will indicate if there is any free ligand or Ig constant region in the supernatant as a result of fusion protein cleavage, and determine if the immunoligand is secreted as a homodimer by the cell.

The immunoprecipitation is carried out by utilizing antisera or monoclonal antibody with specificity for either the ligand or the Ig. In addition, if the Ig isotype used in the immunoligand is one that binds Protein A, this reagent may be used for immunoprecipitation analysis. The antibody/immunoligand complex is then isolated from the supernatant by a solid-phase reagent (e.g. Protein A–agarose), washed free of other labelled proteins, and run on a polyacrylamide gel. Subsequent autoradiography reveals the molecular character of the immunoligand.

Protocol 4. Biochemical characterization by radioimmunoprecipitation

1. 10^7 transfectant cells are incubated from 6 h to overnight in 10 ml of methionine-free medium, containing 1mCi of [^{35}S]methionine. (Dialysing the FCS used in the labelling media can increase the efficiency of labelling by depleting the serum of methionine.) **Note**: volatile breakdown products of [^{35}S]methionine can be released at 37°C and will contaminate the incubator with radioactive vapours, thus labelling should be carried out in a closed flask (or other chamber).
2. Collect the supernatant. Dialyse against two litres of PBS with two changes to remove unincorporated [^{35}S]methionine. (The supernatant may also be concentrated 5–10 ×.)

Protocol 4. *Continued*

3. Divide the supernatant into aliquots for immunoprecipitation. Usually a 1 ml equivalent of neat labelled supernatant per sample is sufficient.
4. Add the antisera/monoclonal antibody to the labelled supernatant (usually ~1 μl of antisera or 500 ng of purified monoclonal antibody is sufficient).
5. Incubate overnight (or a minimum of 3 h) at 4°C.
6. Add 10 μl of Protein A–agarose (Sigma Chemical Co.). **Note**: if the monoclonal antibody employed does not bind Protein A, pre-coat the Protein A–agarose with a rabbit anti-mouse IgG reagent prior to use.
7. Incubate for 1 h at 4°C with agitation.
8. Wash the Protein A–agarose beads three times in 0.025 M Tris buffered saline (TBS) containing 0.5% (v/v) NP40, 0.1% (w/v) SDS, and 0.2% (w/v) Na deoxycholate.
9. Wash one final time in TBS.
10. Dry the pellet (allow to air-dry or dry under a vacuum while spinning).
11. Rehydrate the pellet in 60 μl gel sample buffer, boil, and microfuge. Remove 50 μl for application to a 10–12.5% SDS–polyacrylamide gel. The immunoprecipitates can be analysed using conventional polyacrylamide gel electrophoresis. Analysis under non-reducing conditions will indicate if the immunoligand is secreted in a dimeric (or multimeric) form. The use of an autoradiography enhancer (e.g. Enhance, DuPont) and intensifying screens will optimize detection of the ^{35}S-labelled proteins.

4.3 Biochemical characterization by Western immunoprecipitation

A variation on radioimmunoprecipitation uses supernatants from unlabelled cells. The immunoligand is isolated from the supernatant by binding to *Staphylococcus aureus* cells, eluted and run on a gel. The molecule is detected by Western blotting using an Fc-specific reagent.

Protocol 5. Western immunoprecipitation

1. Harvest supernatants from transfected cultures. Spin out cells and other debris in a table-top centrifuge for 5 min at 500–800*g*.
2. Spin 1 ml aliquot of *S. aureus* cells (Calbiochem Pansorbin #507858) in microfuge for 2–3 min to pellet. Aspirate supernatant. Wash successively in original volume as follows:
   (a) STE-hi (0.15 M NaCl, 0.05 M Tris–HCl, and 1 mM EDTA) pH is adjusted to 7.2 with HCl. Add NP40 to 0.5% (v/v).

(b) STE-lo (same as above, but NP40 is added to 0.05%).

(c) Re-suspend cells in original volume PO_4-RIPAE buffer + 1 mg/ml ovalbumin carrier protein. (PO_4-RIPAE: 0.15 M NaCl, 0.05M $Na_2HPO_4.7H_2O$, 1% (w/v) DOC.Na, 1% (v/v) Triton X-100, 0.1% (w/v) SDS, 5 mM EDTA.) Add 1% aprotinin stock solution, and 30 µg/ml PMSF just prior to use.

3. Add 100 µl cell supernatant to 50 µl washed *S. aureus*. Incubate on ice for approximately 30 min.
4. Pellet cells. Aspirate liquid. Wash once in TNEN (20 mM Tris base, 100 mM NaCl, 1 mM EDTA, and 0.5% NP40; pH = 8.0, adjust with HCl). Re-suspend the final pellet in 30–35 µl SDS-PAGE loading buffer.
5. Boil for 5 min, vortex, then boil for 2 min. Clarify by centrifugation. Load the supernatant on to SDS-PAGE gel.

Gels containing Western immunoprecipitate samples may be transferred to nitrocellulose by published methods, the blots blocked for 60 min in Blotto (PBS, 0.5% (v/v) NP40, 1% (w/v) non-fat dry milk), and incubated for 60 min with alkaline-phosphatase-conjugated goat anti-human IgG1 (usually diluted 1:1000 in Blotto). This reagent is obtained from Boehringer Mannheim Biochemicals (catalogue No. 605 415). Blots are then developed in alkaline phosphatase substrate (substrate = 3.5 mg 4-nitro blue tetrazolium chloride and 6.0 mg 5-bromo-4-chloro-3-indolyl phosphate (Sigma or BMB) per 20 ml alkaline phosphatase buffer (0.1 M Tris pH 9.5, 0.1 M NaCl, 5 mM EDTA)). Alkaline phosphatase buffer is also commercially available as Western Blue from Promega (catalogue No. S384B).

4.4 Purification of immunoligands by affinity chromatography

After a stable or transient transfectant has been isolated and the secreted product has been characterized as being biochemically consistent with the designed molecule, the immunoligand can be easily purified using Protein A for functional studies.

Protocol 6. Purification of immunoligands by Protein A affinity chromatography

1. Accumulate 500 ml of culture supernatant from cultures of the transfectant that have been allowed to overgrow for 2–3 days, or pool harvested culture supernatants from scaled-up transient transfections.
2. Prepare a 1 ml Protein A–agarose column using a reagent such as immobilized Protein A from Repligen (IPA-300).
3. Wash the column with 10 ml PBS or binding buffer (1 M KPO_4 pH 8.0).

Protocol 6. *Continued*

4. Pre-elute column with 2.5 ml of 0.2 M glycine, pH = 2.0 or 0.1 M citrate, pH 2.2.
5. Wash the column with 10 ml PBS or binding buffer (1 M KPO_4 pH 8.0).
6. Pass the supernatant over the column, wash the column with PBS until the $O.D._{280}$ of the column wash is less than 0.1.
7. Elute the bound immunoligand with 4 ml of 0.2 M glycine, pH = 2.0 or 4 ml elution buffer (=0.1 M citrate pH 3.0). Collect 0.5 ml fractions and neutralize the fractions by adding a sufficient amount of 1 M Tris, pH = 9.0 (usually 100 μl) to bring the pH to 7.5–8.0.
8. Assay the fractions for absorbance at 280 nm, and pool appropriate fractions.
9. Dialyse against 2 litres PBS overnight at 4°C.

While Protein A is a convenient purification matrix, it is of course also possible to couple serological reagents with specificity for the Ig or ligand moieties, or the ligand's receptor to Sepharose to serve as an affinity matrix.

4.5 Analysis of the functional activity of the immunoligand

Functional characterization of the immunoligand will indicate to what extent the ligand and Ig moieties have retained their activity. The functional status of the ligand can be examined at the level of binding specificity by a variety of techniques. For example, the status of the IL-2 portion of the IL-2/IgG1 immunoligand was determined by assaying binding to a soluble form of the IL-2 receptor in an ELISA (procedure similar to *Protocol 2* except that the plate was pre-coated with soluble IL-2 receptor instead of goat anti-human IgG). Immunoligands that have binding specificity for cell surface molecules can be conveniently assayed using indirect immunofluorescence and flow cytometry. In this case, the immunoligand is incubated with a target cell that expresses the receptor for the ligand. The unbound immunoligand is washed from the cells and the cells are incubated with a fluoresceinated secondary reagent (e.g. fluoresceinated goat anti-human IgG). The unbound secondary reagent is washed from the cells and they are analysed for immunofluorescence by flow cytometry.

Protocol 7. Analysis of immunoligand binding by indirect immunofluorescence

1. The assay is carried out in 12 × 75 mm polystyrene tubes. Add the immunoligand (in a volume of 10–200 μl) to the tubes. Titration of several dilutions of the ligand may also be performed and compared with a similar

titration of the positive control antibody. There should also be a negative control tube (no immunoligand) to assay autofluorescence and a positive control (antibody known to bind the cell type) to ensure that reagents are working.

2. Add 100 μl of the cells (at a concentration of (2–5) × 10^6 cells per ml) to each tube. The cells should be in a protein-containing liquid (e.g. culture medium or PBS + 0.5–2% BSA).
3. Incubate the tubes on ice (or in the refrigerator) for 20–30 min. Occasionally agitate the tubes. (Keeping the samples cold eliminates the possibility of patching, capping, and subsequent endocytosis of the cell surface marker of interest during the assay.)
4. Wash each sample by adding 2–4 ml cold PBS to each tube and centrifuging for 5–10 minutes at about 200*g*.
5. After centrifugation, pour off the supernatant (blotting any remaining liquid from the lip of the tube on a paper towel) and add the fluorochrome-conjugated detecting reagent (secondary reagent).
6. Incubate the tubes on ice (or in the refrigerator) for 20–30 min. Occasionally agitate the tubes.
7. Wash each sample by adding 2–4 ml cold PBS to each tube and centrifuging for 5–10 minutes at about 200*g*.
8. After centrifugation, pour off the supernatant (blotting any remaining liquid from the lip of the tube on a paper towel). Add 200 μl of 1% paraformaldehyde in PBS to each tube and vortex. This will fix the cells. The samples may be analysed immediately or stored in the dark at 4°C (stored samples are good for several months).

In addition to the analyses described in this chapter, stimulation of proliferation, colony formation, cytotoxicity, or other functions expected of the fusion proteins should be assayed *in vitro*. The type of assay depends on the particular immunoligand constructed. The reader is referred to other chapters in this volume and/or other technique manuals for this purpose. Briefly, the experiment is usually performed in a 96-well microtitre dish, and wells usually include radiolabel, some type of effector cell, target cells if appropriate, dilutions of the immunoligand to be assayed, or dilutions of the native molecules from which they were derived. Incorporation or release of the radiolabelled reagent is then measured at the end of the experiment.

5. Antibody fusions

The other class of Ig fusion proteins are those which make use of the antigen binding site of a particular monoclonal antibody (MAb). Thus, in this case the variable regions are maintained and modifications are directed to the Fc

Table 2. Examples of antibody fusion molecules

Ab specificity	**Fc activity**	**Reference**
Anti-tumour L6	Human IL-2	16
Anti-tumour	TNF	17
Anti-fibrin	Single-chain urokinase	18
Anti-dansyl	Insulin-like growth factor 1	19

region of the molecule (see *Figure 1*, centre). Several examples of fusions of this type are shown in *Table 2*.

These Ig fusions can be used to target biologically active molecules to specific tissues such as tumours. Desired alterations might include immune modulators, sites for specific chemical conjugation of drugs, isotopes, or toxins, or even enzymes which cleave non-toxic prodrugs into chemotherapeutic agents (20). Molecules such as these can be genetically constructed and expressed in two ways. The classical approach has been to clone the Ig variable-region gene segments from the hybridoma expressing the desired specificity, link the segments to constructs encoding modified Fc regions, and transfect them into suitable cell-lines for expression (e.g. Sp2/0 or Ag8.653).

Alternatively, homologous recombination may be utilized to target modifications of the Fc region to the endogenous Ig locus of a hybridoma expressing the desired specificity (21). Modifications are limited to those for which an assay is available (i.e. if an enzyme is desired then an assay for the activity or an antibody-based ELISA must be available). A diagram of two possible strategies is shown in *Figure 3*. Constant-region exons cannot be expressed alone, but require the variable-region exons to provide a transcriptional promoter, translation initiation site, and RNA splice donor site to place the downstream exons in frame. Thus, modified constant regions can be flanked by sequences homologous to the murine heavy-chain Ig locus. When transfected, only those that integrate via a homologous recombination event will result in expression of the modified constant regions, while vectors that insert elsewhere will be silent. A dominant selectable marker is included within the portion of the construct that must be integrated for expression.

The transfection and screening procedures are identical to those described for stable expression (*Protocols 3* and *4*). In practice, one performs a DNA transfection, selects for cells that have incorporated the vector (and are therefore resistant to the appropriate drug), and then screens the surviving transfectants for those that express the desired modification. Frequencies of homologous versus non-homologous integration can vary from 1/1000 to 1/100. There are two basic strategies for directing a modification to the IgH locus. The first is via an insertion vector. This is the simplest to create, in that, all that is required for targeting is a portion of the intron separating the

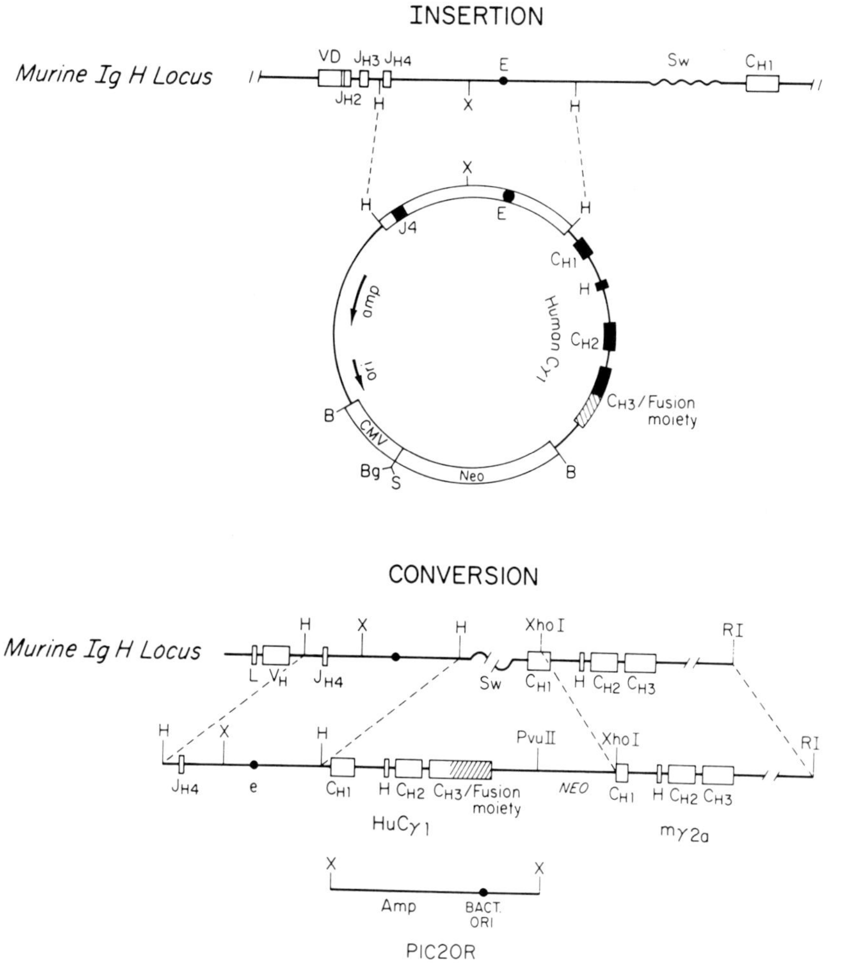

Figure 3. Modification of Ig Fc regions by homologous recombination. The two basic strategies of insertion and conversion are compared. The insertion vector makes use of a single target region of homology represented by the *Hind*III (H) fragment derived from the intron located between the variable- and constant-region exons of the murine IgH locus. The conversion vector bears this homology as well, but in addition, makes use of sequences homologous to the constant-region exons expressed by the specific hybridoma to be targeted.

variable region from the downstream constant regions. Since this region is held in common among all hybridomas regardless of their antigen specificity or heavy-chain isotype, such vectors are essentially 'universal' and can be applied to hybridomas representing a variety of specificities. However, it should be noted that this type of vector, once integrated, results in an effective duplication of the sequences used for targeting (i.e. the intron) and, at a low frequency, can allow for the reverse reaction to occur (i.e. the plasmid can be removed by excision via the duplicated homologous intron), thus reconstituting the original heavy-chain locus (22). This can be avoided by flanking the desired modification by a homologous sequence downstream as well, relying on recombination to occur within both target sequences (i.e. a conversion event). These vectors require more effort, as a separate vector must be created for each of the heavy-chain isotypes to be targeted. However, these vectors consistently result in a high frequency of homologous integration events.

6. Conclusion

Nearly 20 years after the advent of monoclonal antibodies, the predicted therapeutic potential of these agents has not been realized. 'Antibody engineering' has now become a reality. Custom modifications of therapeutically valuable murine monoclonal antibodies, such as 'humanization', will most likely result in agents that will play a future role in the treatment of disease. The role of immunoligands and/or antibody fusion proteins is more speculative at this time; however, it is probable that this type of 'protein design' will play a prominent role in future drug development.

References

1. Winter, G. and Milstein, C. (1991). *Nature,* **349,** 293.
2. Landolfi, N. F. (1991). *J. Immunol.,* **146,** 915.
3. Capon, D. J., Chamow, S. M., Mordenti, J., Marsters, S. A., Gregory, T., Mitsuya, H., *et al.* (1989). *Nature,* **337,** 525.
4. Traunecker, A., Schneider, J., Kiefer, H., and Karjalainen, K. (1989). *Nature,* **339,** 68.
5. Aruffo, A., Stamenkovic, I., Melnick, M., Underhill, C. B., and Seed, B. (1990). *Cell,* **61,** 1303.
6. Watson, S. R., Imai, Y., Fennie, C., Geoffroy, J. S., Rosen, S. D., and Laskey, L. A. (1990). *J. Cell Biol.,* **110,** 2221.
7. Walz, G., Aruffo, A., Kolanus, W., Bevilacqua, M., and Seed, B. (1990). *Science,* **250,** 1132.
8. Aruffo, A., Kolanus, W., Walz, G., Fredman, P., and Seed, B. (1991). *Cell,* **67,** 35.
9. Stamenkovic, I., Sgroi, D., Aruffo, A., Sy, M. S., and Anderson, T. (1991). *Cell,* **66,** 1133.
10. Damle, N. K. and Aruffo, A. (1991). *Proc. Natl Acad. Sci. USA,* **86,** 6403.
11. Damle, N. K., Klussman, K., and Aruffo, A. (1991). *J. Immunol.* (In press.)
12. Linsley, P. S., Brady, W., Grosmaire, L., Aruffo, A., Damle, N. K., and Ledbetter, J. A. (1991). *J. Exp. Med.,* **173,** 721.
13. Linsley, P. S., Brady, W., Urnes, M., Grosmaire, L. S., Damle, N. K., and Ledbetter, J. A. (1991). *J. Exp. Med.,* **174,** 561.

14. Aruffo, A. and Seed, R. (1987). *EMBO J.*, **6,** 3313.
15. Liu, A. Y., Robinson, R. R., Hellström, K. E., Murray, D., Jr., Chang, C. P., and Hellström, I. (1987). *Proc. Natl Acad. Sci. USA,* **84,** 3439.
16. Fell, H. P., Gayle, M. A., Grosmaire, L., and Ledbetter, J. A. (1991). *J. Immunol.,* **146,** 2446.
17. Hoogenboom, H. R., Raus, J. C. M., and Volckaert, G. (1991). *Biochim. Biophys. Acta,* **1096,** 345.
18. Haber, E., Quertermous, T., Matsueda, G. R., and Runge, M. S. (1989). *Science,* **243,** 51.
19. Shin, S.-U. and Morrison, S. L. (1990). *Proc. Natl Acad. Sci. USA,* **87,** 5322.
20. Senter, P. D. (1990). *FASEB J.,* **4,** 188.
21. Fell, H. P., Yarnold, S., Hellström, I., Hellström, K. E., and Folger, K. R. (1989). *Proc. Natl Acad. Sci. USA,* **86,** 8507.

16

Re-shaping human monoclonal antibodies for *in vivo* diagnosis and therapy

M. E. VERHOEYEN

1. Introduction

Until now, the main impact of monoclonal antibodies (MAbs) has been in the *in vitro* diagnostic field, whilst their clear potential as powerful reagents for *in vivo* diagnostic and therapeutic applications remains to be realized. The majority of available and characterized MAbs are of animal origin (often murine) and give rise to a human anti-mouse antibody (HAMA) response when administered to human patients. This response can neutralize the effect of the MAb and can even lead to anaphylactic shock. Furthermore, once patients have been sensitized to murine MAbs and established a HAMA response, repeated dosage schemes and, hence, successful treatment are severely compromised (1, 2). In addition, murine constant regions are not very efficient in interacting with human Complement and ADCC, both of which normally form an excellent line of self-defence against undesired antigens. Human MAbs would be more suitable but, unfortunately, the success in generating rodent MAbs has not been matched by a similar success in the derivation of human MAbs, where many more technical hurdles remain (3). However, an alternative route to obtain human MAbs was established by Dr G. Winter and colleagues, who used protein engineering technology to graft the binding sites of rodent MAbs on to human antibody framework regions. This resulted in so-called re-shaped human antibodies, which had acquired the specificity of the rodent MAbs (4–6).

The rationale behind this technique is as follows. A close examination of antibody sequences reveals that each variable domain contains three hypervariable regions (the complementarity determining regions or CDRs) surrounded by more conserved sequence stretches (the four framework regions or FRs). In the folded protein, each variable domain is found to consist of two disulphide connected β-sheets, formed mainly by the FRs, whilst the CDRs appear as loops on top of the structure. As the heavy- and light-chain variable regions combine, the six CDR loops protrude from the top of the molecule, supported in the correct conformation for antigen binding by a 'scaffold' formed by the FRs. From these observations it was postulated that it should be possible to graft the CDRs of one antibody on to the FRs of another antibody, and the principle has been well proven since. A growing number of human antibodies have been re-shaped successfully (4–12) and preliminary clinical data are available for some, indicating their effectiveness in human patients and the lack of a HAMA response (13, 14).

2. General strategy for re-shaping human antibodies

Firstly, it is necessary to obtain a non-human MAb cell-line which best suits the planned application: the secreted MAb should have the desired specificity and as high an affinity as possible (as some loss of affinity may occur during the re-shaping process). From this cell-line the cDNA encoding the variable regions of the MAb can be cloned, and the nucleotide and amino acid sequences determined. The CDR and framework sequences can be identified according to Kabat by straightforward sequence alignment with other known variable-region sequences (15). Comparison of the new sequences with those already in the Kabat database allows classification into the appropriate variable-region families. This allows identification of non-conserved framework residues which are peculiar to the specific antibody, and different from the 'consensus' residues found in those positions for their particular variable-region families. Such 'unusual' residues could be important for the antigen-binding function of the antibody involved, especially if positioned close to a CDR.

The next step involves the choice of suitable heavy- and light-chain human FRs to accept the non-human CDRs. These do not need to be derived from the same antibody. Ideally the new FRs should belong to a crystallographically solved structure, to facilitate molecular modelling. Practically this is not always possible, as too few antibody structures have been solved to date, so a choice must often be made between either human sequences very similar to those of the original rodent but with unknown three-dimensional structure, or sequences with defined structures, but with more dissimilarities. In the absence of firm rules, final judgement has to be made on a case-by-case basis.

Once suitable human FRs have been chosen and the final sequences designed, the actual construction of the re-shaped antibody can proceed. This is performed at the genetic level: a gene has to be assembled that encodes the newly designed human variable regions, achieved either by *de novo* gene synthesis (4, 7, 12) or, if genes with the required FRs are already available, by site-directed mutagenesis with long oligonucleotides encoding the rodent CDRs (5, 6). The re-shaped variable region genes are then incorporated into expression vectors based on pSV_2gpt (16) or pSV_2neo (17) and linked to suitable human constant-region genes. The choice of constant-region isotype will depend on the application envisaged. For example, for therapy efficient interaction with Complement and good ADCC performance are often desired, in which case γ1 and γ3 human constant-region genes provide the best choice. Finally, the assembled expression vectors are introduced into non-producing myeloma cells by electroporation, to achieve random incorporation into the host cell chromosomes. This is followed by stable expression in a number of transfected cell-lines (transfectomas). Selection of transfectoma colonies is based on the expression of the selective marker genes *gpt* and *neo*, which confer resistance to mycophenolic acid- (MPA) and neomycin-containing media respectively. Surviving transfectoma colonies are screened and tested for functional human antibody production, and single clones are obtained. Further maintenance and treatment of cells is the same as for hybridoma cultures. Re-shaped antibody is harvested from cell supernatants and purified for further characterization, e.g. affinity measurements, achieved by conventional methods.

3. cDNA cloning and sequence determination of antibody variable regions

mRNA can be isolated from antibody-secreting hybridoma cells using established protocols, e.g. as described in reference (18), or using commercial kits (e.g. Invitrogen).

With the mRNA as a template, cDNA can be synthesized following conventional protocols as described by Gubler and Hoffman (19). More recently, reverse transcription of mRNA followed by the polymerase chain reaction (PCR) has been shown to provide an alternative route to obtain large quantities of antibody-specific cDNA (20). Oligonucleotide primers designed to clone antibody variable regions have been described in the literature: they may be complementary to sequences of constant-region genes (e.g. reference (6)), or to consensus sequences corresponding to the relatively conserved termini of variable regions (20), or to consensus sequences derived from antibody signal sequences (21). Primers used in PCR protocols often incorporate restriction sites to facilitate immediate cloning into phage vectors (20). *Table 1* shows six typical examples of primers used for cloning antibody variable regions. Oligonucleotides I and II are complementary to the 5′ ends of the mouse γ1 and κ constant regions respectively, and have been successfully used in our laboratory on a routine basis for conventional cDNA cloning (obviously, if the antibody to be cloned is not of the γ1, κ isotype, other primers will have to be chosen). Oligonucleotides III+IV and V+VI are pairs of universal primers which can be used for PCR cloning of heavy- and light-chain variable regions, respectively. They contain restriction sites to facilitate

Table 1. Examples of primers for cloning antibody variable region genes

I.	5′ GAT AGA CAG ATG GGG GTG TCG TTT 3′
II.	5′ AGA TGG ATA CAG TTG GTG CAG CAT 3′
III.	5′ TGA GGA GAC GGT GAC CGT GGT CCC TTG GCC CCA G 3′[a]
IV.	5′ AGG T(C,G)(A,C) A(A,G)C TGC AG(C,G) AGT C(A,T)G G 3′[b]
V.	5′ GTT AGA TCT CCA GCT TGG TCC C 3′[c]
VI.	5′ GAC ATT CAG CTG ACC CAG TCT CCA 3′[d]

[a,b,c,d] Underlined sequences = *BstE*II, *Pst*I, *Bgl*II, *Pvu*II restriction sites respectively

subsequent cloning for sequencing and expression (20). dsDNA obtained with primers I and II can be cloned in a vector such as pUC9, preferably after adding linkers. Alternatively, when obtained by PCR amplification (using primers III to VI), the vectors described by Orlandi *et al.* can be used (20).

A convenient method for screening *E. coli* colonies (or phage plaques) containing antibody variable-region specific genes is to probe with ^{32}P-labelled ss cDNA made with the same primers as used for the preparative ss cDNA synthesis (this is achieved by adding one or more α-^{32}P-labelled nucleotides to the dNTP mix during the reverse transcription reaction). These probes yield far fewer false positives than ^{32}P-labelled cloning primers, and a high proportion of the clones identified contain a full-sized antibody-specific insert. Nucleotide sequences should be determined for at least three independent clones to rule out possible sequence errors resulting from the initial cloning process. Furthermore, hybridoma lines often produce other Ig mRNAs additional to the ones encoding the secreted MAb, so it is advisable to confirm the resulting amino acid sequences by determining the N-terminal amino acid sequences of both the heavy and light chains of the original MAb. Another advantage of this control is that it allows the identification of the true N-terminal sequence in cases where PCR cloning was performed, and where consequently the N-terminus is force-cloned.

4. Choosing human framework regions for CDR grafting

The process of choosing human FRs compatible with a given set of rodent CDRs can be facilitated greatly by the use of molecular graphics and molecular modelling techniques. Commercial software packages such as InsightII from Biosym Ltd, or academic packages such as FRODO (22) can be used. Protein structural data are available from the Brookhaven Protein Database (Brookhaven National Laboratory, Department of Chemistry, Upton, NY 11973, USA).

Firstly, the sequences obtained by cloning are compared with other sequences in the Kabat database (15) and the V-region family to which they belong is deduced. Then, the new sequences are carefully aligned with the consensus sequences of their respective V-region families (determined from the information in the Kabat database): this may reveal unusual FR residues which, when positioned near a CDR, could play a role in FR–CDR packing, or even in direct antigen binding. It has been shown in crystallographically solved antibody–antigen complexes that, although the main sites of contact with antigen are indeed formed by the CDRs, FR residues near the CDRs can also participate in binding (23).

The next step is to align the rodent sequences of interest with sequences of the different human V-region families in order to decide on the best possible acceptor FRs for the rodent CDRs. Several factors should be taken into consideration when comparing human and rodent antibody sequences. The extent of the differences between the rodent and human antibody frameworks may be critical: the more dissimilar the less likely it becomes that the human frameworks can support the rodent CDR loops in a correct conformation for antigen binding. There are indications that antibody structure is flexible enough to accommodate slight changes and to tolerate 'errors' in assembly of re-shaped antibodies (5), but it is not known what the limitation of such flexibility is. On the other hand it has also been demonstrated that binding can be completely abolished by only one 'wrong' residue (6). Our experience indicates that choosing a very similar human framework gives the best results, even when no defined structure is available as a basis for molecular modelling predictions.

Another important factor is the chemical nature, relative size, and position in the folded proteins of non-conserved framework residues. As it has been shown that certain framework–CDR interactions can be critical to functional binding (5, 6), the possible structural and functional implications for each non-conserved FR residue must be assessed with care. Comparisons with solved structures can be of great help, even in cases where the structure of the antibodies under investigation is unknown: all antibody variable regions share a similar framework structure, and using these known structures it is possible to get a reasonable idea of the position of residues in the molecule. For example, the potential importance of many residues can often be ruled out because they are found to be in positions too far away from the CDRs to have any influence, and/or are likely to be surface residues with their side chains protruding into solution. For some residues, especially residues near CDRs, the impact can be difficult to assess, especially when no structural data are available. Some substitutions could be irrelevant in one case but highly damaging in another. For example, tyrosine and phenylalanine are very similar residues in size and aromatic character and should, therefore, be able to maintain similar van der Waals interactions with neighbouring residues. However, as tyrosine bears a hydroxyl group, it has the potential to take part in strong hydrogen-bond interactions with surrounding residues. This means that, although a tyrosine to phenylalanine substitution may not have serious structural implications, it can have a profound negative effect on the function of the molecule due to the loss of hydrogen bonding. Of course, if in the original rodent antibody the tyrosine is not involved in such an interaction (not usually known), substitution to phenylalanine will probably be irrelevant. Our approach is to incorporate such rodent framework residues into the human frameworks, hoping to retain the potential interactions between those residues and the rodent CDRs. This mostly involves framework residues adjacent to CDRs, and often such residues can be shown to be peculiar to the specific rodent antibody. They may be atypical for the V-region family to which it belongs. Sometimes, residues in the middle of FRs are identified as having the potential to form interactions. In general, though, the aim is to keep the acceptor FRs as 'human' as possible by limiting the number of rodent residues incorporated to a strict minimum. Practically, it may be desirable to design a few alternative structures with a gradually increasing rodent contribution. The CDRs themselves should not be seen by humans as non-human, since they are so hypervariable, and it can be envisaged that antibodies of human origin would use identical sequences to derive the same specificities as the equivalent rodent antibodies.

5. Grafting of rodent binding sites on to human framework regions

5.1 CDR grafting by site-directed mutagenesis with large oligonucleotides

The first successful CDR graft experiments (4–6) made use of FRs based on those of human *VHNEW* (24) and human *VκREI* (25). The initial re-shaped genes were synthesized *de novo*, but subsequent CDR grafts using the same human FRs were achieved by site-directed mutagenesis of these first synthetic genes using large oligonucleotides (5, 6). The oligonucleotides are designed such that they contain a central sequence complementary to, and encoding, the CDR to be grafted, flanked at each side by 12 nucleotides complementary to the human FR sequences immediately adjoining the CDR, to ensure effective annealing during the mutagenesis experiment. Substitutions in the human FRs (to maintain possibly critical rodent residues) occurring near the CDRs can be incorporated in the same mutagenic oligonucleotide, as long as a 12-nucleotide stretch of sequence completely complementary to the adjoining human FR is maintained at each end of the oligonucleotide. Substitutions further away from the CDRs should be made with separate small primers. Although the efficiency is low (≤5%), the three CDRs can be grafted in a single mutagenesis experiment using all three mutagenic primers at the same time. Additional mutagenesis, for example to a residue in the middle of a FR, is better done separately. It is not necessarily critical and provides an alternative gene construct. As explained in the general strategy, it is advisable to keep the number of rodent residues to an absolute minimum, but it can be useful to have a back-up of a few alternative constructs with a gradually increasing number of non-human residues, in case the minimal graft fails to transfer a functional binding site.

Useful templates for this type of CDR graft are the constructs M13mp9-HuVHLys and M13mp9HuVκLys, as described in (5) and (6). These vectors contain re-shaped variable-region genes based on human *VHNEW* and human *VκREI* respectively, incorporated in a gene cassette. The cassette also features a functional Ig heavy-chain promoter and signal sequence (including intron), as well as a splice signal 3′ of the variable region gene to allow functional attachment of a constant-region gene during mRNA formation. The whole cassette can be removed from the M13 vector as a *Hind*III–*Bam*HI fragment for easy incorporation into the final pSV_2gpt- or pSV_2neo-based expression vectors (see *Figure 1*).

Protocol 1 describes how to graft three CDRs simultaneously by using large oligonucleotides, whilst *Protocol 2* describes the screening procedure for correctly mutagenized phage. These protocols are largely based on previously published site-directed mutagenesis methods (26), with some minor adjustments to optimize for this particular procedure. Mutagenesis and screening with small primers (no more than 20 nucleotides) can be done by exactly following the procedures outlined in (26).

To screen for phage containing the desired CDR sequences, the same oligonucleotides as used for the mutagenesis can be utilized. Due to the large size of the primers and the great number of mismatches in the template sequences, a substantial proportion of the mutagenized clones will contain undesired mutations. The number of clones with all three CDRs in place and with the correct sequences is generally low (≤5%). As the highest proportion

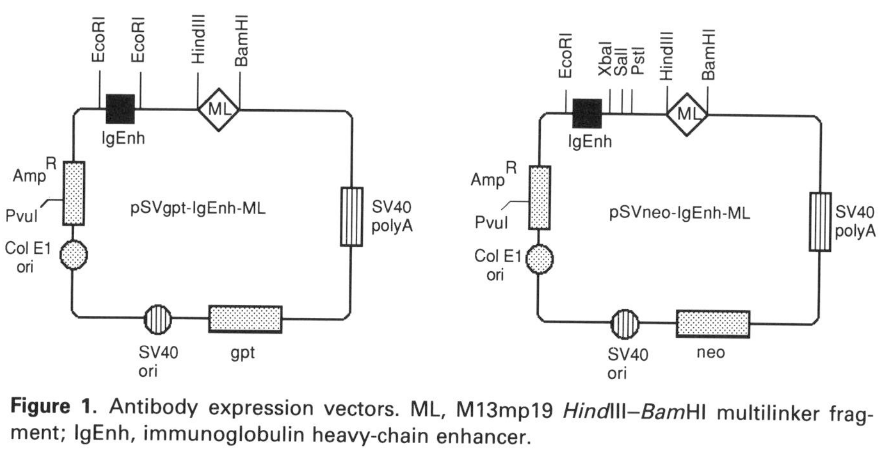

Figure 1. Antibody expression vectors. ML, M13mp19 *Hind*III–*Bam*HI multilinker fragment; IgEnh, immunoglobulin heavy-chain enhancer.

of positives is always obtained for CDR3, 400 plaques are initially grown as colonies and screened for CDR3 only, followed by a secondary round of screening of CDR3-positives for CDR1 and CDR2. It is preferable to re-grow plaques as colonies rather than screening them directly, as better signals are obtained this way.

Positives for all three CDRs are further checked by nucleotide sequencing. It is important to sequence through the whole re-shaped gene of the clone selected for further use (including the surrounding regulatory sequences), as undesired mutations may have been introduced elsewhere in the gene (not necessarily at the intended mutagenic target sites).

Protocol 1. CDR grafting by site-directed mutagenesis

1. Annealing:
   (a) Mix the following in an autoclaved microcentrifuge tube:
   - kinased CDR1, CDR2, and CDR3-primers, 2 μl (5 pmoles/μl) each
   - ss M13 template containing human *V* gene, 1 μl (1 μg/μl)
   - 10× TM buffer,[a] 1 μl
   - H_2O, 2 μl

   (b) Transfer the tube to a small beaker containing water at 80°C and leave to cool down slowly to a temperature below 40°C. This will take 30 min to 1 h.

2. Extension and ligation:
   (a) to the annealed template-primer mix add:
   - 10× TM buffer,[a] 1 μl
   - 5 mM rATP, 1 μl
   - 5mM dNTPs, 1 μl
   - 100 mM DTT, 1 μl
   - H_2O, 4 μl

   (b) Place on ice, then add 1 μl of T4 DNA ligase (10 U/μl) and 1 μl of Klenow enzyme (5 U/μl). Incubate the mixture 16 h at 14°C.

   (c) Stop the reaction by adding 180 μl of 10 mM Tris–HCl (pH 8), 10 mM EDTA. The mixture is kept on ice until used and can be stored at −20°C.

3. Transfections: take 0.1, 1, and 10 μl of the mutagenesis mix to transfect three different aliquots of competent BMH 71-18 mut L cells (27), using BMH 71-18 *E. coli* (28) as lawn cells when plating out (2 × TY plates). Incubate overnight at 37°C. Phage plaques will be clearly visible the next morning.

[a] TM buffer: 10 mM Tris–HCl pH 8.0, 10 mM $MgCl_2$.

Protocol 2. Screening of mutagenized phage

1. Re-grow 400 phage plaques as colonies on fresh 2 × TY plates (overnight; 100 or 200 colonies per plate, create an asymmetric grid).
2. Transfer the phage-infected colonies on to nitrocellulose filters.
3. Position the filters on a sheet of Whatman 3MM paper soaked in 0.5 M NaOH (fresh) with the colonies face up and leave for 3 min. Neutralize by transferring to sheets of Whatman 3MM soaked in 1M Tris–HCl pH 7.4 (2 × for 1 min) and finally to 2 × SSC[a] (5 min).
4. Leave the filters to dry on 3MM paper, then bake for 30 min in a 80°C vacuum oven, sandwiched between sheets of dry 3MM paper.
5. Pre-wet the filters in 6 × SCC for 5 min (room temperature).
6. Pre-hybridize in 10× Denhardt,[b] 6× SSC, 0.2% SDS for 5 min, at 67°C.
7. Rinse the filters in 6× SSC, at room temperature.
8. Place each filter in an 8 cm plastic petri dish containing 3 ml of ^{32}P-labelled oligonucleotide probe (in 6× SSC), with the colonies facing down. Incubate at 37°C for 30 min, then at room temperature overnight. To ensure a homogeneous wetting of the filter during the hybridization, place the petri dish on a slowly rocking platform.
9. Stop the hybridization by removing the filters from the probe solution and wash three times in 6× SSC at room temperature for 1 min.
10. Cover the filters with Saranwrap and autoradiograph (20 min exposure at room temperature is often enough to show up the background, aiding later orientation of the filters with respect to the colonies on the plates).
11. Wash the filters in 6× SSC at 60°C for 1 min and autoradiograph (at −70°C, using pre-flashed film and intensifying screen). If using short oligonucleotides (<20 bases), calculate their dissociation temperature (T_d) first and start washing at T_d −5°C (T_d = 2× number of A, T basepairs + 4× number of G, C basepairs. See (29).)
12. Repeat step **10**, each time incrementing the wash temperature by 3°C, until a satisfactory discrimination between positive and negative signals is obtained. Sometimes this is difficult, even when washing at 72°C or even 75°C, in which case it is better to repeat the wash a number of times under the same conditions or at a lower salt concentration (4× SSC or 2× SSC), rather than further increasing the temperature.
13. Identify the positive colonies on the plates by careful repositioning of the filters and final autoradiograms with respect to the colonies on the plate.
14. Toothpick a number of positive colonies and grow the phage by infecting a culture of *E. coli* host cells (e.g. BMH 71-18).

Protocol 2. *Continued*

15. Prepare ss template from the phage and check the mutagenized gene by nucleotide sequencing.

[a] 20× SSC (1 litre): 175.3 g NaCl, 88.2 g tri Na citrate, H_2O to 1 litre, adjust to pH 7.0 with 10M NaOH, sterilize by autoclaving.

[b] 50× Denhardt (1 litre): 10 g Ficoll 400, 10 g polyvinylpyrrolidone, 10 g BSA (fraction V), H_2O to 1 litre, sterilize by filtering, store in 50 ml aliquots at −20°C.

5.2 CDR grafting by *de novo* gene synthesis

Once the choice of human FRs has been made (see Section 4), a corresponding gene sequence will have to be designed if the gene is not readily available. Optimal codon usage is preferably taken from the sequences of mouse constant-region genes when expression is in a mouse myeloma line. The newly synthesized gene can then be used to substitute the human *VH* or *Vκ* gene in the M13mp9HuVHLys and M13mp9HuVκLys vectors respectively (5, 6), resulting in a vector containing a gene cassette with the same convenience in use as the original one. For practical reasons it is easiest to synthesize the new gene as two or three fragments, flanked by suitable restriction sites, which are then assembled into one complete gene. The synthesized sub-fragments can be cloned in a vector such as pEMBL9 (30) and their sequences checked. To allow this, the fragments should be designed such that they begin and end in pEMBL9-compatible restriction sites (e.g. *Hind*III and *Bam*HI), flanking the restriction sites used for later assembly in a complete gene. This initial cloning allows isolation of the fragments in good yield from the plasmids, and an easy final assembly of the complete gene in a vector of choice. A convenient method is to divide the coding strand of each fragment in oligonucleotides with an average length of 33 bases. The same can be done for the non-coding strand, in such a way that the oligonucleotides overlap approximately 50% with those of the coding strand. Before assembling the fragments, the 5′ ends of the oligonucleotides should be phosphorylated in order to facilitate ligation. *Protocol 3* describes how individual fragments can be assembled.

Protocol 3. Assembly of a synthetic gene fragment from a set of overlapping oligonucleotides

1. Ethanol precipitate the kinased oligonucleotides (25–50 pmol of each).
2. Dissolve the pellet in 30 μl of a buffer containing: 7 mM Tris–HCl pH 7.5, 10 mM 2-mercaptoethanol, and 5 mM ATP. Place the mixture in a water bath at 65°C for 5 min, followed by cooling to 30°C over a period of 1 h.
3. Add $MgCl_2$ to a final concentration of 10 mM.

4. Add 2.5 U of T4 DNA ligase and incubate at 37°C for 30 min (or overnight at 16°C).
5. Stop the reaction by heating for 10 min at 70°C, then ethanol precipitate.
6. Dissolve the pellet in the appropriate restriction digest buffer and cut with the relevant restriction enzymes (corresponding to the chosen pEMBL9 cloning sites flanking the fragment).
7. Separate the mixture on a 2% agarose gel and isolate the fragment with a length corresponding to a correctly assembled fragment.

6. Assembly of re-shaped human V-region genes in functional expression vectors

Using the M13 vectors referred to above, an easy assembly in pSV_2gpt- and pSV_2neo-based expression vectors is possible. These vectors contain the Ig heavy-chain enhancer sequence and have been described elsewhere (4–6). We adapted these vectors slightly for easy cloning, by inserting the *Hind*III–*Bam*HI fragment of the M13mp19 multilinker (see *Figure 1*). The cassette containing the re-shaped V-region can be inserted as a *Hind*III–*Bam*HI fragment, and a suitable constant-region gene can then be cloned in as a *Bam*HI fragment. The pSV_2gpt- and pSV_2neo-type vectors are often used for expressing heavy- and light-chain genes respectively, allowing selective screening of transfected cells for production of either the heavy or light chain or, ideally, both together. This is not critical, however, as both vectors can be used for heavy- and light-chain gene expression. Furthermore, it is not necessary to use two vectors with different selective marker genes. Simultaneous expression of both heavy- and light-chain genes by the same host cell can be achieved equally successfully by assembling them each in a (separate) pSV_2gpt-type vector, and using only the *gpt* selection (see also Section 7).

7. Expression of re-shaped human antibody genes in myeloma cells

Functional expression of the re-shaped human antibody genes can be achieved by co-transfection of non-producing myeloma cells (e.g. NS0 (31)) with linearized expression vectors. Circular DNA can be used as well, but it has been shown that prior linearization yields a higher transfection efficiency. For the vectors used by us, this can be achieved by cutting the unique *Pvu*I site, which is situated in the ampicillin-resistance gene, a selective marker no longer required at this stage (obviously the re-shaped human genes should be checked for the possible presence of *Pvu*I sites first!).

Transfection is achieved by electroporation (32) and a procedure optimized for NS0 cells is described in *Protocol 4*.

Table 2. Recipes for selective media

1. MPA selective medium (for gpt selection).
   To 500 ml DMEM add:
   - 25 ml xanthine (at 5 mg/ml in 50 mM NaOH)
   - 5 ml hypoxanthine (at 2 mg/ml in 10 mM NaOH)
   - 50 ml 10% FCS
   - 0.5 ml 0.5 M HCl
   - 0.2 ml 6.25 mg/ml MPA
2. G418 selective medium (for neo selection).
   To 500 ml DMEM add:
   - xanthine, hypoxanthine, and FCS as in the above recipe
   - 1 g G418 (GIBCO, in 8 ml H_2O + 100 μl of 1M Hepes buffer pH 7, neutralized with 10 M NaOH)

Selection of useful transfectomas is described in *Protocol 5*. The recipes for the selective media used are given in *Table 2*. Selection for *neo* is not strictly necessary, as the majority of transfectomas positive for *gpt* (and expressing the heavy chain) are also positive for *neo*, and produce complete Ig molecules (8). In addition to this, selection for *gpt* is more straightforward and clear cut than selection for *neo*, and is also much cheaper in terms of reagent costs.

Protocol 4. Transfection of NS0 myeloma cells by electroporation

1. Wash 5×10^7 NS0 cells once in PBS buffer, re-suspend in a final volume of 3 ml PBS, and keep on ice.
2. Wash the required number of plastic electroporation cuvettes (one per experiment, keep them in 70% EtOH until used) in PBS and place them on ice.
3. Place 20 μl of DNA (10 μg of each construct in 20 μl TE buffer[a]) on the side wall of the cuvette, add 250 μl of cells and mix with the DNA. Keep the cuvette on ice during these manipulations.
4. Place the cuvette in the electroporation chamber (APELEX, distributor CP Instruments), insert the electrodes and allow the electroporation to take place, applying the following conditions: 1.5 kV, 15 pulses with 1 sec intervals, each lasting 34.9 μsec (using all capacitor settings).
5. Place the electroporated cells on ice for 10 min.
6. Add 1 ml of DMEM,[b] supplemented with 10% serum (foetal calf or horse).
7. Take the mixture out of the cuvette and add to a flask with 25 ml DMEM (+10% serum). Gas the flask with 5% CO_2 and leave 1–2 days at 37°C.

[a] TE buffer: 10 mM Tris–HCl pH 7.5, 1 mM EDTA.
[b] We routinely supplement our DMEM with L-glutamine and sodium pyruvate (2 mM and 1 mM final concentration respectively).

Protocol 5. Selection of transfectomas

1. On day 2 after the electroporation (or day 1 if the cells have sufficiently recovered), add 10 ml of DMEM (+ 10% serum) and 15 ml of MPA selective medium (see *Table 2*), bringing the total volume to 50 ml.
2. Plate the cell suspension out at 1 ml per well in two 48-well plates and add a further 1 ml of the selective medium to each well.
3. Leave the plates for 10–14 days at 37°C, in a 5% CO_2 incubator, until colonies start to appear.

8. Characterization of transfectomas

Supernatants of wells containing transfectomas are tested for human Ig production and antigen binding by standard ELISA assays. This is best done as soon as the colonies appear (approximately two weeks after transfection). Positives for both assays are transferred to small flasks and grown to saturation, after which a simple dilution assay is done to identify the best producers. The yields of the most promising clones can be estimated using standard curves based on known Ig concentrations, and are usually found to be between 10 and 25 μg/ml of culture medium.

The key to estimating the binding capability of the re-shaped antibody compared to the parent mouse antibody lies in the determination of the concentrations of the specific mouse IgG and human IgG in the two samples. For purified antibodies ultraviolet absorption can give a good estimate, whilst IgG concentration can be determined in non-purified samples by calibration with reference standards.

A first and rapid estimate can be achieved by comparing their antibody dilution curves, provided that antigen is available and can be adsorbed on to microtitre wells. The curves are plotted in terms of IgG concentrations. Whilst not directly reflecting any affinity differences between the antibodies, the method is sensitive to them. Any major drop in affinity during re-shaping is detectable with this method. *Protocol 6* provides a method to obtain antibody dilution curves using polystyrene wells as a solid phase for a typical soluble protein antigen. Alternatively, micrometre-sized magnetic beads can be used; they have provided a more stable solid phase for some antigens (Verhoeyen *et al.*, in preparation).

Competition assays provide a means to detect a two- to three-fold difference in affinity which is normally sufficient. The method is simplest with purified antibodies, but impure preparations can be used as outlined above. The method outlined in *Protocol 7* is based on the use of increasing concentrations of unlabelled rodent and unlabelled re-shaped MAb to inhibit binding of ^{125}I-labelled rodent or re-shaped human antibody to antigen adsorbed on to a solid phase. Loss of affinity shifts the curve to higher Ig concentrations.

Additional characterization can be achieved, with suitable antigens, by epitope mapping where again, purified antibody makes the task much easier (Verhoeyen *et al.*, in preparation).

Protocol 6. Antibody dilution curves

1. Coat a multi well plate with antigen by incubation at 37°C for 2 h (100 μl/well; 5 μg/ml in PBS pH 7.4 is often a suitable concentration but this may need optimizing for individual antigens).
2. Rinse the plate four times in PBS before blocking with gelatin (0.02% in PBS) for 1 h at room temperature.
3. Wash four times with PBS + 0.15% Tween.
4. Aliquot the antibody samples (100 μl/well of serial dilutions in PBS +0.01% Thimerosal + 1% BSA, each in duplicate) and incubate at room temperature for 1 h before washing four times in buffer. Note that it is very important to make very accurate dilutions to obtain good curves; weighing can be of benefit for large dilutions.
5. Visualize bound antibody with HRP-conjugated antibodies (anti-human IgG for re-shaped and anti-rodent IgG for the parent antibody). Incubate the conjugate in PBS + 0.01% Thimerosal (1:1000 or another appropriate dilution) for 1 h at room temperature, followed by four washes as above.
6. Develop for 45 min with tetramethyl benzidene (0.01%) and H_2O_2 (1:200 of 100 vols) in citrate buffer pH 6.5 (use 200 μl/well). Stop the reaction with 2 M HCl.
7. Read the O.D.s at 450 nm.
8. Plot the IgG concentration versus percentage maximum binding (highest O.D. = 100%) for both rodent and re-shaped antibodies.

Protocol 7. Competition assay to assess relative affinities

1. Coat the wells of a Terasaki Microtest plate (10 μl capacity, from Nunc, Roskilde, Denmark) with antigen (try 0.2 μg/ml in PBS pH 7.3, optimize if necessary) by incubating at 37°C for 18 h.
2. Wash the wells three times with PBS + 1% casein (washing buffer).
3. Complete blocking of non-specific adsorption sites by incubating with washing buffer for 1 h at room temperature.
4. Add 5 μl aliquots of 'cold' MAb diluted in washing buffer (e.g. 0, 0.1, 1, 3, 5, 10, 20 μg/ml), followed by radioiodinated rodent or re-shaped human

antibody in 5 μl aliquots at 10^5 c.p.m./5 μl/well. Incubate for 90 min at room temperature (see Chapter 13 for iodination protocols).

5. Aspirate the wells and wash six times.

6. Separate the wells with a band saw and determine the radioactivity in each well.

7. Plot the concentration of 'cold' antibody versus percentage binding of radiolabelled antibody.

References

1. Shawler, D. L., Bartholomew, R. M., Smith, L. M., and Dillman, R. O. (1985). *J. Immunol.,* **135,** 1530.
2. Van Kroonenburgh, M. J. P. G. and Pauwels, E. J. K. (1988). *Nucl. Med. Commun.,* **9,** 919.
3. Carson, D. A. and Freimark, B. D. (1986). *Adv. Immunol.,* **38,** 275.
4. Jones, P. T., Dear, P. H., Foote, J., Neuberger, M. S., and Winter, G. (1986). *Nature,* **321,** 522.
5. Verhoeyen, M., Milstein, C., and Winter, G. (1988). *Science,* **239,** 1534.
6. Riechmann, L., Clark, M., Waldmann, H., and Winter, G. (1988). *Nature,* **332,** 323.
7. Queen, C., Schneider, W. P., Selick, H. E., Payne, P. W., Landolfi, N. F., Duncan, J. F., *et al.* (1989). *Proc. Natl Acad. Sci. USA,* **86,** 10029.
8. Verhoeyen, M., Broderick, L., Eida, S., and Badley, A. (1991). In *Monoclonal Antibodies: Applications in Clinical Oncology*, (ed. A. Epenetos), pp. 37–43. Chapman & Hall Medical, London.
9. Co, M. S., Deschamps, M., Whitley, R. J., and Queen, C. (1991). *Proc. Natl Acad. Sci. USA,* **88,** 2869.
10. Tempest, P. R., Bremner, P., Lambert, M., Taylor, G., Furze, J. M., Carr, F. J., *et al.* (1991). *Biotechnology,* **9,** 266.
11. Gorman, S. D., Clark, M. R., Routledge, E. G., Cobbold, S. P., and Waldmann, H. (1991). *Proc. Natl Acad. Sci. USA,* **88,** 4181.
12. Verhoeyen, M. E., Saunders, J. A., Broderick, E. L., Eida, S. J., and Badley, R. A. (1991). *Disease Markers,* **9,** 197.
13. Hale, G., Dyer, M. J. S., Clark, M. R., Phillips, J. M., Marcus, R., Riechmann, L., *et al.* (1988). *The Lancet,* **2,** 1394.
14. Hird, V., Verhoeyen, M., Badley, R. A., Price, D., Snook, D., Kosmas, C., *et al.* (1991). *Br. J. Cancer,* **64,** 911.
15. Kabat, E. A., Wu, T. T., Reid-Miller, M., Perry, H. M., and Gottesman, K. S. (ed.) (1987). *Sequences of Proteins of Immunological Interest*. US Dept. of Health and Human Services, Public Health Service, N.I.H., Bethesda, Maryland 20892, USA.
16. Mulligan, R. C. and Berg, P. (1981). *Proc. Natl Acad. Sci. USA,* **78,** 2072.
17. Southern, P. J. and Berg, P. (1981). *J. Mol. Appl. Gen.,* **1,** 327.
18. Griffiths, G. M. and Milstein, C. (1985). In *Hybridoma Technology in the Biosciences and Medicine*, (ed. T. A. Springer), pp. 103–15. Plenum, London.

19. Gubler, U. and Hoffmann, B. J. (1983). *Gene,* **25,** 263.
20. Orlandi, R., Gussow, D. H., Jones, P. T., and Winter, G. (1989). *Proc. Natl Acad. Sci. USA,* **86,** 3833.
21. Jones, S. T. and Bendig, M. M. (1991). *Biotechnology,* **9,** 88.
22. Jones, T. A. (1982). In *Computational Crystallography*, (ed. D. Sayre), pp. 303–10. Clarendon, Oxford.
23. Amit, A. G., Mariuzza, R. A., Phillips, S. E. V., and Poljak, R. J. (1986). *Science,* **233,** 747.
24. Saul, F. A., Amzel, M., and Poljak, R. J. (1978). *J. Biol. Chem.,* **253,** 585.
25. Epp, O., Colman, P., Fehlhammer, H., Bode, W., Schiffer, M., Huber, R., *et al.* (1974). *Eur. J. Biochem.,* **45,** 513.
26. Carter, P., Bedouelle, H., and Winter, G. (1985). *Nucleic Acids Res.,* **13,** 4431.
27. Kramer, B., Kramer, W., and Fritz, H-J. (1984). *Cell,* **38,** 879.
28. Gronenborn, B. (1976). *Mol. Gen. Genet.,* **148,** 243.
29. Suggs, S. V., Hirose, T., Mijake, T., Kawashima, E. H., Johnson, M. J., Itakura, K., *et al.* (1981). In *Developmental Biology Using Purified Genes*, (ed. D. Brown). Academic, New York.
30. Dente, L., Cesareni, G., and Cortese, R. (1983). *Nucleic Acids Res.,* **11,** 1645.
31. Galfre, G. and Milstein, C. (1981). *Methods Enzymol.,* **73,** 3.
32. Potter, H., Weir, L., and Leder, P. (1984). *Proc. Natl Acad. Sci. USA,* **81,** 7161.

17

Single-chain Fvs

MARC WHITLOW and DAVID FILPULA

1. Introduction

The Fv fragment of an antibody is probably the smallest structural component which retains the binding site characteristics of the parent antibody. The limited stability at low protein concentrations of the Fv fragments may be overcome by using a peptide linker to join the variable domains (V_L and V_H) of an Fv. The resulting single-chain Fv (sFv) proteins have been shown to have binding affinities equivalent to the monoclonal antibodies (MAbs) from which they were derived (1). In addition, catalytic MAbs may be converted to an sFv form with retention of catalytic characteristics (2).

There are a number of differences between sFv proteins and whole antibodies or antibody fragments, such as Fab or Fab'_2. Single-chain Fv proteins are small proteins with molecular weights around 27 kd, which lack the constant regions of the 50 kd Fab fragment or 150 kd IgG. Like a Fab fragment, and unlike an IgG, an sFv protein contains a single binding site, which may be a disadvantage when working with high-avidity binding specificities for repetitive epitopes.

The *in vivo* properties of sFv proteins are different from MAbs and antibody fragments. Due to their small size, sFv proteins clear more rapidly from the blood and penetrate more rapidly into tissues (3). Due to lack of constant regions, sFv proteins are not retained in tissues such as the liver and kidneys. We have postulated that due to the rapid clearance and lack of constant regions, sFv proteins will have low immunogenicity. Thus, single-chain Fv proteins have applications in cancer diagnostics and therapy where rapid tissue penetration and clearance are advantageous.

Monoclonal antibodies have long been envisioned as 'magic bullets' which can deliver a cytotoxic agent to a tumour. Single-chain Fv proteins offer a clear advantage over MAbs when the cytotoxic or therapeutic agent is a protein, for instead of chemically cross-linking the two functionalities, a single-chain fusion protein can be produced. Single-chain immunotoxins have been produced by fusing an sFv-derived cell binding specificity to *Pseudomonas* exotoxin (4). Recently, a single-chain immunotoxin has been shown to cause tumour regression in mice (5). Thus, after describing the design, construction, and purification of single-chain Fv proteins, we will discuss the design of single-chain Fv fusion proteins.

2. Design of the linker between the V_L and V_H domains

In order to design a polypeptide linker that will join the variable domains of an antibody to form an sFv, the extent of the variable domains must first be defined Kabat *et al.* (6) define the variable domain (V_L) to extend from residue 1 to residue 107 for the lambda light chain, and to residue 108 for kappa light chains, and the variable domain of the heavy chain (V_H) to extend from residue 1 to residue 113.

Single-chain Fvs can and have been constructed in either one of two ways. Either V_L is the N-terminal domain followed by the linker and V_H (a V_L–linker–V_H construction) or V_H is the N-terminal domain followed by the linker and V_L (V_H–linker–V_L construction). Both types of sFv proteins have been successfully constructed and purified, and both have shown binding affinities and specificities similar to the antibodies from which they were derived.

Linkers are designed to span the 3.5 to 3.9 nm between the C terminus of V_L and the N terminus of V_H or between the C terminus of V_H and the N terminus of V_L. They should be designed to be flexible, and it is recommended that an underlying sequence of alternating Gly and Ser residues be used. To enhance the solubility of a linker and their associated sFv, three charged residues are included; two positively charged residues (Lys) and one negatively charged residue (Glu). One of the Lys residues is placed close to the N-terminus of V_H, to replace the positive charge lost when forming the peptide bond of the linker and the V_H. We have found that linker lengths of more than 18 residues reduce aggregation. A third property that is important in engineering an sFv protein is proteolytic stability. We found that our 212 linker is susceptible to being clipped by subtilisin BPN′. The proteolytic clip in the 212 linker occurred between Lys8 and Ser9 of the linker (see *Table 1*). By placing a proline at the proteolytic clip site one can protect the linker. *Table 1* shows the 218 linker that incorporates all of these ideas.

Table 1. Linker design

V_L–linker–V_H construction				
V_L	Linker sequence	V_H	Linker name	Reference
–KLEIK	GSTSGSGKSSEGKG	*EVKLD–*	212	Pantoliano *et al.* (20)
–KLEIK[a]	GSTSGSGKPGSGEGSTKG	*EVQLV–*[a]	218	

[a] Consensus sequences, residues L103–L107 and H1–H5.

3. Genetic construction of a single-chain Fv

Single-chain Fv genes may be constructed in a variety of ways, depending on where one first isolated the binding specificity. Traditionally, monoclonal antibodies have been produced by screening hybridoma libraries. At this time, one can screen combinatorial libraries that have been expressed on fd phage as either Fabs or sFv fusion proteins to gene III (7, 8). All genetic cloning strategies for the variable domains of an antibody take advantage of conserved sequences present in signal and constant (C_{H1} or C_L) domains which adjoin the variable domains or, alternatively, use the variable framework regions (FR1 and FR4) which are on the boundary of the variable domains (9, 10).

There are a number of other features one should include in the genetic construction of an sFv gene, in addition to the cloning of the variable-domain genes and the sequence of the linker between them. First, the constructed sFv gene will need to be put into an expression plasmid. Second, one or two stop codons will need to be placed at the 3′ end of the gene. Finally, one may want to put restriction sites on either side of the linker, such that it can be removed and replaced with a new linker. In the examples given below, the sFv gene has an *Aat*II site at the 5′ end, *Hind*III and *Pvu*II restriction sites flanking the linker sequence, and two stop codons and a *Bam*HI site at its 3′ end.

3.1 Genetic construction of a single-chain Fv from hybridoma cell-lines

The PCR (polymerase chain reaction) cloning of sFv genes from hybridoma cells has been reported by Chaudhary *et al.* (9). PCR amplification of first-strand cDNA is performed separately with two sets of primers which hybridize to the ends of either the light- or heavy-chain variable regions. The sFv linker region is incorporated into an upstream segment on the long V_L-3′ PCR primer. *Sal*I sites were also introduced into the V_L-3′ primer and the V_H-5′ primer to allow subsequent ligation of the V_L–linker and V_H segments. In the case of the 218 linker, a *Sma*I site at positions 25–30 of the 54 bp linker may be exploited in similar PCR cloning strategies (see *Table 2*).

Davis *et al.* (11) have described a PCR gene synthesis method using splicing by overlap extensions (see *Protocol 1*). The PCR amplification is performed in a single tube first with all four primers followed by a second PCR synthesis with the two outside primers only and produced completed sFv genes directly from either the isolated V_L and V_H cDNA clones or from total hybridoma first-strand cDNA. The engineered *Hind*III and *Pvu*II sites allow convenient linker interchange and do not alter the protein sequence. The N-terminal *Aat*II site can be fused to the *omp*A signal sequence for expression in *E. coli* (2, 3).

Table 2A. PCR primers used in the splicing by overlap extension construction

```
                         1
G VL                     D  I  V  M  T  Q  S  P
          5'           GACATTGTGATGACACAGTCTCCATC- - -3'
primer 1  5'  AGGTGCAGACGTCGTGATGACACAGTCTCCATC  3'
                         AatII

                                          107
VL               -  -  F  G  S  G  T  K  L  E  I  K
          5'  -  - - TTCGGCTCGGGGACAAAGTTGGAAATAAAA  3'
primer 2  3'          AAGCCGAGCCCCTGTTTCGAACTTTATTTTCCGAGATGAAGGCCAAGTCCTTTCGGGCCCTCACCACTTCCA   5'
                                     HindIII                                      SmaI
                                                     1
VH                                                   Q  V  Q  L  Q  Q  P  G  A  E  -  -
          5'                                        CAGGTCCAACTGCAGCAGCCTGGGGCTGAG - --    3'
primer 3  5'  GGAAAGCCCGGGAGTGGTGAAGGTAGCACTAAAGGTCAGGTCCAGCTGCAGCAGCCTGGGGCTGAG   3'
                  SmaI                                       PvuII

                                   112
VH               -  -  - T  L  V  T  V  S
          5'  -  - - GGACTCTGGTCACTGTGTCT    3'
primer 4  3'          CCTGAGACCAGTGACACAGAATTATCCTAGGCG   5'
                                               BamHI
```

Table 2B. Resulting single-chain Fv gene with 218 linker

```
        1
        D   V   V   M   T  –   –   –
5'     GACGTCGTGATGACA– –   – –
        AatII

                          107                       218 linker                             1
 –   –   T   K   L   E   I   K   G   S   T   S   G   S   G   K   P   G   S   G   E   G   S   T   K   G   Q   V   Q   L   Q   –   –
–   –   –ACAAAGCTTGAAATAAAAGGCTCTACTTCCGGTTCAGGAAAGCCCGGGAGTGGTGAAGGTAGCACTAAAGGTCAGGTCCAGCTGCAG–   –
          HindIII                            SmaI                                     PvuII

                                                                 112
                                                    –   –   –   T   V   S
                                                   – – –   –ACTGTGTCTTAATAGGATCC   3'
                                                                          BamHI
```

Protocol 1. Polymerase chain reaction for single-chain Fv

1. Combine in a 0.5 ml microfuge tube 1 μg of purified hybridoma mRNA, 100 pmol of random oligonucleotide hexamers (Pharmacia), 200 U of Maloney *MuLV* reverse transcriptase, 20 U of RNAsin and 250 μM dNTPs in 1 × PCR buffer (67 mM Tris–HCl, pH 8.8, 6.7 mM $MgCl_2$, 16.6 mM $(NH_4)_2$ SO_4, and 10 mM β-mercaptoethanol) in a total volume of 20 μl.
2. Incubate for 1 h at 42°C, heat to 92°C for 5 min, and cool to 4°C.
3. Add 80 μl volume containing 50 pmol of each of the four PCR primers (*Table 2A*), 250 μM of each dNTP, and 2.5 U Taq DNA polymerase in 1 × PCR buffer. Overlay with 100 μl mineral oil.
4. Perform PCR synthesis in thermal cycler. Each cycle consists of 1 min denaturation at 94°C, 2 min annealing at 60°C, and 1 min extension at 72°C. Each cycle is repeated 25 times and is followed by a 5 min extension at 72°C.
5. Remove a 10 μl aliquot from step **4** and add to 90 μl of a PCR reaction mixture equivalent to the step **3** mixture except that only the outside primers 1 and 4 are included and primers 2 and 3 (*Table 2A*) are omitted. Perform the second PCR synthesis as in step **4**.
6. Extract PCR products with phenol and chloroform and precipitate the DNA with ethanol. Digest the re-suspended DNA with *Aat*II plus *Bam*HI and purify the fragment on NuSieve GTG low-melt agarose (FMC). Ligate 'in gel' (12) the fragment to the desired vector.

3.2 Genetic construction of a single-chain Fv from combinatorial libraries

Variable-domain genes isolated from a combinatorial library in lambda or fd phage as Fabs (8, 10) can be converted to an sFv gene using oligonucleotide-directed mutagenesis (ODM) (see *Protocol 2*). This is a simple alternative to PCR methods, which may also be employed. *Protocol 2* is useful any time that cloned antibody cDNA genes are available (2).

Protocol 2. Oligonucleotide-directed mutagenesis for single-chain Fv construction

1. Prepare plasmid DNA from Stratagene lambda phage/Fab clone (10).
2. Subclone the *Xho*I–*Eco*RI heavy chain (V_H) fragment into *Sal*I, *Eco*RI digested M13mp18. Subclone the *Sac*I–*Xba*I light chain (V_L) fragment into *Sac*I–*Xba*I-digested M13mp19.

3. Prepare standard M13 template DNA preparations of about 0.1 μg/μl from *E. coli* host JM101.
4. Obtain the Amersham Corporation commercial mutagenesis system, version 2 (RPN 1523).
5. Follow the protocol on pages 14–16 of the Amersham manual with the following modifications:
   (a) In step 1, 11.5 μl of the V_L template is combined with 1 μl of 20 pmol of phosphorylated mutant oligomer 1 (*Table 3*) to introduce the 5′ flanking *Aat*II site, 1 μl of 20 pmol of phosphorylated mutant oligomer 2 to introduce the 3′ flanking *Hind*III site. For the V_H template, 11.5 μl of the DNA is combined with 1 μl of 20 pmol of the phosphorylated mutant oligomer 3 (*Table 3*) to introduce a 5′ flanking *Pvu*II site and 1 μl of 20 pmol of phosphorylated mutant oligomer 4 to introduce a 3′ flanking *Bam*HI site. Omit the 6 μl water in step 1.
   (b) Omit the ammonium acetate precipitation in step 6.
   (c) Directly transform 2 μl and 20 μl of the step 6 ligation into competent *E. coli* host JM101.
6. Prepare RF DNA from transformant plaques, of which about 50% will typically be successful double mutants.
7. Digest 10 μg V_H RF DNA with *Pvu*II plus *Bam*HI and purify the V_H fragment by electrophoresis on NuSieve GTG agarose in TAE buffer and excise the gel fragment.
8. Anneal the complementary strands of the *Pvu*II–*Hind*III linker (oligomers 5 and 6 in *Table 3*) by mixing 30 pmol of each phosphorylated oligomer in a 10 μl final volume containing 1 × polynucleotide kinase buffer. Incubate for 5 min at 95 °C and slow-cool to 22 °C.
9. Ligate 1 μl of the linker from step **8** and 50 ng of *Bam*HI, *Hind*III digested, phosphatased M13mp18 with 4 μl of the gel slice from step **7** as described previously (12). Transform JM101 and prepare RF DNA from the resulting plaques.
10. Gel-purify the *Aat*II–*Hind*III V_L fragment and the *Bam*HI–*Hind*III V_H/linker fragments as in step **7**. Ligate these fragments to the desired *Aat*II, *Bam*HI digested vector (2) in a three-way ligation as in step **9**. Transform the desired *E. coli* host.
11. Confirm the correct DNA construction by DNA sequencing around the sites of mutagenesis.

3.3 Expression of a single-chain Fv

Secretion from *E. coli* of functional Fv and Fab fragments as first described by Skerra and Pluckthun (13) and Better *et al.* (14) has also been achieved for an

Table 3. Oligomers for oligonucleotide-directed mutagenesis for single-chain Fv construction

Oligomer 1	5′ – CAGTGAATTCGACGTCGTGATGACCC – 3′ *Aat*II
Oligomer 2	5′ –GGCACCAAGCTTGAAATCAAA – 3′ *Hind*III
Oligomer 3	5′–GCTTGCATGCCAGCTGGTCGAGTCTGGAC – 3′ *Pvu*II
Oligomer 4	5′–GTCACTGTCTCTTAATAGGATCCAACACCCCCATC – 3′ *Bam*HI
Oligomer 5	5′–AGCTTGAAATAAAAGGCTCTACTTCCGGTTCAGGAAAGCCCGGGAGTG GTGAAGGTAGCACTAAAGGTCAGGTCCAG–3′
Oligomer 6	5′–CTGGACCTGACCTTTAGTGCTACCTTCACCACTCCCGGGCTTTCCTGAA CCGGAAGTAGAGCCTTTTATTTCA–3′

sFv (15). Cytoplasmic expression of sFv in *E. coli* followed by re-naturation has also been reported (1, 9). Yeast (11), plants (16), baculovirus (17), and mammalian cells (18) may be other possible expression hosts. Successful expression of active sFv on the surface of phage may allow rapid screening of large antibody libraries (7).

The Genex expression vector used for sFv expression in *E. coli* contains the hybrid lambda phage promoter O_L/P_R and the *omp*A signal sequence (see *Figure 1*). To produce the final expression strains, the completed sFv expression vectors are transformed into *E. coli* host strain GX6712 which has the mutant temperature-sensitive repressor gene cI^{857} integrated into the chromosome. This provides a transcriptional regulation system where induction of sFv synthesis occurs by raising the culture temperature from 32°C to 42°C. Eleven independent murine-derived and one rat-derived sFv proteins have been expressed at 5–20% of total cell protein using this expression system. N-terminal amino acid sequence analysis has confirmed the predicted signal sequence removal. High-level expression of secreted proteins in *E. coli* may result in the formation of protein aggregates in the periplasmic space. Since our expressed sFv proteins accumulate as insoluble aggregates, denaturation and refolding are required for purification (see Section 4). Because expression of sFv proteins fused to the *omp*A signal sequence has resulted in mature sFv production levels of 5–20% of total cell protein for 11 distinct sFv proteins, we have included the signal sequence as part of our standard expression system.

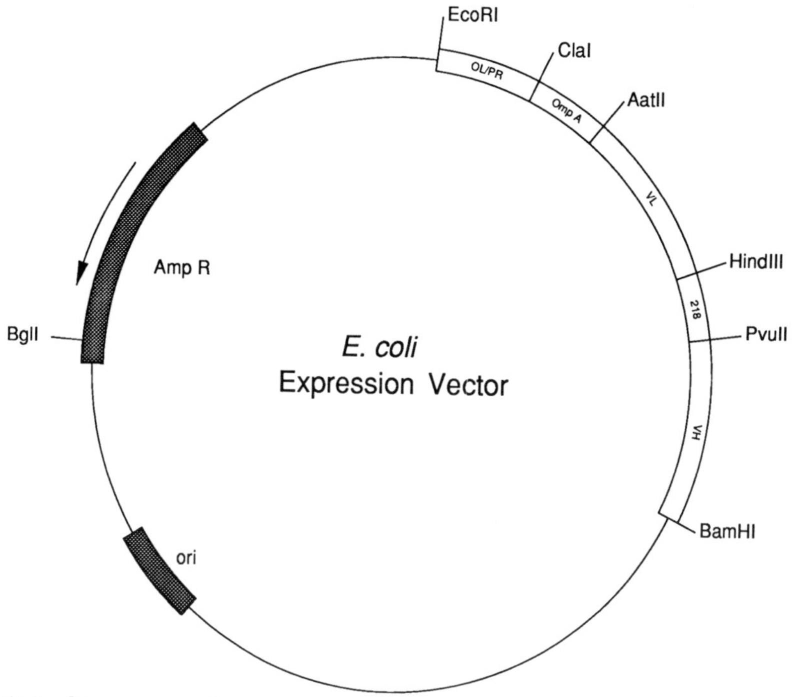

Figure 1. Genex expression vector used for the single-chain Fv expression in *E. coli*. Contains the hybrid lambda phage promoter O_L/P_R, the *ompA* signal sequence and a V_L–linker–V_H sFv gene.

4. Fermentation and purification of a single-chain Fv

As mentioned above, sFv proteins have been produced in a large number of expression systems. We will only briefly describe the *E. coli* fermentation we have used to produce our sFv proteins and will give a detailed protocol for the purification of an sFv protein. A number of sFv proteins have been purified by affinity chromatography. The purification protocol we will describe does not use affinity chromatography, for such purification protocols depend on both the affinity matrix and the sFv protein. Rather we have employed cation exchange HPLC chromatography.

The *E. coli* fermentations are performed at 32°C using a casein digest–glucose-salts medium. At an optical density of 18–20 at 600 nm, sFv expression is induced by a 42°C temperature shock for 1 h. After cooling the fermentation to 10°C the cells are harvested at 7000*g* for 10 min. The wet cell paste is then stored frozen at −20°C. Approximately 200 to 300 g of wet cell paste is normally recovered from one 10 litre fermentation.

Protocol 3 describes the purification of an sFv protein produced from a 10 litre *E. coli* fermentation. Like a number of proteins produced in *E. coli*, sFv proteins are produced as insoluble aggregates. We have used this protocol, or a similar protocol, to purify a dozen sFv proteins. This purification procedure yields sFv proteins that are more than 95% pure as examined by SDS-PAGE (sodium dodecyl sulphate polyacrylamide gel electrophoresis).

The following information is useful when purifying an sFv protein. First, the isoelectric point of most sFv proteins lies between a pH of 8.0 and 9.4. Second, the optical density at 280 nm of most sFv proteins lies between 1.9 and 2.2 $O.D._{280}$ ml/mg. Finally, sFv proteins have molecular weights around 27 kd, thus, we have used commercial 4–20% tris-glycine SDS-PAGE gels (Novex).

Protocol 3. Purification of sFv proteins from *E. coli* cell paste

You will need

- cell lysis buffer: 50 mM Tris–HCl, 1.0 mM EDTA, 100 mM KCl, 0.1 mM PMSF (phenylmethylsulphonyl fluoride), pH 8.0
- denaturing buffer: 6 M guanidine hydrochloride, 50 mM Tris–HCl, 10 mM $CaCl_2$, 50 mM KCl, pH 8.0
- refolding buffer: 50 mM Tris–HCl, 10 mM $CaCl_2$, 50 mM KCl, 0.1 mM PMSF, pH 8.0
- HPLC buffer A: 60 mM MOPS, 0.5 mM Ca acetate, pH 6.4
- HPLC buffer B: 60 mM MOPS, 10 mM Ca acetate, pH 7.5
- HPLC buffer C: 60 mM MOPS, 100 mM $CaCl_2$, pH 7.5

A. *Cell lysis*

1. Thaw the cell paste from a 10 litre fermentation (200–300 g) overnight at 4°C.
2. Gently re-suspend the wet cell paste in 2.5 litres of the cell lysis buffer at 4°C.
3. Pass the cell suspension through a Manton–Gaulin cell homogenizer three times. Because the cell homogenizer raises the temperature of the cell lysate to 25 ± 5°C, the cell lysate is cooled to 5 ± 2°C with a Lauda/Brinkman chilling coil after each pass.

B. *Washing the cell pellet*

1. Centrifuge the cell lysate at 24 300*g* for 30 min at 6°C. Discard the supernatant, for the pellet contains the insoluble sFv.
2. Wash the pellet by gently scraping it from the centrifuge bottles and re-suspending it in 1.2 litres of lysis buffer.
3. Repeat steps **1** and **2** as many as five times. At any time during this washing procedure the material can be stored as a frozen pellet at −20°C.

C. *Solubilization and renaturation of the sFv protein*

1. Solubilize the washed cell pellet in freshly prepared denaturing buffer at 4°C, using 6 ml of denaturing buffer per gram of cell pellet. If necessary, a few quick pulses from a Heat Systems Ultrasonics Tissue Homogenizer can be used to complete the solubilization.
2. Centrifuge the resulting suspension at 24 300*g* for 45 min at 6°C and discard the pellet.
3. Determine the optical density at 280 nm of the supernatant. If the $O.D._{280}$ is above 30, additional denaturing buffer should be added to obtain an $O.D._{280}$ of approximately 25.
4. Slowly dilute the supernatant into cold (4–7°C) refolding buffer (50 mM Tris–HCl, 10 mM $CaCl_2$, 50 mM KCl, 0.1 mM PMSF pH 8.0) until a 1:10 dilution is reached. We have found that the best results are obtained when the supernatant is slowly added to the refolding buffer over a 2 h period, with gentle mixing.
5. Allow the solution to stand undisturbed for at least a 20 h period at 4°C.
6. Filter the solution through 0.45 μm microporous membranes at 4°C.
7. Concentrate the filtrate to about 500 ml at 4°C.

D. *Cation-exchange HPLC purification*

1. Dialyse the renatured sFv solution against the HPLC buffer A, until the conductivity is lowered to that of buffer A.
2. Equilibrate the 21.5 mm × 150 mm polyaspartic acid PolyCAT A column (PolyLC, Inc., Columbia, MD) with HPLC buffer A for 20 min.
3. Load the dialysed sample on the PolyCAT A column. If more than 60 mg is loaded on this column the resolution begins to deteriorate, thus the sample must usually be divided into several PolyCAT A runs.
4. Determine optical density at 280 nm and calculate the protein concentration. Most sFv proteins have an extinction coefficient of about 2.0 mg/ml/cm at 280 nm and this can be used to determine the protein concentration.
5. Elute the sample from the PolyCAT A column with a 50 min linear gradient between HPLC buffers A and B (see *Table 4*). Most of the sFv proteins that we have purified elute between 20 and 26 min using this gradient. We normally collect 3 min fractions.
6. Apply a final salt bump to the PolyCAT A column to remove the remaining contaminants with HPLC buffer C.
7. Analyse the collected fractions on 4–20% Tris-glycine SDS-PAGE gels.

Table 4. Poly CAT A cation exchange HPLC gradients

Time (min)[a]	Flow (ml/min)	Buffers		
		%A	%B	%C
Initial	15.0	100	0	0
50.0	15.0	0	100	0
55.0	15.0	0	100	0
60.0	15.0	0	0	100
63.0	15.0	0	0	100
64.0	15.0	100	0	0
67.0	15.0	100	0	0

Buffer A = 60 mM MOPS (3-[*N*-morpholino]propanesulphonic acid), 0.5 mM Ca acetate, pH 6.4
Buffer B = 60 mM MOPS, 10 mM Ca acetate, pH 7.5.
Buffer C = 60 mM MOPS, 100 mM $CaCl_2$, pH 7.5.
[a] Linear gradients are run between each time point.

5. Design of single-chain Fv fusion proteins

The considerations of solubility, stability, and proteolytic susceptibility which are important in the design of linkers between the variable domains of a single-chain Fv, may also be applied to the design of linkers between an sFv domain and a fusion partner. In the engineering of a diphtherial toxin IL-2 immunotoxin (DAB_{389}-IL-2), amino acids 2 through 8 of IL-2 were duplicated, effectively increasing the linker length between the diphtherial toxin (DAB_{389}) and IL-2 domains by 7 residues (19). The resulting DAB_{389}-$(1–10)_2$-IL-2 immunotoxin is 10-fold more toxic than that of DAB_{389}-IL-2. This result, and the results of our studies on linker length, suggest that it is important to have a sufficiently long linker between functional domains. The longer linker lengths probably allow a domain to function with less interference from the other domains in a fusion protein.

Single-chain Fv fusion proteins may be assembled in a variety of ways, using methods analogous to those described in Section 3. Both the V_L–linker–V_H and V_H–linker–V_L sFv domain constructions have produced active sFv fusion proteins. Single-chain Fv fusion proteins have been constructed with the effector domain at either the N- or C-terminus of the sFv domain.

References

1. Bird, R. E., Hardman, K. D., Jacobson, J. W., Johnson, S., Kaufman, B. M., Lee, S.-M., *et al.* (1988). *Science,* **242,** 423.
2. Gibbs, R. A., Posner, B. A., Filpula, D. R., Dodd, S. W., Finkelman, M. A. J., Lee, T. K., *et al.* (1991). *Proc. Natl Acad. Sci. USA,* **88,** 4001.

3. Colcher, D., Bird, R., Roselli, M., Hardman, K. D., Johnson, S., Pope, S., *et al.* (1990). *J. Natl Cancer Inst.*, **82,** 1191.
4. Chaudhary, V. K., Queen, C., Junghans, R. P., Waldmann, T. A., FitzGerald, D. J., and Pastan, I. (1989). *Nature,* **339,** 394.
5. Brinkmann, U., Pai, L. H., FitzGerald, D. J., Willingham, M., and Pastan, I. (1991). *Proc. Natl Acad. Sci. USA,* **88,** 8616.
6. Kabat, E. A., Wu, T. T., Reid-Miller, M., Perry, H. M., and Gottesman, K. S. (1987). *Sequences of Proteins of Immunological Interest*, (4th edn). US Department of Health and Human Services, Bethesda, MD.
7. McCafferty, J., Griffiths, A. D., Winter, G., and Chiswell, D. J. (1990). *Nature,* **348,** 552.
8. Barbas III, C. F. and Lerner, R. A. (1991). *Methods,* **2,** 119.
9. Chaudhary, V. K., Batra, J. K., Gallo, M. G., Willingham, M. C., FitzGerald, D. J., and Pastan, I. (1990). *Proc. Natl Acad. Sci. USA,* **87,** 1066.
10. Huse, W. D., Sastry, L., Iverson, S. A., Kang, A. S., Alting-Mess, M., Burton, D. R., *et al.* (1989). *Science,* **246,** 1275.
11. Davis, G. T., Bedzyk, W. D., Voss, E. W., and Jacobs, T. W. (1991). *Bio/Technology,* **9,** 165.
12. Dumais, M. M. and Nochumson, S. (1987). *BioTechniques,* **5,** 62.
13. Skerra, A. and Pluckthun, A. (1988). *Science,* **240,** 1038.
14. Better, M., Chang, C. P., Robinson, R. R., and Horwitz, A. H. (1988). *Science,* **240,** 1041.
15. Glockshuber, R., Malia, M., Pfitzinger, I., and Pluckthun, A. (1990). *Biochemistry,* **29,** 1362.
16. Hiatt, A. (1990). *Nature,* **344,** 469.
17. Hasemann, C. A. and Capra, J. D. (1990). *Proc. Natl Acad. Sci. USA,* **87,** 3942.
18. Biocca, S., Neuberger, M. S., and Cattaneo, A. (1990). *EMBO J.,* **9,** 101.
19. Kiyokawa, T., Williams, D. P., Snider, C. E., Strom, T. B., and Murphy, J. R. (1991). *Protein Eng.,* **4,** 463.
20. Pantoliano, M. W., Bird, R. E., Johnson, L. S., Asel, E. D., Dodd, S. W., Wood, J. F., *et al.* (1991). *Biochemistry,* **30,** 10117.

18

Engineering cytokine-secreting tumour cells

POULAM M. PATEL, CLAUDIA L. FLEMMING, SUZANNE A. ECCLES, and MARY K. L. COLLINS

1. Introduction

The ability of tumours to evade the host immune system can be reduced by boosting the anti-tumour response in a variety of ways. Cytokines are soluble growth factors, often produced by antigen-triggered cells during immune stimulation. They serve to co-ordinate and amplify the response to antigen, by acting as autocrine and paracrine stimulators of proliferation and effector function. One cytokine may exert its effects on many different target cells within the haemopoietic system. Systemic cytokine administration might therefore be predicted to boost the immune response to any antigen, including inappropriately expressed or mutated self-antigens found on tumour cells. Clinically, this approach has been used in the treatment of melanoma or renal cell carcinoma with systematic interleukin-2 (IL-2) (1).

However, the response of these patients to IL-2 is not complete, and other human malignancies are refractory to such treatment. Therefore, the determination of the optimal cytokine(s) for the treatment of a variety of human malignant diseases, will require the screening of a number of cytokines, singly or in combination, in appropriate animal tumour models.

In this chapter, we describe a simple assay to test the effect of cytokines on rodent tumour growth. As cytokines are often species-specific, and large amounts of recombinant rodent cytokines are not readily available, systemic administration of cytokines to tumour-bearing rodents is difficult. We, and others, have used the approach of transfer and expression of cytokine genes in rodent tumour cells (summarized in *Table 1*), as a method to identify cytokines which may be effective in the treatment of various tumour types. The secreting tumour cells can often be rejected by syngeneic hosts, whereas the parental cells cannot. The method which we have used for gene transfer and expression is described here, as are simple bioassays for IL-2 and interleukin-4 (IL-4), the most commonly used cytokines. This approach could clearly also be used to assay the effect of any expressed protein upon tumour growth.

Table 1. Studies of cytokine gene transfer to tumours

Tumour model	Cytokine	Rejection		Reference
		i/c	Athymic	
CT26 mouse adenocarcinoma	IL-2	+	n/d	20
B16 mouse melanoma	IL-2	+	n/d	20
CMS-5 mouse fibrosarcoma	IL-2	+	n/d	6
P815 mouse mastocytoma	IL-2	+	n/d	21
HSNLV rat sarcoma	IL-2	+	Slowed	2
FS29 mouse sarcoma	IL-2	+	–	3
J558L mouse plasmacytoma	IL-4	+	+	22
K485 mouse adenocarcinoma	IL-4	n/d	+	22
FS29 mouse sarcoma	IL-4	+	–	3
Renca mouse renal carcinoma	IL-4	+	Slowed	23
C1300 mouse neuroblastoma	γ-IFN	+	n/d	4
CMS-5 mouse fibrosarcoma	γ-IFN	+	n/d	5
SP1 mouse adenocarcinoma	γ-IFN	+	n/d	24
C-26 mouse adenocarcinoma	G-CSF	+	+	25
MCA-205 mouse sarcoma	TNF-α	+	n/d	26
J558l mouse plasmacytoma	TNF-α	+	n/d	27
J558L mouse plasmacytoma	IL-7	+	–	28
TS/A mouse adenocarcinoma	IL-7	+	n/d	28

i/c, immunocompetent; n/d, not done

2. Vectors for cytokine gene expression

In tumourigenicity assays, it is crucial to have long-term, stable, gene expression when the modified tumour cells are inoculated into the animal. Various methods of gene transfer have been used in these studies (*Table 1*); we (2, 3) and others (4–6) have chosen recombinant retroviral vectors. The advantage of such a system is that the vector DNA integrates stably, as a single copy in the tumour cell genome, although its level of expression can be influenced by the chromatin environment. Thus, clones of tumour cells expressing consistent (but different) levels of a given cytokine can be isolated (2, 6). Also, the high efficiency of retroviral gene transfer will allow the use of a bulk-infected, unselected, population if this is desirable.

If selected clones of tumour cells are to be used, a retroviral vector which expresses a dominant selectable marker, as well as the cytokine gene of interest should be used. The earlier vectors of this type, such as pZIPneo (7), or the more efficient N2 (8), encode the bacterial *neo* gene which confers resistance to G418. Both of these vectors have been used successfully to express cytokine genes in tumour cells (2, 6); the only contra-indications for their use would be:

(a) Inability to select tumour cells of interest in G418 due to high intrinsic resistance. In this case vectors of the pBABE series (9), which carry a variety of selectable marker genes, can be used.
(b) Inefficiency of the Moloney murine leukaemia virus (Mo-MLV) long terminal repeat (LTR) to drive expression of the cytokine gene in a particular tumour cell. This promoter works well in a variety of rodent and human cells, but has been shown to work poorly in undifferentiated embryonal carcinoma cells (10). Better levels of cytokine gene expression might be achieved in a given tumour cell by the use of an internal promoter within the retroviral vector (see (11) for example).
(c) The need for high-efficiency infection of a bulk population of tumour cells. In this case, a vector carrying only the cytokine gene may be preferable as it gives increased viral production (12). This would also eliminate any concern regarding potential immunogenicity of the bacterial selectable marker gene product.

Vector construction requires basic molecular cloning techniques to insert a murine cytokine cDNA clone into an appropriate restriction enzyme site of the recombinant retroviral plasmid. This plasmid carries the portions of the retroviral genome required for its incorporation into virions, and integration into target cell DNA, but lacks any genes encoding retroviral proteins. The plasmid is then introduced into retroviral packaging-cells, to generate recombinant retroviral particles which transmit and express the cytokine gene.

3. Packaging cells

To understand retroviral packaging cell-lines, a basic knowledge of the retroviral life cycle is essential. The simplest retroviruses consist of a core containing a diploid RNA genome and viral proteins, which is enclosed in a membrane expressing glycoprotein envelope molecules. Following binding of the envelope to a specific cell-surface receptor on the target cell, the viral core enters the cell. Using viral reverse transcriptase, the RNA genome is converted to double-stranded DNA, which is then incorporated into the host genome. Transcription of this integrated proviral DNA, which is regulated by the viral LTR, then generates new RNA genomes and mRNA which is translated into the viral proteins.

Incorporation of these RNA genomes into retroviral particles is dependent on the presence of an RNA sequence, termed the ψ sequence. ψ is present in retroviral vectors, but absent in the retroviral genomes used to construct packaging cells. Packaging cells are simply murine fibroblasts transfected with plasmids which express the retroviral proteins. Thus, when retroviral vectors are introduced into packaging cells, the vector genome is incorporated into viral particles. Such particles are capable of one round of infection of target cells, but do not carry the viral genes required for further replication.

Several packaging cell-lines have been used for producing recombinant retroviruses for gene transfer (summarized in (13)). For tumourigenicity experiments it is crucial that no retroviral proteins, which are antigenic, be expressed on the tumour cells. Recombination between vector and packaging constructs leading to generation of replication competent helper virus has been observed in the early packaging cell-lines. Therefore the most recent packaging cell-lines, which were designed to prevent this, should now be used. We recommended the lines GPE86 (14) or GPAM12 (15); alternatives would be the ψCRIP and ψCRE cells (16).

The host range of the retrovirus is dependent on the presence of specific cell surface receptors to which the envelope binds. The murine retroviruses have several envelope specificities. The two used in packaging cells are the ecotropic (GEP86 or ψCRE) and amphotropic (GPAM12 or ψCRE) strains of Mo-MLV. Ecotropic receptors are found on murine and other rodent cells. Amphotropic receptors are found on most mammalian cells.

3.1 Care of packaging cells

Although the packaging cell-lines described are on the whole relatively stable there is some loss of packaging function after prolonged passage in culture. This appears to be exacerbated by any severe insults such as mycoplasma infections or inefficient freeze/thawing. Thus when stocks of packaging lines are received they should be expanded and several aliquots (about 15–20) of an early passage should be frozen. For each transfection a fresh one of these stocks should be used. If there is a marked loss of packaging function this may be restored by reselecting the cells in the appropriate selection medium. Packaging cells should be grown in Dulbecco's modified Eagle's medium (DMEM) containing 10% newborn calf serum (NCS).

3.2 Transfecting packaging cells

To obtain stable production of helper-free stocks of retrovirus carrying a cytokine gene, first transfect a packaging cell with a recombinant retroviral plasmid carrying the cytokine gene (*Protocol 1*). The resulting clones of packaging cells are then selected for incorporation and expression of the cytokine gene (*Protocol 9*), and assayed for production of functional virus (Section 3.3) and the absence of helper virus (Section 3.4). The packaging cell clones thus selected are used to make retroviral stocks which will be used to infect the tumour cell-line to be studied. (The generation, care, and maintenance of retroviral vectors is also described in Chapter 20.)

Protocol 1. Transfection of packaging cell-lines

- ×2 HEPES buffered saline (×2HBS): dissolve 2.16 g D-glucose, 16.02 g NaCl, 0.74 g KCl, 0.2 g Na_2HPO_4, and 10.0 g HEPES in water. Adjust pH to 7.05 using 1 M NaOH. Make up to a final volume of 1 litre with water. Store at −20°C in 50 ml aliquots. Filter though a 0.2 μm filter before use.

1. 24 h prior to transfection, plate 90 mm dishes with 2×10^5 packaging cells.
2. Make DNA/$CaCl_2$ solution: 10 μg DNA, 46.5 μl filtered 2 M $CaCl_2$ made up to 375 μl with filtered water.
3. As a control, make $CaCl_2$ solution (as in step **2**) but omit the DNA and proceed as for DNA/$CaCl_2$ solution.
4. Add DNA/$CaCl_2$ solution dropwise to 375 μl × 2 HBS in a clear 5 ml tube, tapping continuously to ensure adequate mixing.
5. Leave to stand for 30 min at room temperature. A fine, barely visible precipitate should form.
6. Drain each 90 mm dish completely of medium and add the 750 μl of DNA solution. Leave for 15 min, rocking regularly to ensure that the whole plate is kept covered with liquid.
7. Add 8 ml of medium and incubate for 4 h.
8. Drain medium. Add 2 ml of 15% glycerol in HBS for 2 min. Drain off glycerol solution carefully. Wash twice with 10 ml of medium. Incubate for 48 h at 37°C in 10 ml of medium.
9. Split confluent plates at appropriate concentrations into selection medium. For GPAM12 and GPE86, at 1/4, 1/8, 1/16, 1/32.
10. Re-feed with selection medium two to three times a week to remove cell debris.
11. When colonies are approximately 100 cells (2–3 weeks) pick 20–30 colonies using a cloning ring and transfer to 24-well plates.
12. When confluent, test supernatant for cytokine secretion (*Protocol 9*).
13. Expand and freeze down aliquots of positive clones.

Protocol 1. *Continued*

14. Titrate supernatant from these clones for virus production and presence of 'helper' virus (*Protocols 3* and *4*).
15. When clones with high titres of helper-free virus are identified, expand and freeze down aliquots (10–20) of an early passage.

3.3 Titration of virus production

The amount of viral production by packaging cell-lines is conventionally expressed as infectious units/ml of supernatant when titred on a given cell. The packaging cell-lines are capable of a maximal virus production of approximately 10^6 U/ml of supernatant. Some vectors appear to be packaged less efficiently than others and multiple genes are packaged less well. Therefore the actual viral production is often much less.

Protocol 2. Harvesting retroviral supernatant

1. Plate 2×10^5 packaging cells per 90 mm dish.
2. After 48 h remove the culture medium and add 5 ml fresh medium.
3. Incubate the cells overnight (16 h) and harvest the supernatant.
4. Filter supernatant through a 0.45 μm filter.
5. Either use immediately to infect target cells, or aliquot and store at −70°C.

Protocol 3. Titrating for viral production

- Giemsa solution: mix together 5 ml neat Giemsa stain, 50 ml methanol and 45 ml water.

1. Harvest the supernatant from packaging cells (*Protocol 2*).
2. Infect the target cells, commonly NIH3T3 cells (*Protocol 5*) with appropriate dilutions of supernatant. For an initial titration, use 1 ml of neat, 1/10, and 1/100 dilution in medium.
3. When colonies are approximately 100 cells in size, drain off medium and add 5 ml Giemsa solution.
4. After 30 min drain Giemsa and leave to dry for 30 min.
5. Count blue colonies. Each colony represents one infectious particle and therefore the titre can be calculated and expressed as infectious particles/ml of supernatant.

3.4 Assaying for helper virus

The assay for helper virus is based on the ability of functional helper virus to rescue a marker gene from a suitable cell-line, e.g. the *HisD* gene from the EH cell-line (16). When EH cells are infected with any virus carrying a functional envelope gene, virus can be detected upon infection of NIH3T3 cells and their selection in histidinol (17).

Protocol 4. Helper assay

1. Harvest test supernatant.
2. Plate 2×10^5 EH cells 24 h prior to assay.
3. Infect EH cells as in *Protocol 5* (steps **1–5**).
4. Grow the cells for 2 weeks, splitting them two to three times a week.
5. Harvest the supernatant from these cells.
6. Infect a dish of NIH3T3s, which were plated at 5×10^5 24 h previously.
7. After 48 h, split these NIH3T3s 1/2, 1/10, 1/20, and 1/50 into selection medium: histidine-free DMEM, 10% NCS, and 100 mM histidinol.
8. Grow the surviving cells for 2–3 weeks, feeding them two to three times a week. The presence of any surviving colonies indicates the presence of helper virus.

---

4. Cytokine-secreting tumours

When stocks of helper-free high-titre supernatants have been obtained, these can be used to infect target tumour cells (*Protocols 5* and *6*). These tumour cells are then assayed for cytokine secretion (*Protocol 9*), and re-checked for the presence of helper virus. Cytokine-secreting cells can be investigated either as clonal or bulk populations. The former has the advantage that clonal populations have less variation and can be better characterized. The latter, however, compensates for any unwanted clonal variations that may occur in the tumour cells, e.g. MHC or tumour antigen expression. Before tumourigenicity assays are carried out, the *in vitro* growth rates should be measured and the absence of pathogens confirmed.

Protocol 5. Infecting adherent cells with retrovirus

- Stock × 1000 polybrene: 8 mg/ml of polybrene in water, filtered through a 0.2 μm filter.

1. 24 h prior to infection, plate 2×10^5 target cells on to a 90 mm petri dish.
2. Drain off the medium.

Protocol 5. *Continued*

3. Add 0.45 μm filtered viral supernatant (a range for the initial titration on NIH3T3 cells, the equivalent of 10^3 infectious particles for tumour cells), 1 ml fresh medium, and 2 μl of × 1000 polybrene.
4. Incubate for 4 h, rocking the dish occasionally.
5. Add 8 ml medium and incubate for 48 h.
6. When the plates are confluent, split them 1/2, 1/10, 1/20, and 1/50.
7. Wash the cells two to three times a week.
8. If clonal populations are required, then pick colonies when they become visible using a cloning ring, and expand them. If bulk populations are required then trypsinize the cells, replate them and expand them as a bulk population.
9. Target cells are then titrated for cytokine secretion (*Protocol 9*).

Protocol 6. Infecting suspension cells with retrovirus

A. *By co-cultivation*

1. Plate 10^5 packaging cells into a 25 cm^2 flask in 5 ml medium.
2. Add 10^5 target cells and 5 μl × 1000 polybrene.
3. Grow cells for 1–2 weeks splitting as necessary. The suspension cells often stick to the monolayer. Gentle tapping of the flask will free them from the packaging cells.
4. Put the suspension cells into selective medium for 2–3 weeks.
5. The resulting cells are either cloned by limiting dilution, or kept as a bulk population, and then assayed for cytokine secretion.

B. *By cell-free infection*

1. Incubate suspension cells at 10^6/ml in high-titre retroviral supernatant plus × 1 polybrene for 4 h.
2. Pellet cells and culture as normal.
3. Repeat every 24 h for 5 days.
4. Proceed as from step **4** in A above.

4.1 Tumourigenicity assays

The tumourigenicity of the modified tumour cells can be measured *in vivo* by assessing the growth of tumours when injected into immune-competent or immune-deficient animals. In *Protocol 7*, we describe the tumourigenicity assay for a subcutaneously injected murine fibrosarcoma monitored by regular measurements of tumour diameter (see also Chapter 2).

Protocol 7. Tumourigenicity assay

1. Trypsinize exponentially growing tumour cells. Count them.
2. Wash the required number of cells in PBS.
3. Re-suspend in 100 μl PBS per injection.
4. Using a 21-gauge needle inject subcutaneously into the shaved flank of an anaesthetized animal.
5. Using calipers measure the largest tumour diameter two to three times a week.

4.2 Assessing cytokine secretion of explanted tumours

Having performed tumourigenicity studies on the cytokine-secreting cells it may be desirable to study any tumours that have grown. We have shown that some IL-2- and IL-4-secreting tumours do grow out and in the former, these tumours have often lost cytokine secretion. The growing tumours are excised and grown *in vitro* as adherent monolayers (*Protocol 8*). These tumour cells can be assayed for cytokine secretion (*Protocol 9*). The assay described measures the proliferation of cytokine-dependent cell-lines (CTLL for IL-2 (18) and HT2 for IL-4 (19)) when exposed to cytokine. In tumours that have lost cytokine secretion a loss of the gene can be determined by Southern blot analysis.

Protocol 8. Explanting tumours[a]

1. Excise the tumour nodule from a freshly killed or anaesthetized animal.
2. Macerate the tumour using a scalpel and place the pieces in a conical flask.
3. Add 25 ml 1% trypsin, 0.01% DNase in serum-free medium and stir for 1 h at room temperature.
4. Filter the suspension through sterile gauze.
5. Add 10% FCS in medium to filtered supernatant and centrifuge at 175*g* for 10 min.
6. Re-suspend pellet in 10 ml fresh medium and pour into a 25 cm^2 tissue-culture flask.
7. Refeed every day initially, until the cell-line is established, to remove debris.

[a] The preparation of cell-lines from solid tumours is also described in Chapter 1.

Protocol 9. Assaying cytokine secretion of tumour cells

A. *IL-2 assay*

1. Plate 10^6 tumour cells on to a 90 mm plate with 10 ml medium.
2. 48 h later harvest 1 ml of supernatant through a 0.2 μm filter and use it in the assay immediately or store at −20°C.
3. Approximately 5×10^4 CTLL cells are required to assay each sample supernatant. (These cells are maintained in 50 U/ml recombinant IL-2 (rIL-2). To reduce background stimulation, these cells should not have been given IL-2 within 2 days prior to the assay.) Cells are pelleted by centrifugation at 175*g* for 10 min. They are then re-suspended in fresh medium and re-centrifuged twice to remove rIL-2. The final cell pellet is re-suspended in 1 ml medium.
4. Cells are counted and diluted in medium to 2.8×10^4/ml. 180 μl are pipetted into the required number of wells of a 96-well plate (18 per sample plus 6 control wells), resulting in 5×10^3 cells per well.
5. Serial ⅓ dilutions of each sample supernatant are prepared with medium.
6. 20 μl of supernatant or dilution are added to the wells in triplicate. Triplicates with 20 μl of medium (negative control) or 20 U of rIL-2 (positive control) are also set up.
7. The 96-well plate is incubated overnight (16 h) at 37°C. 0.5 μCi of methyl [^{3}H]thymidine (in 5 μl of medium) is added to each well and the plate re-incubated for a further 4 h.
8. Cells are harvested on to filter paper using a cell harvester. The dried filter discs are placed in liquid scintillant and counted for 1 min.
9. In this assay, 1/2 of the maximal stimulation (positive control) represents 1 U of IL-2. The amount of IL-2 in each sample can be calculated from the c.p.m. of the dilution that gives sub-maximal proliferation by using the following equation:

$$\text{Units of IL-2 per well} = \frac{\text{c.p.m. of sample} - \text{c.p.m. of negative control} \times 2}{\text{c.p.m. of positive control} - \text{c.p.m. of negative control}}.$$

Therefore units of IL-2 in 1 ml of supernatant equals this value × 50 × the dilution factor.

B. *IL-4 assay*

As for IL-2 assay but use HT2 cells, and rIL-4 (10 U) for the positive control (bioassays for cytokines are described quantitatively in Chapter 11).

References

1. Rosenberg, S., Lotze, M., Yang, J., Aebersold, P., Linehan, W., Seipp, C., *et al.* (1989). *Ann. Surg.,* **210,** 474–85.
2. Russell, S., Eccles, S., Flemming, C., Johnson, C., and Collins, M. (1991). *Int. J. Cancer,* **47,** 244–51.
3. Patel, P. M., Russell, S., Flemming, C., Eccles, S., and Collins, M. (1991). *Horizons in Medicine,* **3,** 214–22.
4. Watanabe, Y., Kuribayashi, K., Miyatake, S., Nishihara, K., Nakayama, E.-I., and Sakata, T.-A. (1989). *Proc. Natl Acad. Sci. USA,* **86,** 9456–60.
5. Gansbacher, B., Bannerji, R., Daniels, B., Zier, K., Cronin, K., and Gilboa, E. (1990). *Cancer Res.,* **50,** 7820–5.
6. Gansbacher, B., Zier, K., Daniels, B., Cronin, K., Bannerji, R., and Gilboa, E. (1990). *J. Exp. Med.,* **172,** 1217–24.
7. Cepko, C., Roberts, B., and Mulligan, R. (1984). *Cell,* **37,** 1053–62.
8. Keller, G., Paige, P., Gilboa, E., and Wagner, E. (1985). *Nature,* **318,** 149–54.
9. Morgenstern, J. and Land, H. (1990). *Nucleic Acids Res.,* **18,** 3587–96.
10. Peries, J., Aves-Cardosa, E., Canivet, M., Debons-Guillemin, M., and Lasnert, J. (1977). *J. Natl Cancer Inst.,* **59,** 463–5.
11. Guild, B., Finer, M., and Houseman, D. (1988). *J. Virol.,* **62,** 3795–801.
12. Ferry, N., Duplessis, O., Houssin, D., Danos, O., and Heard, J. M. (1991). *Proc. Natl Acad. Sci. USA,* **88,** 8377–81.
13. Danos, O. (1991). In *Practical Molecular Virology,* (ed. M. Collins), pp. 17–28. Humana Clifton, NJ.
14. Markowitz, D., Goff, S., and Bank, A. (1988). *J. Virol.,* **62,** 1120–4.
15. Markowitz, D., Goff, S., and Bank, A. (1988). *Virology,* **167,** 400–6.
16. Danos, O. and Mulligan, R. (1988). *Proc. Natl Acad. Sci. USA,* **85,** 6460–4.
17. Hartman, S. and Mulligan, R. (1988). *Proc. Natl Acad. Sci. USA,* **85,** 8047–51.
18. Gillis, S., Ferm, M. M., Ward, O. V., and Smith, K. A. (1978). *J. Immunol.,* **120,** 2027–32.
19. Lichtman, A. M., Kurt-Jones, E. A., and Abbas, A. K. (1987). *Proc. Natl Acad. Sci. USA,* **84,** 824–7.
20. Fearon, E., Pardoll, D., Itaya, T., Golumbek, P., Karasuyama, H., Vogelstein, B., *et al.* (1990). *Cell,* **60,** 397–403.
21. Ley, V., Langlade-Demoyen, P., Kourilsky, P., and Larsson-Sciard, E. (1991). *Eur. J. Immunol.,* **21,** 851–4.
22. Tepper, R., Pattengale, P., and Leder, P. (1989). *Cell,* **57,** 503–12.
23. Golumbek, P., Lazenby, A., Levitsky, H., Jaffee, L., Karasuyama, H., Baker, M., *et al.* (1991). *Science,* **254,** 713–17.
24. Esumi, N., Hunt, B., Itaya, T., and Frost, P. (1991). *Cancer Res.,* **51,** 1185–9.
25. Colombo, M., Ferrari, G., Stoppacciaro, A., Parenza, M., Rondolfo, M., Mavilio, F., *et al.* (1991). *J. Exp. Med.,* **173,** 889–97.
26. Asher, A., Mule, J., Kasid, A., Restifo, N., Salo, J., Reicherb, C., *et al.* (1991). *J. Immunol.,* **146,** 3227–34.
27. Blankenstein, T., Qin, Z., Uberla, K., Muller, W., Rosen, H., Volk, H.-D., *et al.* (1991). *J. Exp. Med.,* **173,** 1047–52.
28. Hock, H., Dorsch, M., Diammemtsein, T., and Blankenstein, T. (1991). *J. Exp. Med.,* **174,** 1291–8.

19

Ex vivo activation of effector cells

K. E. PLATTS

1. Introduction

The last decade has seen the rise of a new approach to the treatment of cancer—immunotherapy. One aspect of this new methodology, adoptive immunotherapy, involves the transfer of immunological cells or signalling molecules (e.g. cytokines) into cancer patients. The patient's cells responsible for immune defence are removed and are either stimulated to recognize cancer target cells or have their native ability to kill tumour cells enhanced. This *ex vivo* activation of cells allows the expansion of cells with potential therapeutic value, whose activation *in vivo* may be impaired.

Cytotoxic cells within the immune system that have the ability to react against and destroy tumour cells include antigen-specific cytotoxic T lymphocytes (CTL) (which recognize tumour antigens in association with membrane products of the major histocompatibility complex (MHC) present on tumour cells) and natural killer (NK) cells (a description of a function rather than a cell type, which morphologically are large granular lymphocytes (LGL), and include CD3− lymphocytes and some activated CD3+ lymphocytes). The latter cells do not recognize tumour-specific antigens, but less-well defined targets on the membrane of target cells. The target cells are killed independently of, or in the absence of, expressed MHC products, and NK cells can kill certain tumour cells spontaneously *in vitro*.

The use of antigen-specific cytotoxic cells as therapeutic agents for the treatment of cancer rests upon the assumption that tumour cells carry surface antigens that such cells can specifically recognize. Some immunogenic experimental murine tumours can generate T cells specifically reactive to antigens found primarily on tumour cells, and in certain models, antigen-specific tumour reactive T cells can induce tumour regression when transferred to tumour-bearing animals. Problems arise when the tumours are non-immunogenic or if tumours arise spontaneously, as they often lack surface antigens which cytotoxic cells can recognize. In humans (with the exception of melanoma) the presence of tumour-specific T-cell reactivity has been difficult to prove. In some human tumours there is loss of MHC class-I molecules and therefore these cells would escape an antigen-specific cytotoxic response.

The generation of low numbers of potentially cytotoxic cells *in vitro*, has little therapeutic value: to realize the possibility of utilizing these cells for immunotherapy they need to be expanded during culture, then infused back into the patient. The discovery in 1976 of T-cell growth factor (TCGF), now termed interleukin 2 (IL-2), eventually led to the description of another population of cells with therapeutic potential. IL-2 is produced by T helper cells and stimulates the proliferation of activated cells of lymphoid lineage including: activated lymphocytes, natural killer cells, lymphokine-activated cells, B lymphocytes, and macrophages.

IL-2 has been shown to generate effector cells derived from peripheral blood mononuclear cells (PBMC), tumour-infiltrating lymphocytes (TIL), and lymph-node lymphocytes from healthy donors and cancer patients, which can recognize and kill cancer cells *in vitro*. This phenomenon has led to the use of this cytokine to activate cells of the immune system *ex vivo* to kill tumour cells *in vivo*.

These lymphokine activated killer (LAK) cells are heterogeneous in phenotype: when generated from the peripheral blood of healthy human donors, they are primarily derived from NK cells (CD3−CD5−CD56+ CD16+) and recognize tumour cells in a non-MHC restricted manner; however, a sub-population of T cells which are CD3+CD56+ and constitute less than 1% of total T cells can also mediate non-MHC-restricted cytotoxicity and are a source of LAK cell precursors.

IL-2 has been utilized to generate populations of cytotoxic effectors which have subsequently been used in human adoptive therapy. Due to a limited clinical success, much research has attempted to improve this alternative approach to the treatment of cancer. This chapter will document protocols for the generation of effector cells suitable for experimental studies and therapeutic applications. Details of effector cells employed to treat experimental animal tumours are summarized in *Table 1*.

Initially, attention focused upon the non-MHC-restricted response mediated by LAK cells; however, more specific responses were sought for the treatment of some human cancers. A number of cell populations generated by different activation protocols have been employed for the treatment of human cancer, and are summarized in *Table 2*.

Table 1. Molecules involved in activating effector cell populations with therapeutic potential in murine systems

Cell type	Source	Activating agent	Reference
LAK	Splenocytes	IL-2	20 (rat (21))
	Splenocytes	IL-2 + OKT3	22
	Splenocytes	IL-2 + tumour	23
TIL	Tumour	IL-2	24
	Tumour	CD3	25

Table 2. Molecules involved in activating effector cell populations with therapeutic potential

Cell type	Source	Activating agent	Cytotoxicity
CTL	Peripheral blood	Mitogen, lectin, antigen	MHC restricted
NK	Peripheral blood	Interferons, interferon inducers, microbial agents	MHC unrestricted
A-LAK	Peripheral blood	IL-2	MHC unrestricted
LAK	Peripheral blood	IL-2	MHC unrestricted
TIL	Tumour	IL-2	MHC restricted MHC unrestricted
TDAC	Tumour	IL-2 + tumour, IL-2 + anti-CD3 MAb	Specific[a]
Macrophages	Peripheral blood		(see references (26, 27))

CTL, cytotoxic T lymphocyte; NK cell, natural killer; A-LAK, adherent lymphokine-activated killer; LAK, lymphokine-activated killer; TDAC, tumour-derived activated cell; MAb, monoclonal antibody.

[a] Specificity is defined as effectors which in *in vitro* assays (i) preferentially react against autologous tumour, rather than (ii) react against autologous and allogeneic tumour of the same histology, or (iii) have broad reactivity against allogeneic cell-lines and tumour irrespective of histology. As mentioned previously, non-MHC-restricted cytotoxicity is not mediated solely by NK cells, cytotoxic T lymphocytes can become activated in the presence of high concentrations of IL-2 to mediate non-specific activity an addition to antigen-primed MHC-restricted cytotoxicity.

2. Isolation of effector populations

Human cell populations which may be activated *ex vivo* for use in immunotherapy include peripheral blood lymphocytes and lymphocytes isolated from within the tumour. Protocols for the isolation of these two populations are given.

2.1 Peripheral blood mononuclear cells (PBMC)

Cells most commonly employed for the generation of cytotoxic effectors of potential therapeutic use are PBMC, as they are easy to obtain in large numbers from healthy blood donors and can also be obtained from patients. Unclotted venous blood from the donor is taken and separated on a density gradient as the method of Boyum *et al.* (1). This initial enrichment procedure depletes erythrocytes, granulocytes, and platelets.

Protocol 1. Isolation of peripheral blood mononuclear cells

1. Obtain sterile blood by venupuncture into sterile syringes, and transfer it immediately into clean sterile glass bottles containing anti-coagulant, e.g. preservative-free heparin at a final concentration of 10 IU/ml blood.[a]
2. Dilute the blood 1:1 with phosphate-buffered saline (PBS).
3. Layer two volumes of blood on to one volume of Lymphoprep—a commercially available lymphocyte separation density-gradient medium (Nycomed Ltd, Middlesex, UK)[b] in a sterile centrifuge tube.
4. Centrifuge at room temperature for 35 min at 420*g*. To prevent disturbance to the interface do not use the brake facility on the centrifuge.
5. Harvest the cells from the interface into fresh plastic universals/centrifuge tubes, and wash by centrifugation at 600*g* for 15 min at 4°C with three volumes of PBS, to remove any separation medium left in contact with the cells.
6. Remove contaminating platelets by centrifugation at 200*g* fo 15 min, 4°C; repeat.
7. Re-suspend the cells in medium and count the number of viable cells by trypan blue dye exclusion (0.1% trypan blue in PBS) using a cell-counting chamber. Viability should exceed 95%. Expected yield, (1–2) $\times$ 10^6 PBMC/ml blood.

[a] Alternatively EDTA or acid citrate dextrose can be used.
[b] Alternative density gradients may be used (1).

2.2 Tumour-infiltrating lymphocytes (TIL)

Infiltrating cells within a tumour are thought to have an increased affinity for the tumour and therefore increased potential to mediate an immune response; it has been demonstrated that in murine models such cells were 50 times more able to mediate tumour regression. There are two procedures for tumour dispersion: mechanical and enzymic. A combination of the two is usually employed. Mechanical digestion may cause damage to the cells by breaking them open, whereas enzymes (usually proteases) may destroy or alter cellular surface molecules. The use of trypsin has been shown to destroy many cellular surface antigens as determined by flow cytometry.

The enzymes commonly employed for tumour digestion, either singly or in combination, include collagenase, dispase, trypsin, and hyaluronidase. DNAse is employed to disperse DNA released from disrupted cells, and the reducing agent dithiothreitol is employed to reduce mucus in those tumours with high mucin content (colon and stomach). Procedures for isolating cells from tumours are described in Chapter 1.

Tumour structure and morphology vary greatly, and there is no single dispersion procedure to follow. Soft tissue will digest easily, whilst hard tissue will need more intense treatment, it is therefore necessary to determine the optimal conditions for tumour digestion empirically. *Protocol 2* has been routinely used in our laboratory to isolate TIL from human colon and breast carcinoma tissue. For the isolation of TIL from colon tissue it is recommended that antibiotics are added to the medium (usually RPMI 1640 or AIMV) to minimize bacterial contamination: penicillin (50 U/ml), streptomycin (100 μg/ml), gentamycin (20 U/ml), and mycostatin (10 U/ml) are present throughout the washing and culturing stages.

The enzyme cocktail used for the dissociation of breast and colon tumour tissue used in our laboratory consists of the following: RPMI 1640 medium containing 200–300 U/ml collagenase IA, 0.02 mg/ml DNase I type IV, and 0.01 mg/ml hyaluronidase VIII (Sigma Chemical Co. Ltd, Dorset, UK).

The specimens should be transported from the operating theatre to the laboratory in ice-cold medium and treated as soon as possible.

Protocol 2. Isolation of TIL

1. Remove all visible fatty and necrotic tissue and mince the tumour into small pieces (1 mm^3) using scalpel blades.
2. Wash the tumour cells in medium (containing antibiotics if necessary—see above), by centrifugation (400*g*, 6 min, room temperature) to remove cellular debris.
3. Weigh the tumour and add enzyme digest (allow 10 ml for 1g of tumour wet weight).

Protocol 2. *Continued*

4. Digest at 37°C for 2 h (the time may vary considerably depending upon the tumour, maximal digestion was 8 h). To ensure maximal digest, gentle mixing of tumour and enzyme digest mixture is carried out using an end-over-end mixer. The use of magnetic fleas is not recommended since shearing forces may damage the cells.
5. Wash the cells twice in medium to dilute out the digestion cocktail (serum can be added at this stage to stop the enzyme digestion process).
6. Re-suspend the cells in medium and count (as in *Protocol 1*). Cell viability varies greatly depending upon the tumour type and the digestion process.

In our experience, the majority of cells obtained are mononuclear cells (60–96% viable) with few, mainly non-viable tumour cells. The range of cell yields was from (0.6–40.0) $\times$ 10^6 cells per gram wet weight of tumour (see also Chapters 1 and 7).

The cellular infiltrate may be separated by density-gradient centrifugation, as described in *Protocol 1*, alternatively TIL can be separated from tumour cells (using a 75:100% discontinuous density gradient in PBS), tumour cells will be enriched for at the 75% interface, whilst the lymphocytes will be enriched for at the 75–100% interface.

3. Separation techniques to isolate enriched or purified populations of effector cells

In most activation procedures, unseparated PBMC are employed in the generation of LAK cells; however, additional procedures may be used to isolate purified populations including LGL, T lymphocytes, and macrophages in order to generate more efficacious effector cells. Using such highly purified effector cells, less IL-2 may be required for the activation and maintenance of these cells, and fewer cells needed to mediate greater therapeutic efficacy. The protocols for these separation techniques are beyond the scope of this chapter; the reader is referred to protocols and references for further details (*Table 3*).

4. Activation of effector populations

Populations of effector cells can be maintained in culture in the presence of stimuli which confer upon the activated cells the ability to mediate a specific or non-specific response. The latter has been well documented in the treatment of human neoplasms; protocols for activating such non-specific cytotoxic cells will be given, as well as some improvements in the generation of potential effectors.

Table 3. Methods employed for the enrichment or purification of precursor populations: which include natural killer cells (NK), T lymphocytes, (T) and large granular lymphocytes (LGL)

Type of selection	Property of cells	Technique	Reference
Enrichment	Adherence	Plastic/glass adherence	Chapter 6
Enrichment	Adherence	Nylon wool	28
Enrichment	Density	Percoll	Chapter 5
Enrichment	Density	Centrifugal elutriation	29
Enrichment	Chemical	Phenylalanine methyl ester	30
Purification	Surface phenotype	SRBC rosette formation	31
Purification	Surface phenotype	Panning	32
Purification	Surface phenotype	Antibody + complement-mediated lysis	33
Purification	Surface phenotype	Lymphokwik T	34
Purification	Surface phenotype	Flow cytometry	Chapter 3
Purification	Surface phenotype	Immunomagnetic beads	35

4.1 Generation of IL-2-activated human peripheral blood mononuclear cells

Initially, natural IL-2 was obtained from the Jurkat cell-line; however, subsequent cloning and expression of the gene sequence facilitated the production of recombinant DNA-derived material which was indistinguishable from the naturally occurring protein. There are many commercial sources of IL-2 and it should be noted that the specific activity of each IL-2 may differ. Unless otherwise stated in the protocols, the IL-2 used was a generous gift from Glaxo, Geneva, Switzerland, with a specific activity of 8.3×10^6 U/mg (MTT colorimetric assay, CTLL-273 cells).

Early experiments generating LAK cells involved culturing $(1–2) \times 10^6$ cells/ml for three or four days in the presence of high concentrations of IL-2; however, LAK cells can be generated at much lower concentrations, without loss of LAK activity particularly in the presence of IL-12. The concentration of IL-2 should be determined empirically: in these protocols, the IL-2 concentration for each particular system is reported. The use of low concentrations of IL-2 has led to the generation of effector cells using potentially synergistic combinations of different activating molecules (see Section 4.3.5).

Traditionally, LAK cells were cultured in RPMI 1640 medium containing 2–10% AB serum (which should be heat-inactivated by heating to 55 °C for 30 min, and stored in amounts at −20°C for single use). With the need to transfer effector populations back into the patient, a more defined medium was sought. A variety of serum-free media are commercially available including AIM V (Gibco Ltd, UK), HB-LAK (DuPont, Wilmington, Delaware), HL-1 (Ventrex, Portland, Maine), and X-VIVO 10 (MA Bioproducts,

Walkersville, Maryland), all of which support the generation of LAK cells (AIM V is routinely used in our experiments). The use of serum-free, defined medium provides consistency to culture techniques, is safer, and more readily available than human serum; however, the precise constituents of AIM V medium are not disclosed, therefore variations in activation responses may occur.

In general, with an unpurified population of cells there is no overall expansion in lymphocyte numbers recovered following four day activation *in vitro*, due to a low proliferation rate, and PBMC which adhere to the tissue-culture flasks.

The length of culture affects the phenotype of effector cells generated: short-term LAK activity has been shown to be generated by NK precursors; longer incubations in the presence of IL-2 increases the numbers of T-cell derived (CD3+ CD56+) LAK effectors.

Protocol 3. Generation of human IL-2-activated lymphocytes

1. Isolate PBMC (*Protocol 1*).
2. Initiate cultures at 1×10^6 cells/ml in RPMI 1640 medium (containing 10% AB) or AIM V medium containing 125 U/ml IL-2 (Glaxo) in tissue-culture plates or flasks at 37°C, 5% CO_2.[a]
3. Add fresh medium containing 125 U/ml IL-2 every 4–5 days. Keep the cell concentration at, or below 1×10^6 cells/ml.[b]
4. Assess the activation of the cells (see Section 5) periodically during the initial week, then at weekly intervals.

[a] For short-term generation of LAK tissue-culture plates are used; however, when cell cultures are to be expanded *in vitro* tissue-culture flasks are preferred, and are incubated lying on their side.

[b] The viable cell count (non-adherent cell number) will decrease initially due to cell adherence to the culture vessel.

4.2 Generation of IL-2-activated human TIL

The cells present in solid tumours that can be cultured in the presence of IL-2 are heterogeneous, and include T cells (both cytotoxic T lymphocytes, and non-MHC restricted), NK cells, macrophages, and granulocytes. It was thought that these cells may provide an excellent source of effector cells as they may be reactive within the tumour *in vivo*.

Protocol 4. Generation of IL-2-activated human TIL

1. Dissaggregate tumour (*Protocol 2*).
2. Initiate the culture at 1×10^6 cells/ml in RPMI 1640 medium (containing 10% AB) or AIM V medium in the presence of 125 U/ml IL-2 (Glaxo).

3. Add fresh medium containing 1000 U/ml IL-2 every 3–4 days until the culture begins to expand.
4. Sub-culture when the lymphocytes reach a cell count of 1×10^6 cells/ml, or every 4 days.[a]
5. Assess for activation (see Section 5).

[a] Viable cell number will decrease initially.

4.3 Modifications to the procedures for the generation of human effector cell populations

Following limited success treating human neoplasia with *ex vivo*-activated cells, alternative procedures were explored to enhance the potency of effector cells including the isolation of more specific populations and, increasing the capacity of activated cells to mediate a cytotoxic response.

4.3.1 Generation of specific cytotoxicity by TIL

Activation of TIL with IL-2 leads to a functionally diverse effector population, which depends largely upon the tumour from which the cells are derived: TIL generated from melanomas show specific cytotoxicity; however, TIL generated from other tumours including ovarian, renal cell, breast, colon, and head and neck carcinoma, generate effector cells which display non-MHC-restricted cytotoxicity. Alternative approaches to the generation of TIL with a view to greater specificity have been developed, these include culturing TIL with IL-2 in combination with tumour necrosis factor, to promote the growth of CD8+ cells some of which may be specific for autologous tumour, and culturing TIL in the presence of tumour (tumour-derived activated cells—TDAC).

i. Generation of tumour-derived activated cells (TDAC)

Tumour-infiltrating lymphocytes are activated in the presence of IL-2 and tumour pieces in an attempt to generate effector cells which are specific for the patient's own, as yet, undefined tumour associated antigens. For specific details of the procedure refer to Yanelli *et al.* (2).

Protocol 5. Generation of TDAC

1. Mince the tumour and place the pieces in the cell culture medium RPMI 1640 containing 10% human AB serum and 1000 U/ml IL-2 (Cetus).
2. Leave the tumour chunks in the cell suspension and culture with the TIL in order to stimulate antigen specificity. Supplement the TDAC cultures with supernatant derived from LAK cell cultures (this provides a source of lymphokines and growth factors).

Protocol 5. *Continued*

3. Add fresh medium containing 1000 U/ml IL-2 every 5–7 days, or when the cell concentration reaches a density of (1.5–2) $\times$ 10^6 cells/ml. The tumour disappears within 2–3 weeks and it is necessary to restimulate cultures with tumour or plastic-bound anti-CD3 monoclonal antibody once the tumour cells have been lost from culture.

4.3.2 Generation of purified populations of effectors

Most studies generating effectors for cancer therapy employ unfractionated populations. Recently, interest has focused upon using purified populations, with a view to decreasing toxicity caused by large numbers of cells being infused back into the patient, and activating cells which are more potent, therefore utilizing less IL-2.

i. Generation of adherent lymphokine-activated killer (A-LAK) cells

A proportion of human PBMC incubated in the presence of high concentrations of IL-2 become adherent to glass and plastic. These cells are phenotypically NK cells (CD3−CD56+CD16+) and have been named 'adherent LAK' (A-LAK) cells. Separation of the NK cells from T cells is dependent upon the fact that the former are activated more rapidly than the latter, and attach to the plastic or glass first, leaving the T cells present in suspension. A-LAK cells can be generated from both healthy donor and tumour-bearing patient peripheral blood mononuclear cells. The prominent phenotype is CD3−, CD56+ (NK cells) and continued expansion over 2–3 weeks *in vitro* culture yields large numbers of highly purified NK cells (80–90% purity). For full details of the activation procedure refer to Melder *et al.* (3).

Protocol 6. Generation of human A-LAK cells

1. Deplete PBMC of monocytes by nylon wool adherence.
2. Suspend cells in RPMI 1640 medium containing 10% AB serum in the presence of 1000 U/ml IL-2 (Cetus).
3. Incubate for 24 h, 37°C, 5% CO_2 in a plastic flask.
4. Remove non-adherent LAK cells and keep the supernatant.
5. Culture the cells in 50% conditioned medium (from 24 h culture—see step 4) in fresh medium containing 1000 U/ml IL-2.
6. Expand in culture for 10–14 days.
7. Assess for activation (see Section 5).

4.3.3 Increasing effector cell numbers

A large number of cells are required for adoptive transfer immunotherapy and methods have been developed to increase cell numbers without the loss of cytotoxic activity, these include culturing cells for a longer period of time and using T-cell mitogens.

i. Expansion of human LAK cells by increased culture time

PBMC cultured at 1×10^6 cells/ml in the presence of IL-2 for 10–12 days, generate primarily CD3+CD16−CD56− LGL which displays strong non-MHC restricted cytotoxicity (4). The following protocol increases the percentage of CD3+, CD16+, and CD56+ cells; however, the non-MHC restricted cytotoxicity detected following four day activation is not always maintained throughout extended culture periods.

Protocol 7. Generation of long-term cultured IL-2-activated PBMC

1. Isolate PBMC (*Protocol 1*).
2. Initiate cultures at 1×10^6 cells/ml in AIM V medium containing 125 U/ml IL-2 (Glaxo).
3. Incubate at 37°C, 5% CO_2.
4. Determine cell proliferation by viable cell counts every 48 h.
5. Add fresh medium containing 125 U/ml IL-2 every 3–4 days. Keep the cell concentration at, or below, 1×10^6 cells/ml.[a]
6. Assess activation (see Section 5).

[a] The viable cell count (non-adherent cell number) will decrease initially due to cell adherence to the culture vessel.

---

ii. Expansion of lymphokine-activated killer cells with IL-2 in combination with OKT3 monoclonal antibody

The mouse anti-human CD3 monoclonal antibody OKT3, is a mitogen for T cells which extends culture periods compared to IL-2-stimulated LAK cell culture (14–21 days), increasing effector yield, and maintaining LAK activity (5). The following protocol generates more effector cells than IL-2 activation alone (*Figure 1*), primarily CD3+ cells; however, the cytotoxic activity is not always maintained.

Protocol 8. Expansion of peripheral blood mononuclear cells cultured in the presence of IL-2 in combination with OKT3

1. Isolate PBMC (*Protocol 1*).
2. Culture cells in RPMI 1640 medium containing 10% AB serum, in the presence of 125 U/ml IL-2 at 1×10^6 cells/ml. Incubate in 5% CO_2 at 37°C.

Protocol 8. *Continued*

3. Add 10 ng/ml OKT3 monoclonal antibody (Ortho Diagnostics Systems Ltd) for the first 48 h.
4. Remove excess antibody by washing twice in medium (400*g*, 6 min).
5. Re-culture cells at (0.1–0.2) $\times$ 10^6 cells/ml in fresh medium containing 125 U/ml IL-2.
6. Sub-culture every 48 h at 0.5 $\times$ 10^6 cells/ml.

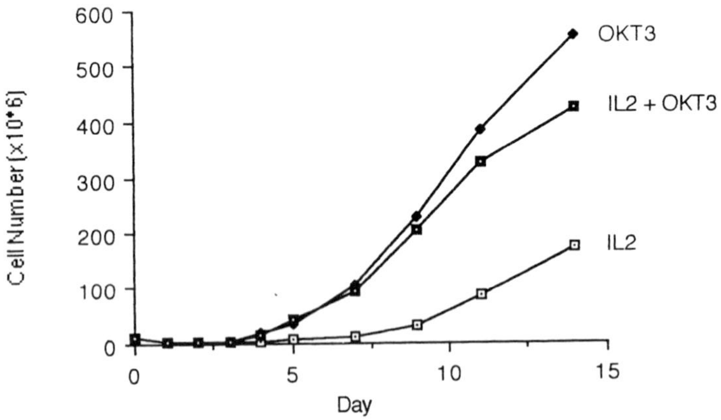

Figure 1. Proliferation of PBMC cultured in the presence of 125 U/ml IL-2 following activation with 125 U/ml IL-2 in combination with 10 ng/ml OKT3 monoclonal antibody, determined by viable cell count.

4.3.4 Reduction of *in vitro* stimulation

Traditionally the generation of effector cells for reinfusion into the patient requires long-term culture which has a number of disadvantages: expense, possible contamination, time. An alternative procedure which minimizes these problems requires a short culture period whilst maintaining the cytotoxic capacity of the effector cells.

i. Generation of LAK cells by pulsing

Extensive culturing of cells may not be necessary for the generation of cytotoxic LAK cells, instead a brief 15 to 60 min pulse with high-dose IL-2 (1000 U per 3 $\times$ 10^6 PBMC) allows the generation of LAK cells, thus overcoming some of the problems associated with culturing PBMC for use in therapy (6). *Protocol 9* has been used by C. Carter, Institute of Cancer Studies, University of Sheffield Medical School, UK, to generate cytotoxic activity from cultured cells (see *Figure 2*).

Protocol 9. Generation of LAK cells by pulsing

1. Isolate PBMC (*Protocol 1*) and adjust cell density to 4×10^6 cells/ml in AIM V medium.
2. Incubate cells for 60 min in the presence of 500 U/ml IL-2 (Glaxo or Cetus).
3. Wash the pulsed PBMC in cold PBS by centrifugation (400*g*, 6 min), three times.
4. Adjust the cell density to 4×10^6 cells/ml in AIM V medium and culture in 24-well tissue-culture plates in 1 ml cultures.
5. Incubate for 4 days in 5% CO_2 at 37°C.
6. Assess activation (see Section 5).

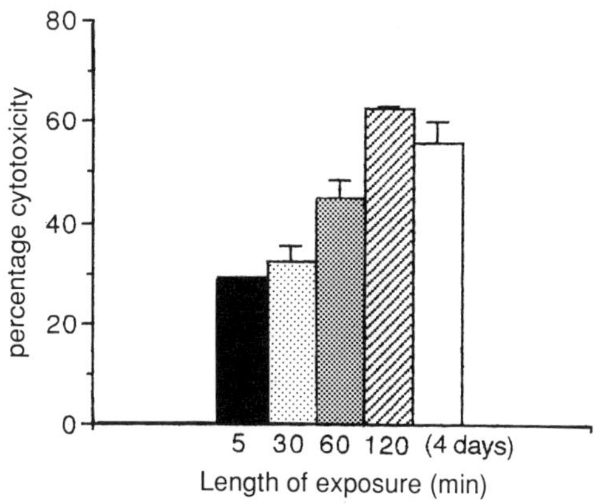

Figure 2. Cytotoxicity of PBMC activated by short-term pulsing with IL-2 against SW742 at a target to effector ratio of 10:1.

4.3.5 Synergy with other immunologically relevant molecules

To increase the cytotoxic capacity of activated effector populations, IL-2, in combination with other cytokines, has been shown to have synergistic effect upon activation: these additional cytokines include interferon gamma (IFN-γ), tumour necrosis factor alpha (TNF-α), IL-1, IL-4, IL-6, IL-7, and IL-12, all of which have been shown to increase the ability of effector populations to mediate cytotoxicity *in vitro*. The procedures for synergy experiments are based on those already given, for more details the reader is referred to the following papers: IFN-γ (7), TNF-α (8), IL-1 (9), IL-4 (10), IL-6 (11), IL-7 (12), IL-12 (13).

5. Assessment of activation

Methods for the detection of activated cells include the measurement of proliferation, cytotoxicity, cytokine expression, and cytokine gene expression. These are briefly discussed.

5.1 Cytotoxicity assays

The chromium release assay is the main method for determining *in vitro* cytotoxicity; the protocol is described in Chapters 5 and 7. Tumour targets may be derived from tumours and used to determine specificity against autologous tumour and non-related tumours, alternatively cell-lines may be employed to determine non-MHC-restricted cytotoxicity. With the exception of SW742 (an adenocarcinoma cell-line), cell-lines can be obtained from the American Type Culture Collection and include K562 an erythromyeloid leukaemia cell-line which is NK and LAK sensitive, and a range of relatively NK-insensitive LAK-sensitive targets including: Daudi (Burkitt's lymphoma-derived B-lymphoblastoid cell-line), Colo205 (human adenocarcinoma cell-line), Molt 4 (T-cell leukaemia cell-line), FeMX (melanoma cell-line), and Raji (Burkitt's lymphoma cell-line). Cell-lines should be routinely tested for mycoplasma, by one of the following methods: isolation of the organism by culture, Hoescht staining, or DNA hybridization (GEN-PROBE rapid detection kit (Laboratory Impex Ltd, Middlesex, UK)) (see Chapter 1).

For further information about the assessment of cell-mediated cytotoxicity refer to Loudon and Grimm (14).

5.2 Proliferation

The simplest assessment of proliferation is by viable cell counting (trypan dye exclusion). The commonest procedure is the uptake of [^{3}H]thymidine by stimulated cells (see Chapter 7); alternatively flow cytometry can be performed (see Chapter 3).

5.3 Cytokine production

Activation of populations of cells can be determined by the production of cytokines, which can be assayed by the following:

(a) Detection of cytokines present in a supernatant, by radioimmunoassay (RIA), immunoradiometric assay (IRMA), enzyme immunoassay (EIA) (15), or bioassay (16).

(b) Detection of cytokines located within a cell, using reverse haemolytic plaque assay, the cell-blot assay and elispots (17).

5.4 Cytokine gene expression

Activation of population of cells may be determined by the production of messenger RNA, the detection of which includes Northern blotting, *in situ* hybridization (18), and message amplification phenotyping (MAPPing), using the polymerase chain reaction (PCR) (19).

Acknowledgement

The support of the Yorkshire Cancer Research Campaign is gratefully acknowledged.

References

1. Boyum, A., Berg, T., and Blomhoff, R. (1981). In *Iodinated Density Gradient Media, A Practical Approach*, (ed. D. Rickwood), p. 147. IRL Press, Washington, D.C.
2. Yannelli, J. R., Crumacker, D. B., Good, R. W., Friddell, C. D., Poston, R., Horton, S., *et al.* (1990). *J. Immunol. Meth.,* **1,** 91.
3. Melder, R. J., Whiteside, T. L., Vajanovic, N. L., Hiserodt, J. C., and Herberman, R. B. (1988). *Cancer Res.,* **48,** 3461.
4. Roussel, E., Gerrard, J. M., and Greenberg, A. H. (1990). *Clin. Exp. Immunol.,* **82,** 416.
5. Ochoa, A. C., Gromo, G., Alter, B. J., Sondel, P. M., and Bach, F. (1987). *J. Immunol.,* **138,** 2728.
6. Horton, S. A., Oldham, R. K., and Yannelli, J. R. (1990). *Cancer Res.,* **50,** 1686.
7. Itoh, K., Shiiba, K., Shimiza, Y., Suzuki, R., and Kamagai, K. (1985). *J. Immunol.,* **134,** 3124.
8. Yang, S. C., Owen-Schaub, L., Grimm, E. A., and Roth, J. A. (1989). *Cancer Immunol. Immunother.,* **29,** 193.
9. Crump, W. L., Owen-Schaub, L. B., and Grimm, E. (1989). *Cancer Res.,* **49,** 149.
10. Higuchi, C. M., Thompson, J. A., Lindgren, C. G., Gillis, S., Widmer, M. B., Kern, D. E., *et al.* (1989). *Cancer Res.,* **49,** 6487.
11. Gallagher, G., Stimson, W. H., Findlay, J., and Al-Azzawi, F. (1990). *Cancer Immunol. Immunother.,* **31,** 49.
12. Stotter, H., Custer, M. C., Bolton, E. S., Guedez, L., and Lotze, M. T. (1990). *J. Immunol.,* **146,** 150.
13. Gately, M. K., Desai, B. B., Wolitzky, A. G., Quinn, P. M., Dwyer, C. M., Podlaski, F. J., *et al.* (1991). *J. Immunol.,* **147,** 874.
14. Loudon, W. and Grimm, E. (1991). In *Cytokines, A Practical Approach*, (ed. F. R. Balkwill), p. 171. IRL Press, Oxford.
15. Meager, A. (1991). In *Cytokines, A Practical Approach*, (ed. F. R. Balkwill), p. 299. IRL Press, Oxford.
16. Wadhwa, M., Bird, C., Tinker, A., Mire-Sluis, A., and Thorpe, R. (1991). In *Cytokines, A Practical Approach*, (ed. F. R. Balkwill), p. 309. IRL Press, Oxford.
17. Lewis, C. E. (1991). In *Cytokines, A Practical Approach*, (ed. F. R. Balkwill), p. 279. IRL Press, Oxford.
18. Naylor, M. S. and Balkwill, F. R. (1991). In *Cytokines, A Practical Approach*, (ed. F. R. Balkwill), p. 31. IRL Press, Oxford.
19. Brenner, C. A., Daniel, S. L., and Adler, R. In *Cytokines, A Practical Approach*, (ed. F. R. Balkwill), p. 51. IRL Press, Oxford.

20. Rosenberg, S. A. (1986). *Important Advances in Oncology*, 55.
21. Vujanovic, N. L., Herbermann, R. B., Olszoy, M. W., Cramer, D. V., Salup, R. R., Reynolds, C. W., *et al.* (1988). *Cancer Res.*, **48,** 884.
22. Loeffler, C. M., Platt, J. L., Anderson, P. M., Katsanis, E., Ochoa, J. B., Urba, W. J., *et al.* (1991). *Cancer Res.*, **51,** 2127.
23. Chen, W., Reese, V. A., and Cheever, M. A. (1990). *J. Immunol.*, **144,** 3659.
24. Topalian, S. L. and Rosenberg, S. A. (1990). *Important Advances in Oncology*, 19.
25. Yoshizawa, H., Sakai, K., Chang, A. E., and Shu, S. (1991). *Cell. Immunol.*, **134,** 473.
26. Andreesen, R., Scheibenbogen, C., Brugger, W., Krause, S., Meerpohl, H-G., Leser, H-G., *et al.* (1990). *Cancer Res.*, **50,** 7450.
27. Higashi, N., Nishimura, Y., Higuchi, M., and Osawa, T. (1991). *J. Immunother.*, **10,** 247.
28. Julius, M. H., Simpson, E., and Hertzenberg, L. A. (1973). *Eur. J. Immunol.*, **3,** 645.
29. Yasaka, T., Wells, R. J., Mantich, N. M., and Boxer, L. A. (1982). *Immunology*, **46,** 613.
30. Leung, K. H. (1989). *Cancer Immunol. Immunother.*, **30,** 247.
31. Londei, M., Clayton, J., and Feldman, M. (1991). In *Cytokines, A Practical Approach*, (ed. F. R. Balkwill), p. 151. IRL Press, Oxford.
32. Wysocki, L. J. and Sato, V. L. (1978). *Proc. Natl Acad. Sci. USA*, **75,** 2844.
33. Shortman, K. (1974). *Contemp. Top. Mol. Immunol.*, **3,** 161.
34. Clouse, K., Adams, P., Sheridan, J., and Orosz, C. (1987). *J. Immunol. Meth.*, **105,** 253.
35. Funderud, S., Nustad, K., Lea, T., Vartdal, F., Gaudernack, G., Stenstad, P., *et al.* (1987). In *Lymphocytes, A Practical Approach*, (ed. G. G. B. Klaus), p. 55. IRL Press, Oxford.

20

Genetic immortalization of human lymphocytes using retroviral vectors

CHRIS DARNBROUGH

1. Introduction

Despite advances in the understanding of the role of oncogenes in cell immortalization and tumorigenesis, little progress has been made in applying genetic approaches to the generation of permanent cell-lines from primary cells of the immune system. This is particularly true of human cells, where the practical problems of obtaining tissues and cells are often compounded by the reluctance of human cells to take up and integrate DNA, whether introduced by transfection, electroporation, or virus infection. Even in those species and cell types from which immortalized cell-lines have been isolated, the resulting cell-lines often fail to retain their differentiated phenotypes and are of limited value as sources of differentiated products or for applications in research or therapy. Additional problems are encountered in the case of highly differentiated cell types. Lymphocytes, at various stages of development, become committed to death by apoptosis. There are indications from transgenic mice that susceptibility to tumorigenesis *in vivo* varies during different stages of development. In the specific context of B cells, pre-B cells may provide a developmental window for susceptibility to immortalization. Therefore the approaches most likely to succeed are those which aim to immortalize pre-B or pre-T cells in such a way that differentiation may be induced subsequently. However, if *myc* is used as an immortalizing gene, it must then be possible to down-regulate its expression in the target cells, since constitutive expression of *myc* blocks differentiation. It may also be necessary to introduce a genetic block to apoptosis.

Work with rodent cells has resulted in the immortalization of only early stages of the B-cell lineage by oncogenes, and T cell-lines have been isolated only from cells with unexpressed TcR genes and in one instance from cytotoxic T cells. Tumours arising from infection *in vivo*, or in transgenic mice carrying *myc* on lymphoid-specific promoters, develop predominantly as early B-cell lymphomas and only pre-B tumours have been established as culture cell-lines. Although the isolation of pre-B cell-lines from mouse bone marrow cells infected with *myc* in combination with other oncogenes has been reported, expression of v-*raf* in immortalized pre-B cells has resulted in a lineage switch to cells with a macrophage phenotype which retain Ig gene rearrangements. The only indication that mature B cells may become immortal consists in the existence of human and murine myelomas and plasmacytomas, where it is not clear at which stage the initial immortalizing event occurred.

2. Immortalization mechanisms

The mechanisms of tumorigenesis and the physiological stimulation processes which maintain proliferating clones of cells *in vivo* yield clues as to which oncogenes may be involved in cell immortalization. Similarly, appropriate growth factors and receptors, when expressed in an autocrine fashion, will provide continual growth stimulation. *Table 1* summarizes the roles of those oncogenes and growth factors which have been implicated in lymphocyte immortalization *in vivo* or *in vitro*.

2.1 Oncogenes

Tumorigenesis in B and T cells is often associated with translocations in which the enhancer of an immunoglobulin or T-cell receptor gene is brought into proximity with a proto-oncogene such as *myc, abl*, or *bcl-2*. The consequent deregulation of oncogene expression leads to cell transformation by disrupt-

Table 1. Genes and growth factors involved in lymphocyte immortalization

Gene	Function	T/B cells	*in vitro/in vivo* effects[a]	References
myc	Competence	B	Tc, Tm, Lp, Im, Tg	1, 2, 36, 37
		T	Tc, Tm, Im	38
bcl-2	Anti-apoptosis	B	Tc, Tg, Ap	39–41
		T	Ap	42, 43
abl	Progression	B	Tc, Tm, Im	44, 45
ras	Progression	B	Tm, Lp, Im	2, 36, 37
		T	Tm, Lp, Im	38
raf	Progression	B	Im	2, 46
fms	Progression	B	Im	47
bcl-3	?	B	Tc	48
PK-C	Protein kinase	T	Im	49
IL-2, IL-2R	Cytokine	T	Im	50
HTLV-1:tat	Transactivation	T	Tm, Im	51, 52
HIV:tax, etc.	Transactivation	T(CD4+)	Im	53
EBV:LMP-1	(*bcl-2*)	B	Tm, Im	52, 54

[a] Tm, tumorigenesis; Tc, translocations; Lp, lymphoproliferation; Tg, transgenics; Im, immortalization; Ap, anti-apoptosis.

ing cell cycle control or, in the case of *bcl-2*, by preventing apoptosis (*Table 1*). In no case, however, is it clear that the translocation is the sole or primary event required for tumorigenesis. Indeed, there is considerable evidence that cell immortalization is a multistep process requiring at least co-operation between two or more oncogenes, and possibly further genetic events not as yet defined. This is borne out in experiments with transgenic animals and by attempts to immortalize primary cells *in vitro* with combinations of oncogenes.

Oncogenes (and growth factors) may be divided into two complementation groups, related to their role in progressing a cell through the cell cycle (*Table 1*). Competence factors act to bring resting (G_0) cells into G_1 and progression factors act to cycle competent cells through S, G_2, and M. Thus, maintenance of cells in the cell cycle requires overexpression or constitutive expression of *myc* (or perhaps other nuclear oncogenes), along with an oncogenic (normally mutated) version of a progression gene. This conclusion has been found to be valid in many experimental systems, both *in vivo* and *in vitro*. Transgenic mouse experiments have also demonstrated the involvement of *bcl-2* in immortalization of both B and T lymphocytes.

2.2 Autocrine loops

The transactivation of growth factor and receptor genes by certain oncogenic viruses suggests the possibility of generating cell-lines by establishing constitutive expression of growth factors to induce continuous proliferation by an autocrine mechanism. In such cases the activation of the appropriate receptor(s) may occur either by factor secretion and binding to cell surface receptors or by an intracellular interaction. Examples include the transactivation of IL-2, IL-2R and other genes by HTLV-1 or HIV. *In vitro*, IL-2-independent T cell-lines have been isolated following transduction with IL-2/3 and introduction of the protein kinase C gene into T_c cells resulted in immortalization with retention of specific cytotoxic function. The use of such quasi-physiological routes to immortalization is an attractive option, since a specific growth factor is likely to stimulate a range of events normally involved in the growth and proliferation response. However, autocrine stimulation depends also on efficient expression of the growth factor receptor genes, which may require to be introduced along with the growth factor. Many receptors contain multiple polypeptide chains or are large and complex molecules, and this is a serious obstacle to the use of retroviral vectors. In addition, autocrine stimulation may negate the possibility of using cytokines to modulate cell growth and function. A number of viral proteins, such as the *tat* and *tax* gene products of HTLV-1 and HIV, function by transactivating both growth factor and receptor genes. LMP-1 of EBV (Epstein–Barr virus), which activates *bcl-2* expression, probably has a role in the immortalization of B cells by EBV. These are shown in *Table 1*.

2.3 Imponderables

The probability that additional genetic changes, beyond those introduced by experimental intervention, are required for immortalization, is strongly suggested by the pathway to immortality taken by primary cells in empirical systems. In many reports of *in vitro* immortalization, particularly of human cells, proliferating cells arise at low frequency from a crisis in the transfected culture. Most of the viable crisis-stage cells, which carry the introduced immortalizing gene, fail to survive. Transgenic Eμ*myc* mice expressing v-*myc* at high levels in the entire B-cell population acquire B-cell lymphomas which are often clonal and arise at a frequency of only 10^{-10} per cell per generation (1). The additional genetic events are not defined, although immortalization of Eμ*myc* primary cells may be accomplished by infection with certain other oncogenes *in vitro* (2). The crisis phase *in vitro* may be partially relieved by simultaneous or sequential infection with more than two oncogenes (3), or by maintenance in growth-factor-dependent culture before infection (4). This probably allows genetic changes which pre-dispose a sub-population of the cells to oncogenesis by the infecting genes.

2.4 Immortalization strategies

Any genetic strategy for lymphocyte immortalization must therefore address the following considerations:

- Overcoming apoptosis. In both B and T cells, *bcl-2* appears to prevent apoptosis in at least early stages of differentiation.
- Provide constitutive signals for proliferation. Conventionally, cell cycle competence has been induced by a deregulated *myc* gene, and cycling maintained by a (mutated) progression gene such as *raf, ras*, or *abl*.
- Further undefined genetic changes. These may occur during a crisis phase after infection or in *in vitro* culture before infection. A second progression gene may achieve a similar result.
- The possibility of autocrine stimulation using growth factor and/or receptor genes or transactivating viral genes. Such a route is more likely to be applicable to T cells.

3. Introducing genes

The introduction of DNA into cells by $CaPO_4$ or liposome-mediated transfection or electroporation suffers from a very low efficiency of transduction, especially in human and primary cells, along with a high frequency of aberrant integration and expression. Retroviruses overcome most of the disadvantages of transfection methods.

3.1 Retroviral vectors

Retroviral infection is very efficient; in tissue culture up to 90% of cells may be transduced by a selectable marker or other gene carried on a retroviral vector, and in the majority of these the provirus is integrated in a site allowing efficient expression. Normally a single copy of the provirus is integrated, reducing the probability of recombination events in the target cell. The method involves no physical disruption to the target cells and, once retrovirus stocks have been generated, is technically simple. Retroviruses have been used successfully to transduce human cell types which have proved resistant to transfection. However, safety considerations demand that handling of cells and virus stocks is subject to higher levels of physical containment and to routine testing for biological containment, particularly in the context of viruses which infect human cells.

3.2 Retroviral vector systems

Retrovirus vector systems achieve delivery of a cloned sequence into a target cell without transfer of retroviral functions. Two essential components need to be considered. The vector, in which the expressed sequence is cloned, carries the viral long terminal repeats (LTRs) required for integration and the packaging signal (Ψ), required for viral RNA transcripts to be packaged into virions. The packaging cell contains an integrated viral genome which expresses in *trans* the viral functions necessary for encapsidating vector RNA transcripts into infective virus particles, while the packaging genome itself cannot be incorporated into virions. On infection of a target cell the vector genome is integrated and expressed, but should not give rise to infective virus. However, recombination between the vector and packaging genomes, or with endogenous retrovirus-related sequences, may result in the secretion by packaging cells or infected target cells of replication-competent helper virus (RCV). It is therefore necessary to test viruses and cells periodically to ensure that no RCV are produced. *Figure 1* summarizes the steps involved in delivering a cloned sequence in a retroviral vector into a primary target cell. The following sections are designed to assist the choice of vectors and packaging systems for the required application.

3.2.1 Vector design

Most vectors are derived from Molony murine leukaemia virus (MoMLV) and related viruses. For a full description of the different types of vectors see (5). The majority allow the insertion of two coding sequences, one of which may be a dominant selectable marker gene, such as *neo*. In spliced vectors all transcription is initiated and terminated at the viral 5′ and 3′ LTRs and individual mRNAs are generated by splicing at the retained viral splice sites. In vectors utilizing an internal promoter one of the inserted genes is expressed from the LTR, utilizing the entire viral transcript as mRNA, while the other is

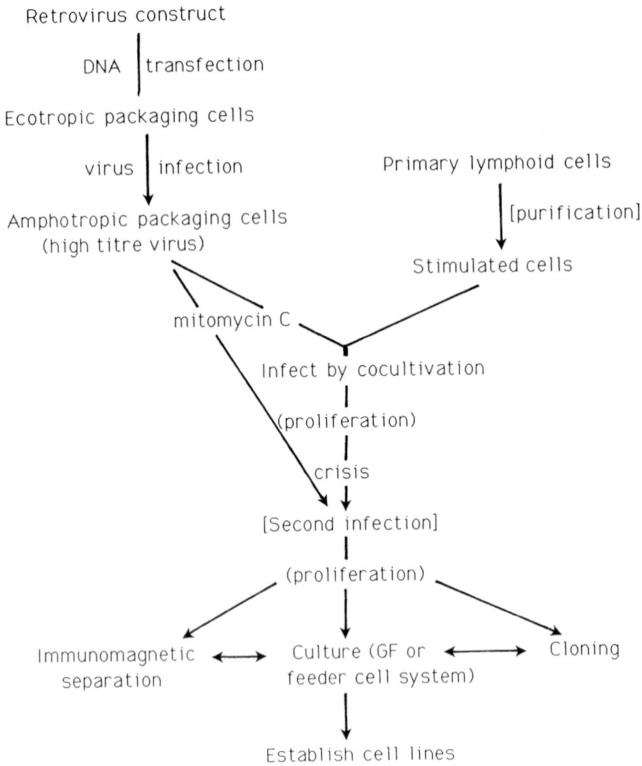

Figure 1. Schematic route to lymphocyte immortalization.

cloned on a separate promoter, resulting in a separately transcribed mRNA. Either the selectable marker or the inserted gene may be driven by the internal promoter. Internal promoters allow the possibility of regulated or tissue-specific expression of a cloned gene, but interactions between the internal promoter and the LTR promoter/enhancer make such regulation difficult to achieve. In self-inactivating (SIN) vectors (6–8), deletion of viral enhancers on transfer to the target cell allows regulated expression from inducible promoters and also appears to abolish epigenetic effects on non-inducible internal promoters. However, no SIN constructs showing regulated expression of oncogenes have been reported.

3.2.2 Internal promoters

Viral LTRs are expressed constitutively with little tissue specificity, although transcription rates and the relative abundance of different spliced transcripts do vary. Internal promoters can be chosen to give specific characteristics. The most widely used are the Herpes Simplex virus *tk* promoter (weak) and the human cytomegalovirus immediate early promoter (strong). Ig and TcR promoters show partial specificity for B and T cells, which is increased in combination with the corresponding enhancers. The inducible MMTV (induced by glucocorticoids) and metallothionein (induced by heavy metals) promoters have shown regulated expression in SIN vectors. However, in the current context, strong promoters may be neither necessary nor desirable, since many oncogenes are effective in immortalization when expressed at low levels. Moreover, if *myc* is expressed from an inducible promoter in an SIN vector, even uninduced levels of *myc* may be high enough to block differentiation.

3.2.3 Selectable markers

On transfection of a vector into packaging cells it is essential to introduce a selectable marker in order to allow isolation of the small number of cells which have integrated the vector genome. This can be done either by incorporating the marker gene into the vector as described above, or by co-transfection of a separate plasmid carrying the marker. The latter route does not result in the transfer of the marker into target cells subsequently infected with the recombinant virus, so it is necessary to apply selection criteria related to the inserted gene function. This may be problematic when infecting established cell-lines but for the immortalization of primary cells the only selection criterion may be cell immortality. In most vectors and constructs which do contain a selectable marker this is the *neo* gene, which confers resistance to the antibiotic G418 (geneticin). Because sequences within *neo* act as transcriptional silencers by repressing nearby promoters (9), it would appear that *neo* is not an ideal selectable marker. Nevertheless, a number of constructs carrying *neo* have been effective in primary cell immortalization despite the demonstrated low transcription levels of the immortalizing oncogene(s). Other dominant selectable markers include puromycin resistance, multidrug resistance, and selectable cell surface markers (10–12). Note that selectable marker genes already introduced into packaging cell-lines along with the packaging provirus cannot be used as a marker in vectors. *Table 2* provides a summary of vectors and constructs which should prove useful in the context of lymphoid cell immortalization. Those wishing to pursue the design and construction of their own vectors should seek guidance from another volume in this series (5).

3.2.4 Packaging cells and host range

Packaging cells are normally mouse fibroblast (NIH3T3) cells into which has been transfected one or more viral genomes which provide the viral functions necessary for processing and encapsidating RNA molecules containing the Ψ sequence. The degree of biological containment depends on the extent to which the packaging genome is disabled to prevent transfer of viral function to a target cell. Recently, packaging cells have been developed in which complementation between two separate packaging genomes is required for

Table 2. Retrovirus constructs

Construct	**Gene(s)**	**Promoter(s)**	**neo**	**Used in immortalization of**	**References**
pmyc309	Fe-v-*myc*	*tk*	+	Macrophage	3, 55
raszip6	v-Ha-*ras*	LTR	+	Macrophage	3, 56
J2	avian v-*myc* + v-*raf/mil*	LTR	−	Pre-B, macrophage	3, 57
deltaRM	avian v-*myc* + v-Ha-*ras*	LTR/SV40	−	Pre-B, T	36, 38
RIM	c-*myc* + v-Ha-*ras*	IgH/LTR	+	B	37
MPZen(bcl-2)	*bcl-2*	LTR	−	B	40
pZipSVIL2	*IL-2*	LTR	+	T	50
(Several)	*HIV:tax, IL-2*	(HIV)	+	T	53
pZipneo.PKC-γ	*PK-C*	LTR	+	T	49
pmycE517	Fe-v-*myc*	*tk* + IgH enh.	+	(B)	Darnbrough, unpublished
pXEP (vector only)	–	IgH + enhancer	+	(B)	58

Table 3. Packaging cell-lines

Cell-line	Tropism	No. of packaging genomes	Selectable markers	References
Ψ2	eco	1	*gpt*	59
PA317	ampho	1	*tk* (HAT)	60
Ψcre	eco	2	*gpt/hygro*	61
Ψcrip	ampho	2	*gpt/hygro*	61
GP + E-86	eco	2	*gpt/hygro*	62
GP + envAM12	ampho	2	*gpt/hygro*	62

viral function. The species specificity of a recombinant virus is dependent on the *env* protein expressed by the packaging cell-line; ecotropic viruses infect murine cells only, while amphotropic viruses recognize receptors on a range of species including mouse and human. For infection of human cells, viral constructs must be introduced into amphotropic cells. In order to avoid the introduction of defective proviral genomes which can arise during transfection, amphotropic virus-producing lines should be generated by infection with helper-free virus from a stable virus-producing ecotropic cell-line (Section 3.3.2). Note that packaging cells cannot be infected by virus of the same tropism (eco–eco or ampho–ampho). *Table 3* lists some available packaging cell-lines. Of these, all have shown very low levels of RCV, with the possible exception of Ψ2, the most widely used ecotropic line.

Most viral constructs are likely to be obtainable as ecotropic cell-lines, but those obtained as DNA must be transfected into the ecotropic line. If a construct is procured as a cell-line, ensure that the cloned proviral DNA, or at least a DNA probe to detect it, is also obtained.

3.2.5 Handling amphotropic retroviruses

The containment category for the work to be undertaken will be determined by the local safety committee with reference to the appropriate regulatory body. However, it may be assumed that the work will require preferably separate facilities for genetic manipulation of bacterial cells to ACGM category 2 and for tissue-culture cells to ACGM category 3. The latter should include a dedicated class-II laminar flow cabinet and CO_2 incubator. Workers in countries other than the UK are advised to consult their local Safety Officer.

3.3 Transfection of packaging cells

In order to introduce a DNA construct into packaging cells, follow the outline below. Detailed protocols for plasmid preparation and transfection may be found in standard laboratory cloning manuals.

(a) Isolate DNA as supercoiled plasmid free from chromosomal DNA using a gentle triton lysis method, such as that described by Gorman (13). If a commercial RPC column-based kit is used, include a CsCl gradient centrifugation as a final purification step.

(b) Maintain packaging cell-lines in DMEM/10% FCS or NCS. In some packaging lines, NCS appears to be necessary to prevent loss of the packaging genome. If necessary, select periodically for the dominant marker which was co-transfected with the packaging genome.

(c) In order to be able to select transfectants for the marker carried on or with the vector, titrate each line with the selective reagent to determine the minimum concentration required to kill 100% of the cells. For G418, this will be between 400 and 800 μg/ml for most NIH3T3-derived lines. Use this concentration plus 200 μg/ml to select for stably transfected clones.

(d) Transfect packaging cells using a standard calcium phosphate method such as that described by Gorman (13).

(e) If the vector does not contain a selectable marker, co-transfect a *neo*-expressing plasmid, such as pRSVneo (13), with the vector.

(f) Reseed transfected cells at approx. 1:6 dilution into medium containing G418 at the concentration required for selection. Subsequently change the medium (including G418) weekly. Cell growth should cease in 24–48 h and colonies of G418-resistant cells appear in 2–3 weeks. Pick colonies into 24-well plates initially, and later transfer to flasks.

(g) After one passage in flasks determine virus titre by dot blotting or marker transduction. Typically only 25% of G418-resistant clones derived by transfection yield high-titre cell-lines ($>10^5$ c.f.u./ml).

3.3.1 Determination of virus titres

High-titre virus-producing clones can be identified rapidly and reliably using the dot-blot method (*Protocol 1*), which yields results in 2–3 days. Actual titres (c.f.u./ml) are determined by transfer of the selectable marker to infected target cells, a method which requires 2–3 weeks for colonies to grow. Since there is a neither linear nor stoichiometric relationship between viral RNA concentration and experimental virus titre, the dot-blot method should not be used to predict actual titres. High-titre clones detected by dot blotting should be titrated if possible using a biological assay (*Protocol 2*). Alternatively, dot blots may be compared with those from virus stocks of known titre determined by selectable marker transduction. The dot-blot method may be used to determine the concentrations of different viruses in a mixed stock, by using probes specific for each virus.

Determine titres on virus stocks harvested from cells in late exponential growth. At 25–50% confluence, change the medium, grow for a further 24 h and harvest supernatant medium. Filter through a 0.45 μm filter to remove cell debris.

Protocol 1. Identification of high-titre clones by dot blotting

This method requires:

- a DNA probe to detect the entire viral vector sequence or the cloned coding sequence, labelled to high specific activity with ^{32}P
- for quantitation, a standard cloned DNA, preferably the entire cloned provirus. Supercoiled DNA must be linearized using a suitable restriction enzyme
- virus from the original packaging cell-line as a negative control

A. *Isolation of viral RNA*

1. It may be convenient to accumulate samples by storing the pelletted virus (step **2**) at −20°C for up to 4 weeks.
2. From 2–10 ml of supernatant, pellet virus by centrifugation at 200–400 000*g* for 60–30 min at 4°C. Remove as much supernatant as possible from the viral pellet.
3. To each pellet add 20 µl of 1 mg/ml *E. coli* tRNA and 200 µl proteinase K (10 µg/ml, pre-digested for 10 min at 37°C) in STE buffer (100 mM NaCl, 10 mM Tris–HCl, pH 8.0, 1 mM EDTA) containing 0.2% SDS. Re-suspend the pellet and incubate for 30 min at 37°C.
4. Transfer to a microfuge tube and extract with 250 µl phenol/chloroform (1:1). Re-extract the aqueous phase with 500 µl chloroform.
5. Precipitate the RNA by adding 25 µl 3 M sodium acetate pH 7.0 and 2.5 volumes ethanol. Cool to −70°C for 30 min and spin for 5 min in a microfuge. Decant the supernatant, spin again for a few seconds, and remove remaining supernatant with a micro tip.
6. Re-suspend RNA in 5–20 µl TE (10 mM Tris–HCl, 1 mm EDTA, pH 8.0).

B. *Dot-blot hybridization*

7. Make serial five-fold dilutions of the viral RNA samples, containing RNA equivalent to 1, 0.2, 0.04,. . . ml of original supernatant (step **2**), in 50 µl DEPC-treated water. Set up similar dilutions of DNA standards containing 100, 20, 4,. . . pg of cloned proviral DNA. Incubate the RNA samples at 65°C for 5 min and chill on ice. Denature DNA standards in a boiling water bath for 2 min and chill on ice.
8. To each tube add 50 µl 20 × SSC, and dot samples on to a nylon membrane such as Hybond-N (Amersham), using a miniblot manifold.
9. If no manifold dotting system is available, make up the samples in smaller volumes, and without the addition of 20 × SSC, such that 2 µl aliquots may be spotted with a micropipette on to a nylon filter prewetted with 20 × SSC.

Protocol 1. *Continued*

10. Dry the filter at 65 °C, then cross-link by exposure of the RNA side of the filter to a 312 nm UV source for a pre-calibrated time (0.5–5 min for most transilluminators). Alternatively, bake the filter for 2 h at 80 °C.

11. Hybridize the filter to the appropriate probe, labelled with ^{32}P by random priming to a specific activity of (1–2) $\times 10^9$ d.p.m./μg. It is worthwhile to invest in a commercial kit (Amersham or BCL) for this stage. All the protocols needed will be supplied with the kit.

12. Expose the hybridized filter to X-ray film. Autoradiography should require only overnight exposure to detect high-titre clones.

13. Viral RNA concentrations can be estimated by comparison with the standards, either visually, by densitometry, or by a suitable scintillation counting method applied to the filter. It is more difficult to obtain accurate quantitation using non-radioactive probes.

14. 10^5 virions contain approximately 1 pg of viral RNA. However, a viral RNA concentration above 20 pg vRNA/ml medium may be taken to indicate a titre of at least 10^5 c.f.u./ml (Darnbrough *et al.* submitted).

Protocol 2. Determination of titres by marker transduction

This method requires an adherent cell-line which is susceptible to infection by the virus to be titrated.

1. Plate exponentially growing cells in flasks at 10^4 cells/cm^2 the day before infection.
2. Prepare serial ten-fold dilutions of the virus to be titrated, down to 10^{-4} or 10^{-5} dilution, in DMEM/10% FCS/8 μg/ml polybrene. Pre-warm to 37 °C.
3. Pipette medium off the cells and add virus in a minimal volume (2 ml in a 25 cm^2 flask). Incubate with virus for 2 h then change the medium.
4. After 24 h trypsinize and reseed the entire culture in 75 cm^2 flasks.
5. Add G418 or other selective reagent to required concentration (Section 3.3(c, f)) and incubate for 10–20 days until colonies appear.
6. Count colonies and determine titres (c.f.u./ml original supernatant) from the lowest dilutions yielding statistically significant colony counts.
7. As soon as possible after identifying high-titre clones, prepare substantial liquid nitrogen stocks of chosen line(s).

3.3.2 Infection of packaging cell-lines

Infect amphotropic packaging lines with helper-free virus from ecotropic cell-lines (or vice versa) using *Protocol 4*. If the virus carries *neo* it may be possible to isolate high-titre amphotropic lines by G418 selection without cloning, since the majority of infected cells will produce virus at high titre. However, titres may change during culture of uncloned lines. Alternatively, isolate clones by G418 selection and determine titres as in *Protocol 1* or *2*.

If the virus does not contain a selectable marker, proceed as follows:

(a) On day −1, seed the amphotropic line at a density of 10^4 cells/cm^2. Change the medium on a culture of high-titre virus-producing ecotropic cells at 25–50% confluence.

(b) On day 0, infect the amphotropic cells with filtered virus-containing supernatant from ecotropic cells, as in *Protocol 4*, at a multiplicity of infection of at least 2 c.f.u./target cell.

(c) On day 1, split the infected culture at several dilutions into 75 cm^2 flasks. When colonies appear, pick at least 12 into 24-well plates. When the clones reach 25–50% confluence, change the medium and harvest the following day for determination of viral RNA by dot blotting. If possible estimate titres by comparison with a virus stock of known titre.

3.3.3 Testing for infective helper virus

Recombination resulting in replication-competent helper virus may occur at any stage during transfection and propagation of packaging cells or during infection and propagation of target cells. Although no involvement of endogenous target cell sequences in the generation of replication-competent helper virus has been demonstrated (14, 15), since hybridoma cell-lines secrete retrovirus-like particles the possibility of infective virus arising from lymphoid cells infected with oncogene-carrying viruses should not be discounted. All virus stocks and infected target cells maintained in culture for any length of time should be routinely tested for the presence of helper virus at intervals of about 2–3 months. This safety requirement is particularly strong when a virus has been carried through an amphotropic cell-line.

Testing for ecotropic virus utilizes an assay based on the formation of syncitia by XC cells infected with a retrovirus (16). Because XC cells are not susceptible to infection by amphotropic virus, an alternative assay using S+L− cells must be used (17). Suitable cell-lines for the S+L− assay are not now obtainable, and testing may need to be referred to a commercial facility such as Quality Biotech. Other indicator lines may be available (15). Cell-lines intended for therapeutic use in humans will require more stringent tests, such as a marker rescue assay for the detection of RCV in target cells (18) (Section 3.3.4). Target cells or virus harbouring sequences derived from the packaging cell genome can be detected with great sensitivity by a PCR-based assay (19).

Protocol 3. The XC assay for replication-competent ecotropic virus

1. Day 0: seed NIH3T3 cells in DMEM/10% FCS at a density of 10^4 cells/cm^2 in 50 mm dishes or 6-well plates.

Protocol 3. *Continued*

2. Day 1: remove medium from cells and add 5 ml 0.45 μm-filtered virus-containing medium and polybrene to a final concentration of 20 μg/ml.
3. Day 2: change medium, omitting polybrene. Day 4: change medium.
4. When cells are fully confluent (day 5–6), withdraw the medium, remove the lid from the plate and expose cells to 1600 erg/mm^2 of 260 nm UV light (60 sec at 15 cm from a standard germicidal UV lamp). Work in a sterile hood and protect your eyes.
5. Add 10^6 XC cells (trypsinized from a late exponential culture) per well.
6. Change the medium after two days.
7. The following day, wash plates with PBS. Fix/stain with methylene blue (3.3. g/litre)/basic fuchsin (1.1 g/litre) in methanol for 10 min. Wash with water.
8. Examine under the microscope and score for the presence of syncitia, which appear as clear areas of giant cells often enclosing an empty space. A negative control with both 3T3 and XC cells should be included to check for spontaneous syncitia: if necessary clone the XC cells to obtain a low background line.

3.3.4 Marker rescue assay for helper virus

(a) This method requires:

- a cell-line A which contains an integrated *neo*-encoding provirus and is susceptible to infection by the virus to be tested
- a naive cell-line B, also susceptible to infection (e.g. 3T3, HeLa)

(b) Infect cell-line A with the virus stock to be tested. Passage for 2 weeks to allow any helper virus to spread.

(c) Harvest the supernatant from near-confluent cells, and infect cell-line B. Select for G418-resistant colonies indicating the presence of helper virus in the original stock.

3.3.5 Infection of target cells

When using a virus-producing cell-line for the infection of primary cells, it may be advantageous also to infect an established cell-line of the same species and cell type as the intended primary target cells. Determine the titre by transduction of the selectable marker, if any, and assess integration and expression of the cloned gene, if possible using a functional assay as well as Southern and Northern blotting. Although titres are more readily determined using an adherent target cell-line such as HeLa, a hybridoma may be more appropriate for studying expression in lymphoid cells.

Protocol 4. Infection of target cell-lines

1. Prepare 0.45 μm-filtered virus stocks from cells in late exponential growth as in Section 3.3.1.[a]
2. Immediately before infection, dilute virus if required to the desired titre and add polybrene to a final concentration of 8 μg/ml, in DMEM/10% FCS. Pre-warm to 37°C.
3. Adherent target cells: plate exponentially growing cells in flasks at 10^4 cells/cm^2 the day before infection.
4. Pipette the medium off the cells and add virus in a minimal volume (2 ml in a 25 cm^2 flask). Incubate with virus for 2 h then change the medium.
5. Suspension cells: pellet cells in exponential growth and re-suspend in the virus suspension at a density of 10^5 cells/ml. Incubate for 2 h then change the medium by sedimentation and re-suspension.
6. Grow for a further 24 h before applying selection.

[a] This supernatant may be stored at −70°C if required, but substantial loss of titre will occur at each freeze–thaw cycle. The virus from low-titre stocks may be concentrated by centrifugation as in *Protocol 1*, step **2** and re-suspension in fresh medium, but this may not yield significant benefits due to the high levels of empty virions present in low-titre stocks.

3.4 HIV-based vectors

Recent reports (20) have described the efficient delivery of a *neo* marker into CD4+ T cells using a vector system derived from HIV. The system, which appears to be highly specific for cells bearing the CD4 antigen, did not result in detectable transfer of HIV helper function and promises to be a powerful tool for introducing genes into CD4+ cells.

4. Primary cells

The introduction of oncogenes into any human cells may result in cell-lines which are tumuorigenic to the individual from whom the cells were obtained, and which may secrete oncogenic viruses that infect other individuals.

- Never use cells obtained from personnel associated with the immortalization work in any way.
- Observe containment requirements scrupulously.
- Test resulting cell-lines stringently for helper virus.

4.1 Sources

Primary lymphocytes may be isolated from a number of lymphoid organs, and the tissue used will be determined by considerations beyond the scope of this chapter. The source of human pre-B cells is likely to be bone marrow (BM), which also contains a T-cell population although no functional T cells have been demonstrated. Work on long-term bone marrow cultures (LTBMC) has indicated that BM B cells may be blocked at an early stage of B-cell differentiation (21). LTBMC conditions can be manipulated to favour growth of B cells at different stages from stem cells to pre-B cells (22–24). Mature B cells may be isolated from spleen, tonsil, or peripheral blood. Peripheral blood lymphocytes (PBL) are likely to be least susceptible to immortalization. The ideal source of early T cells is the thymus, while the above comments on spleen and PBL apply to mature T cells. Thus it may well prove possible to generate early B or T cell-lines from BM or thymus, but immortalization of lymphocytes from spleen or PB is likely to be difficult. The range of methods for isolating primary cells from lymphoid organs is well described in (25).

4.1.1 Cell purification

In the case of rodent cells, myeloid cells are more susceptible to immortalization *in vitro* than are lymphoid cells, and macrophage lines have been readily isolated from both bone marrow and spleen. This raises the question of whether purification of B or T cells should be undertaken before or after attempting to introduce immortalizing genes. Most workers have chosen to use freshly isolated primary cells without purification, since viability and infection efficiency decline rapidly following isolation. Moreover the presence of accessory cells from the primary tissue is likely to be beneficial in maintaining viability and cell cycling. Infection of purified splenic B cells has resulted in proliferation of G418-resistant cells, indicating efficient infection and provirus integration, but these could not be established as cell-lines. Extensive cell purification at this point is therefore unlikely to yield benefits. However, depletion of adherent cells by a panning or G-10 method is advisable, in order to remove readily immortalized fibroblasts. A rapid immunomagnetic separation may also be considered (*Protocol 7*).

4.2 The cell cycle

Only target cells which are replicating at the time of infection are able to integrate viral DNA (26). Thus in a population of primary cells, resting or quiescent cells in G_0 are not susceptible to immortalization and the immortalization route must take account of the need for the target cell population to be stimulated into cell division during the infection. This is attained in part by the co-cultivation method, because the fibroblast virus donor cells exert a feeder effect which stimulates cell division in the primary cell overlayer. It is also likely that accessory cells from the primary tissue will provide a stimulatory effect. However, in addition it is probably necessary to include a specific activation regime for the cell type which is the desired target of infection.

4.3 Stimulation of primary lymphocytes

If specific stimulation of the desired target cells maintains these cells in proliferation for extended periods, enrichment of target cells may also result from the death of other non-required cell types. Infection of cultures containing large numbers of dead cells should be avoided, however. The stimulation regime will depend on the cell type to be infected.

4.3.1 Polyclonal activators

Mitogens such as LPS, PHA, and ConA induce a burst of cell proliferation leading to terminal differentiation and cell death. Attempts to infect spleen cells in the presence of mitogenic levels of LPS did not rescue any cells from early death (3). It is in any case likely that at these concentrations the mitogen interferes with virus infection. By contrast, mouse BM cells stimulated with ConA prior to infection with J2 virus did yield immortalized monocyte cell-lines (27).

4.3.2 Activation by cytokines

Primary lymphocytes, including mature B cells, may be maintained in proliferating cultures for extended periods by applying cocktails of cytokines. B cells stimulated with anti-Ig and cultured with IL-4 and IL-5 (28) can be maintained in proliferation for at least 14 days (3) (*Protocol 5*). T-cell stimulation may also be achieved using cytokines, although the situation is complicated by the possible requirement for antigen-presenting cells. Details of T-cell activation regimes may be found elsewhere in this volume and in (29). Any such regime will stimulate sub-populations of B and T cells to different extents, and will not necessarily be T- or B-cell specific. Because this method may be applied concurrently with infection by co-cultivation, freshly harvested cells can be infected, avoiding any selective effects of apoptosis or specific growth selection prior to infection.

4.3.3 Long-term culture systems

Culture systems utilizing feeder cells cannot be combined concurrently with any infection route. Apart from the effects of competition for virus between lymphocytes and feeder cells, there is the possibility of immortalization of fibroblasts or myeloid cells. If such culture systems are employed prior to infection it may be necessary to purify or clone lymphoid cells before attempting infection. Such systems may, however, be effective following infection, giving a growth advantage to the lymphoid cells in the infected population, and a growth advantage to infected cells over the feeder cell population. Alternatively, the use of conditioned medium from a LTBMC may be considered. Immortalized murine pre-B cells have been isolated by strategies involving the use of Whitlock–Witte BM cultures (30–32) before or after infection.

Protocol 5. Stimulation of B cells with anti-IgG/IL-4/IL-5 (3)

Materials required

- affinity-purified polyclonal $F(ab')_2$ of anti-IgM or IgG, depending on the B-cell subset to be stimulated. Antibody immobilized on polystyrene or dextran beads (33) is effective at 10–100-fold lower concentrations. Note that Fc regions down-regulate B cells and stimulate macrophages via Fc receptors
- IL-4, IL-5 (recombinant grades)

Method

1. Determine optimal concentrations of cells and reagents in RPMI/10% FCS/50 μM 2-ME for stimulation of TdR uptake over 10–14 days. (For unpurified murine spleen cells, in range: cells, $(1–5) \times 10^6$/ml; anti-Ig, 10–100 μg/ml; IL-4 and IL-5, 1–10 U/ml each.)
2. Prior to infection, incubate cells with optimum concentrations of reagents.
3. Infect cells on day 1 or later of stimulation. Immediately before infection, dilute cells to a maximum density of 10^6/ml.
4. Replenish IL-4 and IL-5 in medium changes up to day 14.

4.4 Infection of primary cells

No proven route for the immortalization of human lymphocytes has been described. Therefore the scheme shown in *Figure 1* is given as a guide to be adapted as appropriate. Briefly, freshly isolated primary cells are stimulated using a lymphokine-based regime concurrently with infection by co-cultivation. The subsequent handling of infected cells involves selection by a purification step and/or growth selection using a feeder-cell culture system or conditioned medium.

4.4.1 Infection by co-cultivation

Experience has shown that a single exposure of primary cells to a high-titre virus stock results in a low level of infection. Co-cultivation of the primary cells with the virus donor cells allows a prolonged time of contact with the virus and an increase in the effective titre, greatly increasing the infection efficiency in a cell population which may be slowly dividing or contain many resting cells. The donor cells are killed prior to infection by brief incubation with mitomycin-C, and primary cells remain in contact with the donor cells, which continue to secrete virus, for at least 3 days. If primary cells are to be infected with two or more separate viruses, co-cultivation with two virus donor cell types concurrently has been shown to yield immortalized cells carrying at least one copy of each virus (3). Sequential infections, however, may prove to be more effective, since at 10–14 days post-infection the surviving cells are predominantly those which have integrated the virus(es) acquired in the first infection. Re-infection by a second co-cultivation at this stage will generate a high proportion of doubly infected cells. A second infection has been shown to effect immediate rescue from crisis in the case of murine splenic macrophages immortalized by three viruses carrying *myc*, *ras*, and *raf* (3).

Protocol 6. Infection by co-cultivation

1. Infections are conveniently carried out in 6- or 12-well plates. Wrap the plates in clingfilm to reduce evaporation.
2. On day −1: seed virus donor cells in DMEM/10% FCS to give about 50% confluence after cells have spread out ($(0.5\text{–}1) \times 10^5$ cells/cm^2). Two different cell-lines may be co-seeded.
3. On day 0: prepare primary cells, including any purification steps and finally resuspend at $(2\text{–}10) \times 10^6$ cells/ml in DMEM/10% FCS/50 μM 2-ME/5 μg/ml polybrene plus reagents required for stimulation.[a]
4. Remove the medium from the donor cells and add 3 ml DMEM/10% FCS/20 μg/ml mitomycin-C.[b] Incubate for 1 h at 37°C.
5. Remove medium and wash cells twice with 5 ml DMEM[c] and once with DMEM/10% FCS. Dispose of mitomycin-C safely (it is a carcinogen).
6. Add primary cells at $(2\text{–}5) \times 10^5$ cells/cm^2.[d] Incubate for 3 days.
7. Day 3: change medium to DMEM/10% FCS/50 μM 2-ME plus stimulation reagents.
8. Day 4 onwards: transfer non-adherent infected cells from donors into 24-well plates. Cells remaining on the donors will continue to divide, and transfers at different times after infection may each yield different cell populations. After transfer, replace 50% of the medium, using RPMI instead of DMEM.
9. If a second infection is to be carried out, start on day 10–14. Repeat steps **2–7** with the different donor cells, adding about 10^5 primary cells from the first infection to each well.
10. As proliferating cells grow out of crisis transfer initially to 24-well plates. Characterize by immunofluorescence/cell sorting and perform purification and selection as necessary.

[a] Infection may be performed in RPMI or DMEM. RPMI may enhance the survival and growth of lymphocytes, but will yield lower virus titres than DMEM.

[b] To allow for batch-to-batch variation and cell-line sensitivity, optimize mitomycin-C concentration and incubation times to obtain 100% kill. In each infection include control wells with treated donor cells only, and incubate for up to 2 weeks to check that no viable fibroblasts grow out.

[c] Some lines tend to sheet off the wells in serum-free medium. Handle the cells gently and if necessary perform all washes with DMEM/10% FCS.

[d] Gentamycin may be added to reduce the risk of bacterial contamination.

4.4.2 Crisis management

Following initial proliferation of blast cells during the co-cultivation stage, most infected primary cells enter a crisis in which cells remain viable but non-dividing. Subsequently a small proportion of the viable cells begin to proliferate, perhaps clonally. The action taken at this time may be the essential factor in determining which cell types can be recovered as immortalized cell-lines. A relatively small number of founder cells contribute to the proliferating cell population and if crisis-stage cells are simply pooled and established as cell-lines, the culture will quickly be dominated by one rapidly growing cell type. Murine spleen cells stimulated with anti-Ig/IL-4/IL-5 concurrently with infection failed to yield immortalized B cell-lines, despite the presence of mature B cells at times up to 28 days post-infection, indicated by the accumulation of secreted IgG (S. Slater and C. Darnbrough, unpublished work). The cultures were subsequently dominated by rapidly growing immortalized macrophages. Attempts to clone cells growing out of crisis have generally been unsuccessful, except in the case of transformed macrophage lines, or when foetal cells have been immortalized. Two other options remain:

(a) Place the cells at this stage into a culture system utilizing feeder cells or growth factors which will stimulate the proliferation of the desired cell type. Soft agar cloning may be combined with this;

(b) Carry out a selection/purification step. Such a step should be capable of being performed rapidly and with minimal disruption to the cells. The following immunomagnetic separation can be undertaken in 2–3 h (34, 35).

Protocol 7. Immunomagnetic separation of human lymphocytes using Dynabeads

- Obtain or prepare Dynabeads-450 linked to the appropriate monoclonal antibody (MAb) (Dynal):
  B cells—Dynabeads M450-Pan B (CD19)
  T cells—Dynabeads M450-Pan T (CD2) or CD4 or CD8
- Beads are removed rapidly from rosetted cells by incubation with anti-mouse F(ab) antibodies (34). Determine the optimum antibody concentration for release using a suitable cell-line.

1. Cool cells to 4°C. If target cell number is known (e.g. from cell profiling), add Dynabeads to a bead:target cell ratio of 3:1. Otherwise use a ratio of 1:1. Mix gently for 5 min at 4°C. Check rosette formation by microscopy.
2. Isolate rosetted cells magnetically and wash twice in RPMI/10% FCS.
3. Re-suspend in medium containing anti-mouse F(ab) at the pre-determined concentration. Incubate at room temperature for 30–60 min until beads detach.

4. Remove beads and remaining rosetted cells magnetically.
5. Sediment released cells by centrifugation and re-suspend them in medium.

4.4.3 Establishing cell-lines

The ease with which cells grow out of crisis and can be established and passaged varies enormously. Appropriate culture conditions for immortalized cells growing out of crisis must be determined empirically, but the following points should be noted:

- Once proliferating cells appear at sufficient densities, seed cells at different densities and culture under different regimes on 24-well plates until a consistent growth pattern is established.
- G418 selection may be used to select for virus-infected cells, but should not be applied to the entire culture. Since the threshold concentration for uninfected cells will not be known, use G418 at concentrations up to 1–2 mg/ml. Do not increase the G418 concentration gradually.
- Immortalization is the primary selection criterion.
- Analyse oncogene integration and expression by Southern, Northern, or Western blotting as part of the characterization of the cells, along with studies of cell surface and functional markers.
- Test established cell-lines for replication-competent helper virus.

5. Conclusion

Although the emphasis of this chapter has been on the application of retroviral techniques to human cells, it should be recognized that considerable progress remains to be made in the generation of functional lymphocyte lines from rodent primary cells, some of which may prove to have therapeutic value. The techniques described here are equally, and more easily, applicable to rodent cells. The limitations of current knowledge preclude the possibility of clearly prescribing the genetic elements required for lymphocyte immortalization. However, advances in understanding of the genetics of lymphoid cell growth and differentiation will yield guidance as to appropriate immortalization routes using the techniques described here.

Acknowledgements

While developing the expertise described here, I was supported by grants from the SERC Biotechnology Directorate. I am grateful to Caroline MacDonald for support, advice, and encouragement.

References

1. Harris, A. W., Pinkert, C. A., Crawford, M., Langdon, W. Y., Brinster, R. L., and Adams, J. M. (1988). *J. Exp. Med.*, **167,** 353.
2. Alexander, W. S., Adams, J. M., and Cory, S. (1989). *Mol. Cell. Biol.*, **9,** 67.
3. Darnbrough, C., Slater, S., Vass, M., and MacDonald, C. (1992). *Exp. Cell Res.* (In press.)
4. Robertson, S. M. and Walker, W. S. (1988). *Cell. Immunol.*, **116,** 341.
5. Brown, A. M. C. and Scott, M. R. D. (1987). In *DNA Cloning: A Practical Approach*, (ed. D. Glover), pp. 189–212. IRL Press, Oxford.
6. Engelhardt, J. F., Kullum, M. J., Bisat, F., and Pitha, P. M. (1990). *Virology*, **178,** 419.
7. Mee, P. J. and Browen, R. (1990). *Gene*, **88,** 289.
8. McGeady, M. L., Arthur, P. M., and Seidman, M. (1990). *J. Virol.*, **64,** 3527.
9. Artelt, P., Grannemann, R., Stocking, C., Friel, J., Bartsch, J., and Hauser, H. (1991). *Gene*, **99,** 249.
10. Strair, R. K., Towle, M. J., and Smith, B. R. (1988). *J. Virol.*, **62,** 4756.
11. Pastan, I., Gottesman, M. M., Ueda, K., Lovelace, E., Rutherford, A. V., and Willingham, M. C. (1988). *Proc. Natl. Acad. Sci. USA*, **85,** 4486.
12. Vara, J. A., Portela, A., Ortin, J., and Jimenez, A. (1986). *Nucl. Acids Res.*, **14,** 4617.
13. Gorman, C. (1985). In *DNA Cloning, Vol. 2: A Practical Approach*, (ed. D. Glover), pp. 143–90. IRL Press, Oxford.
14. Scarpa, M., Cournoyer, D., Muzny, D. M., Moore, K. A., Belmont, J. W., and Caskey, C. T. (1991). *Virology*, **180**, 849.
15. Muenchau, D. D., Freeman, S. M., Cornetta, K., Zwiebel, J. A., and Anderson, W. F. (1990). *Virology*, **176,** 262.
16. Rowe, W. P., Pugh, W. E., and Hartley, J. W. (1970). *Virology*, **42,** 1136.
17. Miller, A. D., Law, M. F., and Verma, I. M. (1985). *Mol. Cell. Biol.*, **5,** 431.
18. Belmont, J. W., Hawkins, D., Villalon, D., Chang, S. M., and Caskey, C. T. (1988). *Mol. Cell. Biol.*, **8,** 5116.
19. Morgan, R. A., Cornetta, K., and Anderson, W. F. (1990). *Hum. Gene Therapy*, **1,** 135.
20. Shimada, T., Fujii, H., Mitsuya, H., and Nienhuis, A. W. (1991). *J. Clin. Invest.*, **88,** 1043.
21. Dorschkind, K. and Phillips, R. A. (1982). *J. Immunol.*, **129,** 2444.
22. Peschel, C., Green, I., and Paul, W. E. (1989). *J. Immunol.*, **142,** 1558.
23. Rennick, D., Jackson, J., Moulds, C., Lee, F., and Yang, G. (1989). *J. Immunol.*, **142,** 161.
24. Dorschkind, K., Johnson, A., Harrison, Y., and Landreth, K. S. (1989). *J. Immunol. Methods*, **123,** 93.
25. Hurst, S. V. (1987). In *Lymphocytes: A Practical Approach*, (ed. G. G. B. Klauss), pp. 1–34. IRL Press, Oxford.
26. Miller, D. G., Adam, M. A., and Miller, A. D. (1990). *Mol. Cell. Biol.*, **10**, 4239.
27. Gandino, L. and Varesio, L. (1990). *Exp. Cell Res.*, **188,** 192.
28. Wetzel, G. D. (1991). *Cell. Immunol.*, **137,** 358.
29. Taylor, P. M., Thomas, D. B., and Mills, K. H. G. (1987). In *Lymphocytes: A Practical Approach*, (ed. G. G. B. Klauss), pp. 133–48. IRL Press, Oxford.

30. Whitlock, C. and Witte, O. N. (1982). *Proc. Natl. Acad. Sci. USA*, **79,** 3608.
31. Palumbo, G. J., Ozanne, B., and Kettman, J. R. (1991). *Leukaemia Res.*, **15,** 847.
32. Denis, K. A. and Witte, O. N. (1987). *Int. Rev. Immunol.*, **2,** 285.
33. Allison, K. C., Strober, W., and Harriman, G. R. (1991). *J. Immunol.*, **146,** 4197.
34. Rasmussen, A. M., Smeland, E. B., Erikstein, B. K., Caignault, L., and Funderud, S. (1992). *J. Immunol. Methods*, **146,** 195.
35. Funderud, S., Nustad, K., Lea, T., Vartdal, F., Gaudernack, G., Stenstad, P. *et al.* (1987). In *Lymphocytes: A Practical Approach*, (ed. G. G. B. Klauss), pp. 55–64. IRL Press, Oxford.
36. Overell, R. W., Weisser, K. E., Hess, B., Namen, A. E., and Grabstein, K. H. (1989). *Oncogene*, **4,** 1425.
37. Clynes, R., Wax, J., Stanton, L. W., Smith-Gill, S., Potter, M., and Marcu, K. B. (1988). *Proc. Natl. Acad. Sci. USA*, **85,** 6067.
38. Cattermole, J. A., Crosier, P. S., Leung, E., Overell, R. W., Gillis, S., and Watson, J. D. (1989). *J. Immunol*, **142,** 3746.
39. Williams, G. T. (1991). *Cell*, **65,** 1097.
40. Vaux, D. L., Cory, S., and Adams, J. M. (1988). *Nature*, **335,** 440.
41. Strasser, A., Harris, A. W., Bath, M. L., and Cory, S. (1990). *Nature*, **348,** 331.
42. Strasser, A., Harris, A. W., and Cory, S. (1991). *Cell*, **67,** 889.
43. Sentman, C. L., Shutter, J. R., Hockenbery, D., Kanagawa, O., and Korsmeyer, S. J. (1991). *Cell*, **67,** 879.
44. Dhut, S., Gibbons, B., Chaplin, T., and Young, B. D. (1991). *Leukemia*, **5,** 49.
45. Engelman, A. and Rosenberg, N. (1990). *Mol. Cell. Biol.*, **10,** 4365.
46. Kurie, J. M., Morse, H. C., Principato, M. A., Wax, J. S., Troppmair, J., Rapp, U. R., *et al.* (1990). *Oncogene*, **5,** 577.
47. Borzillo, G. V. and Sherr, C. J. (1989). *Mol. Cell. Biol.*, **9,** 3973.
48. Bhatia, K., Huppi, K., McKeithan, T., Siwarski, D., Mushinski, J. F., and Magrath, I. (1991). *Oncogene*, **6,** 1569.
49. Finn, O. J., Persons, D. A., Bendt, K. M., Pirami, L., and Ricciardi, P. (1991). *J. Immunol.*, **146,** 1099.
50. Yamada, G., Kitamura, Y., Sonoda, H., Harada, H., Taki, S., Mulligan, R. C., *et al.* (1987). *EMBO J.*, **6,** 2705.
51. Yoshida, M. and Seiki, M. (1987). *Ann. Rev. Immunol.*, **5,** 541.
52. Ambinder, R. F. (1990). *Hematol. Oncol. Clin. North Am.*, **4,** 821.
53. Shapiro, I. M., Meier, C., Vlach, V., McDonald, T. L., Wigzell, H., and Stevenson, M. (1990). *Somatic Cell Mol. Genet.*, **16,** 1.
54. Henderson, S., Rowe, M., Gregory, C., Croom-Carter, D., Wang, F., Longnecker, R., *et al.* (1991). *Cell*, **65,** 1107.
55. Darnbrough, C. and MacDonald, C. (1991). *Exp. Cell Res.*, **195,** 263.
56. Dotto, G. P., Parada, L. F., and Weinberg, R. A. (1985). *Nature*, **318,** 472.
57. Rapp, U. R., Cleveland, J. L., Brightman, K., Scott, A., and Ihle, J. N. (1985). *Nature*, **317,** 434.
58. Blankenstein, T., Winter, E., and Muller, W. (1988). *Nucl. Acids Res.*, **16,** 10939.
59. Mann, R., Mulligan, R. C., and Baltimore, D. (1983). *Cell*, **33,** 153.
60. Miller, A. D. and Buttimore, C. (1986). *Mol. Cell. Biol.*, **6,** 2895.
61. Danos, O. and Mulligan, R. C. (1988). *Proc. Natl. Acad. Sci. USA*, **85,** 6460.
62. Markowitz, D., Goff, S., and Bank, A. (1988). *Virology*, **167,** 400.

21

Modifying the specificity of T cells using chimeric *Ig/TCR* genes

ZELIG ESHHAR, GIDEON GROSS, and JONATHAN TREISMAN

1. Introduction

The specific immune recognition of foreign antigens has evolved two major systems; of T cells and of antibody-producing cells. Recognition of antigen by T cells requires that antigenic molecules are displayed on the cell surface of antigen-presenting cells or target cells in association with self-major histocompatibility complex (MHC) molecules. Usually, the antigenic determinants recognized by T cells are formed as a result of intracellular digestion processes resulting in the presentation of short peptides (about 9 or 13–17 amino acids) by either MHC class-I or class-II molecules. This recognition, which is of low affinity (1×10^{-5} to 5×10^{-6} M), is mediated by the T-cell receptor (TCR). In contrast, antibodies recognize both soluble or cell-bound antigens independently of a cellular or MHC-associated context and in high affinity (usually between 10^{-7} and 10^{-9} M).

Despite these fundamental differences in recognition requirements, the TCR and the antibody (Ab) molecules are quite similar. Both Ab and TCR are disulphide-linked heterodimers consisting of light (L) and heavy (H) chains for Ab and α and β (or γ and δ) chains for the TCR. Each chain is divided into variable (V) and constant (C) regions. The V regions of the two chains associate to form the antigen-binding domain. The C region of the Ab molecule is associated with effector function while in the TCR it provides an anchor to the cell surface, the site of interaction with other cell-surface molecules, and is involved with the triggering of T-cell activation. The *TCR* and *Ig* gene loci are also similar, both containing large and diverge clusters of V domains which are formed as a result of recombination. These recombinatorial events provide a major proportion of the immense repertoire of antigen recognition by the immune system.

While the fine molecular mode of antibody–antigen interaction and the physicochemical parameters that underlie it are well known, we are still far from delineating the sub-molecular structure of the TCR:Ag:MHC complex and the role that parameters such as affinity, rigidity, valency, and others play in the TCR–ligand interaction and subsequent T-cell triggering. This shortcoming is due to the facts that the TCR has not yet been crystallized for structural analysis and the practical difficulty in obtaining homogenous and purified complex of Ag:MHC ligand in sufficient amounts. To overcome these problems, and in order to establish a system which will allow us to manipulate the specificity of the T-cell receptor at will, we and others (1–7) have designed a new approach in which we endowed T cells with antibody-type specificity by replacing the V region of the TCR molecule with that of an antibody. In this approach we took advantage of the similarity in structure and genomic organization of the antibody and TCR molecules to construct chimeric *TCR* (c*TCR*) genes composed of segments of the antibody Fv linked to the C region of the TCR. Upon transfer of such c*TCR* genes and their expression in T cells they recognized antigen in affinity and specificity of antibodies and transmitted efficient signal for T-cell triggering.

The scheme for generation of c*TCR* (we nicknamed 'T body') is outlined in *Figure 1* and a summary of the main reported studies which utilized the c*TCR* approach is presented in *Table 1*. From a structural point of view, it seems that there was no preference in terms of expression to any combination of V_H and V_L with either $C\alpha$ or $C\beta$ and the different c*TCR* associated with the CD3 to give functional receptor. All the studies reported so far utilized c*TCR* made of Fv of anti-hapten antibodies. Interestingly, in all the cases the V_H of

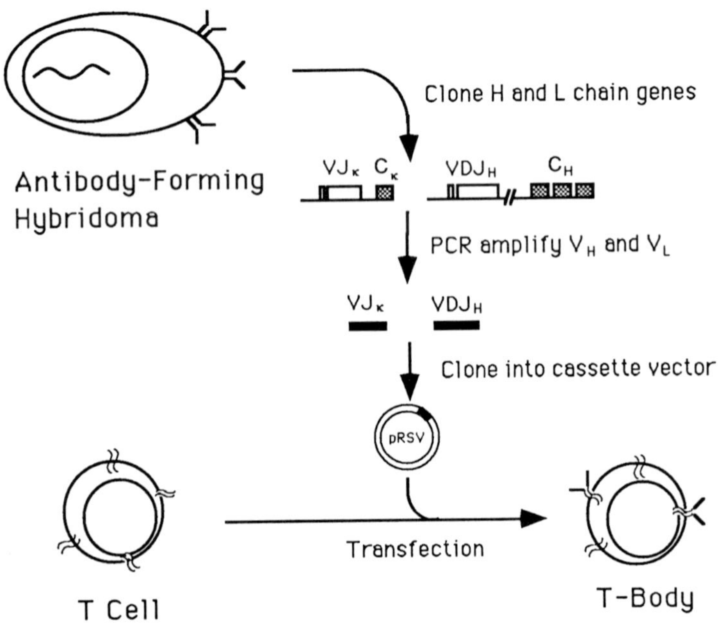

Figure 1. Schematic diagram of the generation and expression of chimeric T-cell receptors.

Table 1. Studies using the chimeric TCR approach

Group (reference)	Antibody specificity	Cell	Transfection method	Promoter	Chimeric gene	Activity
Kurosawa (1)	PC	EL-4	Protoplast fusion	Maloney LTR	$V_H C\alpha + V_L C\beta$ $V_H C\beta + V_L C\alpha$	Increased intracellular Ca^{2+}
Eshhar (2–5, 14)	TNP 38C13-idiotype	MD.45 Jurkat	Protoplast fusion Electroporation	RSV LTR	$V_H C\alpha + V_L C\beta$ $V_H C\beta + V_L C\alpha$	IL-2 secretion in response to antigen Non-MHC-restricted cytolysis of TNP cells. Inhibition of activation by soluble antigen
Hedrick (6)	Digoxin	Transgenic T cells	Transgenic mice	Ig	$V_H C\alpha$	Surface association of c*TCR* with CD3. Activation of T cells by antigen or anti-id. Allelic exclusion of endogenous TCRα
Hood (7)	PC	EL-4 J.RT-T3.1	Electroporation	Maloney LTR	$V_H C\alpha$ $V_H C\beta$	Surface association of c*TCR* with CD3. IL-2 secretion in response to antigen. Expression of β TCR dimers

the monoclonal antibody (MAb) (in association of either $V\alpha$ or $V\beta$) was sufficient to account for the hapten binding. This was not the case when we used Fv of an anti-idiotypic antibody, recognizing a more complex epitope wherein both V_H and V_L were required (8). The major new structure–function related aspects gained so far by the T-body approach are that the TCR can mediate its functions through MHC-independent interactions, and that the β TCR chains can be expressed as a homodimer independent of the α chain (7). These studies also provided further supportive evidence for the need for antigen immobilization for effective T-cell triggering and that cross-linking of adjacent TCR molecules is most likely not sufficient for signalling. These and other findings just illustrate some of the potential embodied in the T-body approach. Although intriguing, it is beyond the scope of this chapter and readers are referred to the references indicated in *Table 1* for further reading.

The potential application of the chimeric T-cell receptor approach is wide and versatile. The main features of the approach that make it attractive for basic research are the ability to manipulate the specificity of the TCR and the TCR:Ag interaction in a controlled and defined manner, and the ability to endow T cells with non-MHC-restricted specificity. *Table 2* outlines the potential application of the T bodies. Particularly exciting is the potential use of the T body in a new immunotherapeutic approach to confer on T cells antibody specificity in order to direct effector and helper cells to their pre-defined target. Along this line, a challenging application is to endow *in vitro* propagating lymphocytes of a tumour patient with anti-tumour specificity by transducing them with c*TCR* genes composed of Fv of anti-tumour MAb.

In this chapter we set out to provide practical information for the construction, expression and functional characterization of chimeric T cell receptors. In doing so, we based the detailed information on our own experimental experience, and review and discuss additional and alternative procedures when pertinent. The field is still evolving and there is certainly more than one

Table 2. Potential applications of the 'T-body' approach

In basic research
- Study the physicochemical parameters underlying the antigen-mediated T-cell activation
- Study the interactions between the TCR and accessory and adhesion molecules under non-MHC associated recognition
- Study the selection and maturation of T cells bearing c*TCR* in transgenic mice

In immunotherapy
- Develop a new immunotherapeutical modality that will allow us to design the specificity of T cells against any pre-defined antigen in a non-MHC restricted fashion
- Such 'designer-lymphocytes' can be then infused into any appropriate patient whose malignant cells express the target antigen

approach. In this article, we hope to put at the reader's disposal and consideration, sufficient guidelines and background to select his own approach to match his needs.

2. Design and construction of the c*TCR* genes

2.1 Antibody selection

In addition to the choice of the antibody specificity (which is at individuals' prerogatives according to with their objectives), there are few points that should be considered in selecting an antibody for use in the c*TCR* context.

For targeting T cells *in vivo* the antibody of choice should:

- be specific to a surface antigen expressed preferentially on the target cells to avoid potential damage to normal tissue
- recognize antigen which is an integral cell surface component and absent from circulation, since soluble or shed antigen may block binding to cellular targets

The effect of the antibody affinity on the T-cell function is as yet unclear. Our preliminary results indicate that high-affinity interactions through the c*TCR* might lead to inefficient target cell lysis, probably due to lack of detachment and recycling of the effector cells. In addition, we believe that low- to moderate-affinity antibodies might be a better choice also, because they can be inhibited to a lesser degree by low concentrations of circulating antigens. Potential antigens for anti-tumour targeting by the T-body approach are oncofoetal surface proteins, membranal oncogene products, or any tumour-specific component toward which antibodies have been raised. Of special interest are viral antigens expressed on the surface of infected cells. These can be either viral components bound to surface receptors or exposed on the cellular membrane while budding out. Even more intriguing is the use for the c*TCR* Fv of antibodies directed at viral core antigens which are presented on the cell surface in association with MHC class-I. This design will avoid blocking of the c*TCR* by free viral particles.

Finally, it has to be emphasized that the few successful attempts to construct c*TCR* does not guarantee that each Fv of an antibody will conform to its native antigen-binding structure upon grafting onto the C region of the TCR. Although no deforming constraints have been observed in the reported cases, one can foresee in certain combinations some structural changes imposed by the slightly different angle between the antibody and the TCR V–C interface (see discussion in (7)). When such difficulties arise, it might be beneficial to change the combination of V_L and V_H with the C region of the second TCR chain. In many antibodies the V_H can associate with different V_L without causing drastic change in the antigen binding properties. Such V_H should be excellent candidates to be used in the context of the c*CTR* because they most likely will assume active binding site in association of *V*α or *V*β upon mixed pairing with the endogenous TCR chains (7). The lower binding affinity usually resulting from such combination can be advantageous in light of the aforementioned discussion.

2.2 The chimeric gene construct

The design of the chimeric *Ab*/*TCR* genes composed of the rearranged DNA encoding either the V_L or V_H and either the *C*α or *C*β in its genomic organization has been described with slight modifications by different groups (1–3, 6, 7). Its advantage over cDNA constructs is that it contains all the authentic genetic elements needed for correct expression and maintenance of the correct reading frame. However, because of their relatively large size, genomic constructs are more difficult to handle and transfect. The fact that cDNA is better expressed using retroviral vectors (which are the vehicle of choice for gene expression in human T cells, see below), makes it the preferred design for the clinical application. Here we shall describe the genomic constructs which proved useful for our studies.

The basic outline for construction of the c*TCR* vectors is shown in *Figure 2*. The essential components of the c*TCR* gene include; a leader sequence of the antibody, the antibody V region and the C region of the TCR. In our initial studies, the V region of the antibody was first cloned into the expression vector, followed by the constant region of the TCR. In subsequent studies, vectors which contain the constant region of the TCR were synthesized. These vectors allow the direct insertion of any antibody V region into a unique cloning site at the 5′ end of the TCR. A further refinement of this technique was the development of 'cassette' type vectors which contain both the TCR C region as well as a generic antibody leader sequence at the 5′ end. Thus, the V region of the antibody may be cloned directly into these genomic expression vectors to produce the chimeric TCR of interest. In this chapter we have given protocols that we have modified for our specific use. The reader is referred to any of the comprehensive laboratory manuals for general methodologies (8, 9).

2.3 Expression vector systems

A large array of expression vectors exist and are presented in a number of reviews (9). For the currently described studies, vectors are chosen which allow for stable integration and expression of the c*TCR* gene in T cells and antibiotic selection. We routinely utilize derivatives of the pSV series of vectors (10, 11). The systems utilized for the c*TCR* has been based on plasmid vectors which contain the RSV (2) or the Moloney leukaemia virus (MLV) (1, 7) LTRs to drive transcription. These are strong and ubiquitous promoter/enhancer sequences and their use eliminates the effect of *cis*-acting elements on *Ig* or *TCR* gene expression in T cells (12, 13). The promoter site in these

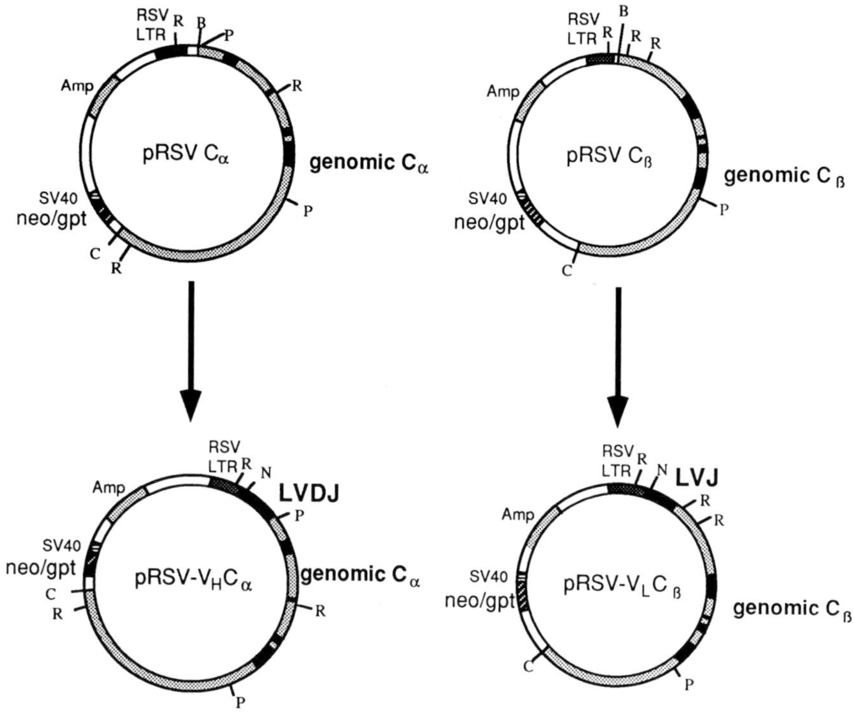

Figure 2. Scheme of expression vectors. The upper vectors contain the genomic Cα and Cβ and either the *neo* or *gpt* antibiotic resistance gene. Following linearization at the *Bam*HI site (B), the V_H (*LVDJ*) or (*LVJ*) gene segments are inserted to yield the cTCR expression vectors. Restriction sites: B, *Bam*HI; C, *ClaI*; N, *NcoI*; P, *PvuII*; R, *Eco*RI.

plasmids is followed by a cloning site for gene insertion, then a polyadenylation signal. In addition, the vectors contain an antibiotic selection gene under control of a second promoter, usually the SV-40 one. Because two genes, corresponding to the two complementary TCR chains, have to be transfected in two separate vectors, we use two different selection markers such as the *neo* resistance (11) and the *gpt* (10) genes. The vectors also contain plasmid sequences which allow for growth in bacteria and resistance to ampicillin. These vectors offer a large host range, yet efficiency of transfection is relatively low. The introduction of retroviral vector systems may provide a way to increase this efficiency and possibly the level of expression. However, they are limited in terms of the size of inserts that may be used for expression.

2.4 Cloning of c*TCR* into mammalian expression vectors

The genomic construction used for the c*TCR* is based on the similarity in gene structure between the TCR and immunoglobulins. Thus, the c*TCR* is produced by combining the VDJ_H or VJ_k gene segment of an antibody with the gene segment encoding the C region of either the TCR α or β chains. Thus far no particular combination of V_H or V_k with Cα or Cβ is preferential; both yielded functional receptors with active Fv. Here we shall describe in detail expression vectors composed of genomic DNA of the TCR constant region in front of which the rearranged DNA of the antibody variable region is introduced. We used these vectors for the expression of c*TCR* of a few antibodies (1–4, 14).

2.4.1 Expression cassettes containing TCR constant region genes

In our initial studies using the chimeric TCR, the vectors were constructed by the sequential insertion of the V and then the TCR C region genes (2, 3). In order to simplify cloning, a set of cassette vectors has been designed (*Figure 2*) by the initial insertion of the TCR C region (Cα and Cβ) into the pRSV vectors, and these can then be used to introduce the antibody V sequence of interest. The cassettes contain a unique *Bam*HI site 5′ to the TCR which is used for insertion of the V_H and V_L region sequence. To construct the c*TCR* expression vectors, genomic murine TCR Cα and Cβ chains were cloned from a mouse embryonic DNA library in the bacteriophage vector Charon 4A (15). The 9.0 kb *Bam*HI fragment contains all the Cα exons and the 6.3 kb *Bam*HI fragment containing $C\beta_2$ were inserted into the *Bam*HI site of the $pRSV_2$ *neo* and $pRSV_3$ *gpt* mammalian expression vectors. In order to obtain vectors with the unique *Bam*HI site, a partial digestion was done, the ends made blunt with Klenow, and the plasmid self-ligated. The plasmids described are illustrate in *Figure 2*. It should be noted that in both the TCR and Ig, the last base of the *J* gene segment is the first base in the first codon of the constant region. This renders Ig and TCR rearranged V genes interchangeable with regard to the reading frame, which also applies to the chimeric gene constructs. In both, the last two bases of the first codon in the first constant exon are AG. The first base of the codon, which resides in the *J* segments is spliced to the AG on the RNA level. In the case of the TCR and Ig V_H this first base is a G, and codes for Glu. In the J_k sequence this first base is a C and codes for Gln. This change is 'permitted', as chimeric genes harbouring it were functionally expressed in the previous systems.

2.4.2 Cloning of rearranged V_H and V_L gene segments

Basically, the V_H and V_L genes of the antibody molecule may be isolated from cDNA or genomic libraries made from hybridoma producing the antibody of interest. Our original studies used restriction sites found at the 5′ and 3′ ends of the VDJ_H and VJ_k to clone these regions into the expression vectors. In order to simplify the cloning of the chimeric genes and allow the rapid insertion of any particular V from the antibody of interest, cDNA sequences of the V region genes may be used. Recently described cloning of immunoglobulin genes using polymerase chain reaction (PCR) to amplify cDNA reverse-transcribed from hybridoma RNA provides a convenient way to rapidly prepare such V region DNA. This technique relies on the presence of conserved regions in the 5′ and 3′ of the Ig V regions (16), and oligonucleotides of these consensus sequences are prepared and serve as primers to amplify the rearranged gene segments (17). The 3′ primers take advantage of the high sequence homology shared by the four functional mouse J_H germ-line segments. Similarly, the five J_k germ-line segments also share sequence homology. These universal primers were designed as the reverse complementary sequence which bears the minimal number of mismatches to the 3′ end of the relevant *J* members. In addition they contain, at their most 5′ end, the six-base pair (ACTTAC) stretch which is the reverse complement sequence of the consensus donor splice signal. This splice signal is essential as the TCR C genes in the cassettes are in their genomic configuration and harbour a splice acceptor signal 5′ to their first exon (see above). The 5′ primers for the V_H and V_k sequences were designed according to the corresponding leader sequences of S1C5 antibody (14, 18). Because of the variability within the 5′ leader sequences, these primers are not considered universal, and must be designed according to the sequence of the antibody of interest. They must contain an ATG starting codon and we have utilized primers which harbour an *Nco*I restriction site which allows confirmation of the insert orientation. The primers we have used for the cloning of antibody chains are shown in *Table 3*, and the final constructs are shown in *Figure 2*.

Table 3. Nucleotide sequence of the oligonucleotide primers used for PCR amplification of antibody *V* gene

5′ LV_H	CCATGGATTTTCAGGTGCAGATTTTCAGCTTCCTC *Nco*I
5′ *LVk*	CCATGGAATGGAGCTGGATCTTTC *Nco*I
3′J_K	ACTTACGTTTGATCTCCAGCTTGGTCCC splice
3′J_H	ACTTACCTGAGGAGACGGTGACCGTGGTCCCTTGGCCCCAG splice

2.4.3 PCR amplification of cloned V_H and V_L genes

This approach can be used with cloned V_H and V_L, or with RNA from the antibody-producing hybridoma which must then be reverse transcribed (see (17)). The 5′ oligonucleotide primers must be designed according to the sequences of the 5′ L_H and L_k in accord to the description in *Table 3*.

Protocol 1. PCR amplification

Because of the outstanding sensitivity of the PCR, extra care must be exercised in using clean reagents, pipetors, and disposable plastic-ware. To avoid contamination, always use freshly made media solutions made from unused stocks. The principles and details of the PCR procedure are described in (18).

1. In a PCR tube, mix 1 μg of DNA template, 50 pmol of both the 5′ and 3′ primers, 200 mM of each deoxynucleotide triphosphate (dNTP), 10 μl of 10× commercial buffer (Perkin–Elmer) and 2.5 units of Taq polymerase (Perkin–Elmer) in a total volume of 100 μl. The oligonucleotide primers used in this stage should be phosphorylized using T4 polynucleotide kinase.
2. Amplify in an automated thermal cycler with an initial 2 min denaturation at 95°C followed by 35 cycles with 1 min denaturation at 95°C, 2 min annealing at 56°C, and 3 min extension at 72°C.
3. Add 6 units of Klenow (large-fragment DNA polymerase I) with 80 μM of each dNTP to the reaction mixture and incubate an additional 30 min at room temperature to complete the full length extension of the strands.
4. Isolate and purify the DNA fragments (approximately 400 bp) obtained from preparative electrophoresis on 1.5% agarose gel.

Protocol 2. Insertion of the *V* gene into the cassettes

The cassettes used in this protocol were constructed using the genomic Cα and Cβ as described in Section 2.4.1 and shown schematically in *Figure 2*.

1. Digest the cassettes with *Bam*HI, and purify the linearized DNA by preparative gel electrophoresis. Dephosphorylate the plasmid using calf intestinal phosphatase for 30 min at 37°C.
2. Inactivate the phosphatase by adding EDTA to a final concentration of 5 mM and heating it to 75°C for 10 min. Phenol/chloroform extract and ethanol precipitate the vector. Blunt the ends using Klenow fragment for 30 min at room temperature.
3. Insert the V_H or V_L PCR fragment into the opened cassette using T4 DNA ligase. A typical reaction is carried out in 10–20 μl of 0.5× commercial buffer supplemented with 5 mM DTT and T4 DNA ligase (BRL) with an insert to vector ratio of 0.5–1:1 for 6–18 h at 14°C.
4. Transform competent bacteria with the ligation mixture, plate, and select colonies. Because of the low efficiency of transformation with the large plasmids, we recommend selection of colonies by Southern hybridization of bacterial lifts on to nitrocellulose filters, using the appropriate V_H or V_k gene probe.

5. Prepare Mini-prep DNA samples from positive colonies and analyse them for proper orientation by restriction endonuclease digestion (e.g. *Eco*RI/*Nco*I digest of the vectors described in *Figure 2* should yield in correct orientation a 150 bp fragment and a large fragment (14.5 kbp for constructs with Cα or 11.9 for those with Cβ)).
6. Prepare from the selected bacterial clones highly purified plasmid DNA (CsCl gradient fractionation) for both sequencing and subsequent transfection.

Note: Sequencing of the V region and the junctions is recommended because of the incidence of PCR and cloning errors (19).

---

3. Transfection and selection of cells expressing the c*TCR* genes

3.1 Choosing cells for transfection

The choice of an effector T cell into which the c*TCR* is inserted is somewhat limited by the relatively low efficiency of transfection. In fact, due to objective difficulties for efficient transgene expression in T cells, the c*TCR* genes have been successfully introduced so far only into T-cell hybridomas and tumours. This is the major factor impeding the testing of the feasibility of usage of the 'T-body' approach as an anti-tumour therapy *in vivo*. Experiments along these lines are in progress using retroviral vectors which have been proved to be potent vehicles for DNA mediated gene transfer into human T cells (20). In the framework of this chapter, we shall focus on procedures to stably express the c*TCR* gene as a functional moiety in T cells as a means to prove its proper construction.

In general, the cells into which the c*TCR* genes are planned to be transfected, should be rapidly dividing and easy to propagate in culture. It is also important that the cells should provide detectable means to confirm functional insertion of the c*TCR* gene. We routinely use the murine allo-specific cytotoxic T-cell hybridoma, MD45 (21), since it secretes large amounts of interleukin-2 (IL-2) upon stimulation as well as being able to lyse target cells. A mutant, MD45.27J which is TCR α−, CD3− is very useful for these studies, since it re-expresses the CD3/Ti complex upon transfection with chimeric α chain. The murine T-cell lymphoma cell-line EL-4 was also used successfully for transfection of c*TCR* genes IL-2 (1, 7). The human T-cell leukaemia line, Jurkat, has also been demonstrated to functionally express the c*TCR* (5). Jurkat is a CD3+, CD4+ line and secretes a variety of lymphokines, particularly IL-2, upon stimulation. Several CD3− mutants of the Jurkat line have also been described, including J.RT–T3.1 which expresses only low levels of message for the TCR α chain, and J.RT3–T3.5 which is TCR β− (22).

3.2 Sequential transfection versus co-transfection

Because of the heterodimeric nature of the antibody and the TCR molecules, the presence of both chains in the cTCR is necessary for function and for proper antigen binding. Both chimeric TCR chains must therefore be transfected into the target cell in order to confer the expected antigen recognition. Although the most straightforward approach would be to place both of the cTCR chains on the same plasmid, currently this presents a variety of logistical problems because of the size of the inserts and negative interaction of various promoters. The alternative is to insert the two cTCR chains either together or in sequential order. The co-transfection of the two chains would appear to be the most direct and easiest route. Co-expression of the transgenes by co-transfection requires that both genes are simultaneously inserted into the same cell and that no interference will occur between the two plasmids. In addition, the achievement of similar levels of stable expression requires the use of two selection markers, each on different vector. Most of the agents used are toxic to cells, and their combination could potentially inhibit the growth of cells which might otherwise survive a single selection agent. The alternative, sequential transfection, involves the initial screening of the cells for the presence of the individual chain inserted. In most of the cases expression of a single chain cannot be followed by functional assay, thus restricting us to selection according to the presence of RNA, and it may require that several clones be chosen for the second transfection.

3.3 Methods of DNA transfection

For stable expression, the transgene should be integrated into the genome of the recipient cell and obey the cellular replication control. The site of integration is random and usually a large concatamer of DNA is being introduced. To minimize damage to coding sequences during this event, linearization of the plasmid in a non-essential locus is recommended. For transient expression, the vector resides as an epigenetic unit which is independently transcribed and diluted upon replication of the cell.

The introduction and expression of plasmid vectors has relied on physical methods for entry into mammalian cells. These methods have included calcium phosphate precipitate uptake, protoplast fusion, liposomal complex fusion (lipofection), and electroporation of cells. These methods contrast with retroviral mediated gene transfer which relies upon the infectious viral particles to introduce the desired gene. All the four last methods have been used to introduce foreign genes into lymphocytes and can be used for transient and stable gene transfer. Although we initially used protoplast fusion to insert the c*TCR* genes into T cells, we currently use electroporation or lipofection which are simpler methods for the generation of stable transfectants.

In electroporation, cells are placed in a strong electrical field of varying strength and duration. Additional parameters which may affect efficiency include temperature, media, and linearized versus circular DNA. A variety of companies now manufacture instruments specifically designed for cell electroporation, although these experiments were originally carried out in disposable spectroscopic cuvettes using foil on either side as electrodes, and electrically shock-pulsing the cells with an electrophoresis power supply. To maximize efficiency, a trial should be conducted with the specific cells used for transfection, varying both the pulse duration (or capacitance) and intensity. A general guide for DNA incorporation is the viability of the cells, with a 50–60% viability generally giving reasonable transfection efficiency. Linearizing the plasmid is reported to give approximately twice the efficiency of transfection (23); however, care must be taken to avoid digest in an essential area of the plasmid.

Another method which has been used for DNA-mediated gene transfer into lymphocytes utilizes lipofectin (GIBCO/BRL) (24) which has the advantage of lower toxicity to the transfected cells and does not require sophisticated instrumentation (transfection techniques are also discussed in Chapters 16 and 20).

Protocol 3. Transfection of cells

A. *Electroporation*

1. Wash cells twice in PBS (Ca^{++} and Mg^{++} free).
2. Re-suspend the cells (40×10^6 viable cells/ml) in ice-cold phosphate-buffered saline (PBS) + 10 mM Hepes buffer.
3. Transfer 0.5 ml cells to an electroporation cuvette (BRL catalogue No. 1601AB) and keep on ice.
4. Add DNA (approximately 20 μg), mix, and keep on ice for 10 min.
5. Place the cuvette in an ice-cold electroporation chamber and shock at predetermined conditions (for the T-cell hybridoma, we use 350 V, 800 μF in a BRL electroporation unit).
6. Allow the cells to stand on ice for 10 min.
7. Transfer the cells to a culture flask using a Pasteur pipette and dilute in an appropriate medium (RPMI or DMEM with 10% FCS, glutamine, and antibiotics), to a concentration of 10^5/ml.
8. Aliquot the cells, 1 ml/well, into 24-well plates and incubate at 37 °C in a humidified incubator.
9. When cells appear to have recovered from electroporation, as witnessed by their proliferation in culture (usually 48–72 h), add to each well 1 ml of selective medium containing the final concentration of antibiotic as predetermined for each cell-line.

Protocol 3. *Continued*

B. *Protoplast fusion*

Preparation of protoplasts

1. Grow *E. coli* containing the plasmid in Luria broth in a 37°C shaker to an absorbance of $O.D._{600}$ = 0.6–0.8 units.
2. Add chloramphenicol to a final concentration of 125 μg/ml and incubate for an additional 12–16 h.
3. Harvest 25 ml of bacteria by centrifugation at 5000g for 10 min.
4. Re-suspend bacteria in 1.25 ml of a chilled solution containing 20% sucrose, 0.05 M Tris pH 8. Add 0.25 ml of 5 mg/ml lysozyme solution (freshly made in 0.25 M Tris pH 8) and incubate on ice for 6 min.
5. Add 0.5 ml of 0.25 M EDTA, pH 8 and incubate for an additional 5 min.
6. Add 0.5 ml of 0.05 M Tris, pH 8 and incubate in a 37°C water bath for 10 min. A microscopic examination at this point should show the majority of bacteria converted to protoplasts.

Protoplast fusion

1. Re-suspend 3×10^7 of viable cells in 1 ml of DMEM without serum.
2. Add 3 ml of the protoplast suspension and centrifuge the mixture for 8 min at 500*g*.
3. Aspirate the supernatant and gently re-suspend in 1 ml of polyethylene glycol (45% PEG diluted w/v in plain medium) and allow to stand for 1 min.
4. Slowly and gently, add 9 ml of plain medium.
5. Centrifuge for 10 min at 500*g*, and remove the supernatant.
6. Re-suspend the cells in medium with 10% FCS and gentamycin 0.1 mg/ml to kill the remaining bacteria.
7. Plate the cells in 24-well plates, 1 ml/well, at 1×10^5 cells/ml.

3.4 Selection of cells using antibiotic resistance

The relatively low efficiency of DNA transfer presents a problem for detecting expression, since only a small minority of the cells will actually bear the DNA and an even smaller fraction of these express the gene of interest. In order to select for cells with the DNA of interest, a reporter gene may be included. The most often used of these is an antibiotic resistance gene, which allows the growth of cells in an otherwise toxic medium. *Table 4* gives a list of some resistance genes currently utilized for cell selection. The most commonly used is neomycin ribosyl phosphotransferase (*neo*^{r}) which allows growth of cells in media containing the neomycin analogue, G418 (11). Another is

Table 4. Preparation of selective media

Drug	Stock solution	Working solution[a]
G418 (Genticin, Gibco/BRL)	100 mg/ml in PBS	1.0 mg/ml[d]
Mycophenolic acid (Sigma)	2 mg/ml[b]	0.5 μg/ml
Xanthine (Sigma)[b]	10 mg/ml in 0.1 M NaOH	250 μg/ml
Hypoxanthine (Sigma)[c]	10 mg/ml in PBS	15 μg/ml

[a] Working concentrations are pertinent to Jurkat and the T-cell hybridomas studied by us.
[b] Dissolve in 0.1 Mn NaOH, and neutralize to pH 7 by dropwise addition of 0.1 M HCl.
[c] Dissolve at 60°C.
[d] Concentration of active drug.

Another is xanthine guanine phosphoribosyl transferase (GPT), a gene present in many prokaryotic but not mammalian cells (10). This allows the growth of cells in media containing mycophenolic acid, a drug which interferes with the purine salvage pathway. Since two complementary chains are used to form the cTCR, each of the chains is combined with a different resistance gene. The incorporation of these antibiotics kills those cells which do not contain plasmid DNA and/or do not express the gene. Although it does not directly select for those cells which express the gene of interest, drug selection is a rapid way to eliminate the background of non-transfected cells. Most of the cell death will occur fairly rapidly, and thus only resistant cells should be alive after 7–10 days in the presence of the drug. Nevertheless, to ensure retention of the inserted gene it is best to maintain selective pressure on the population by continuing to grow cells in antibiotic-containing medium even after cell death has occurred.

The optimal concentration of antibiotic for selection must be determined for each cell-line in use. This represents the concentration which prevents growth of the untransfected cells yet allows growth of the transfectants. In our experience, the sensitivity of various cell-lines to the antibiotics used for selection varies quite significantly. In some cases, the concentrations of drug needed for selection are beyond the useful range of the drug. (See (9) for a comprehensive list of the antibiotics used for selection.)

To reach clonality (following electroporation or lipofection our routine transfection efficiency is around 1 in 5×10^4 out of which 5–20% express the c*TCR*). A convenient way of culturing the cells right after transfection is to distribute them in a 24-well plate at a concentration of approximately $(1–5) \times 10^4$ cells/well. The viability of cells is low, especially following electroporation, so cells are allowed to grow for a few days (2–4) in regular medium, and only when extensive growth is apparent should medium containing the selective drug be added. At early stages, cells usually are resistant to otherwise effective concentration of the drug. To counter this, the gradual addition of drug may be used. An initial concentration of selection marker which is half of the final concentration is achieved practically by initially culturing the cells in medium without selective drug, then adding an equal volume of selection medium. This will usually result in massive cell death within 1–4 days (dependent on the selective drug; most cells will die within a day in mycophenolic acid; however, it takes about 4–6 days for cells to die in G418). When cells appear to have recovered from the drug, increase its concentration to full strength.

4. Selection of cells expressing the c*TCR*

4.1 Molecular analysis of transfectants

Following drug-selection, transfectants expressing the c*TCR* must be identified. The use of antibiotic resistance is an effective way to select for transfectants. However, the drug-resistance gene is under the control of a separate promoter and thus its expression does not necessarily mean that the gene of interest has been introduced nor does it indicate that the cell will function properly. Quite often cells may be resistant to antibiotic, yet fail to express the desired transgene. Screening may be done at several levels; transcription, translation, and activity expression. For the c*TCR*, protein analysis and functional demonstration require coexpression of both chains, therefore these methods usually are not as useful for initial screening, unless co-transfection of both genes has been carried out.

4.1.1 Detection of transcription

The demonstration of specific mRNA transcription may be used as a rapid method for the selection of transfectants expressing the desired c*TCR* transgene. Because the initial phase requires the screening of large numbers of clones, a procedure for rapid extraction and identification of RNA is obligatory. The protocol described below, using guanidinium thiocyanate (25) enables the processing of many samples containing relatively small numbers of cells such as are available in this early phase. To rapidly test the RNA, dot-blot analysis may be performed using V region DNA probes. The cell-lines which appear positive by dot blot should be verified by electrophoresis and Northern analysis for the correct size of the transcript (approx. 1.4 kb for the c*TCR* bearing Cβ and 1.6 kb for those bearing Cα).

Protocol 4. Rapid extraction of cellular RNA

All reagents should be prepared in diethylpyrocarbonate (DEPC)-treated water and autoclaved whenever possible.[a]

1. Wash (1–5) × 10^6 cells twice with TBS (Tris 0.025 M, pH 7.4, NaCl 0.14 M).
2. Transfer the cells to Eppendorf tubes, pellet, and re-suspend the cells in GIT solution composed of 4 M guanidinium isothiocyanate, 0.025 M sodium citrate, pH 7, and 0.5% Sarkosyl, by vigorous vortexing.

3. Add 50 μl 2.0 M sodium acetate, pH 4.0, 0.5 ml of phenol and 100 μl of chloroform:isoamyl alcohol 50:1 and vortex vigorously to achieve a homogeneous 'milky' suspension.
4. Allow to stand on ice for 10 min, then centrifuge 12 000*g* for 15 min.
5. Transfer the upper aqueous phase to fresh Eppendorf tubes, taking care not to disturb the interphase. If the separation is not clear, the samples should be re-vortexed and centrifuged again.
6. Add an equal volume (0.5 ml) of isopropanol to each sample, mix, and allow to precipitate for at least 1 h at −20°C.
7. Centrifuge the tubes at 12 000*g* for 15 min and carefully aspirate the supernatant using a capillary Pasteur pipette.
8. Re-suspend the RNA pellet in 500 μl of GIT solution, vortex, and precipitate again as in steps **6** and **7**.
9. Wash the RNA pellets with 75% ethanol and dry (not too excessively).
10. Re-suspend the RNA pellet in 25–50 μl of sterile water. Samples should be stored at −70°C to minimize degradation.

[a] See also Chapter 10 for a discussion of precautions when handling RNA.

4.1.2 Immunodetection of the cTCR molecule

To express a functional receptor, the two nascent chimeric chains have to be glycosilated, pair, and combine in a proper conformation with the various CD3 complex molecules and be transported to the cell membrane. The presence of heterodimeric cTCR may be detected using specific antibodies by either immunoblotting (Western) analysis and/or immunofluorescence staining. Anti-idiotypic antibodies directed at the Fv of the MAb represent the most specific probe. However, idiotopes usually require the presence of both V_H and V_L and anti-idiotypic antibodies are not always available. Alternative probes are those directed against the T-cell receptor α or β chains, MAb# #H28 and #H57, specific to the murine TCR (26), or Identi-TαF1 (27) and Identi-TβF1 (28) (T Cell Sciences) specific to the human TCR α or β chains are very useful for this purpose. These antibodies can recognize the single chain and offer an advantage when transfection takes place into cell which do not express the native TCR, or express TCR from different species. These techniques detect both surface and intracellular proteins.

i. Surface expression of cTCR

Appearance of the cTCR on the cell surface of transfected cells is one of the most convenient methods to prove the expression of the c*TCR* genes. This can be readily tested following transfection of a single c*TCR* gene into TCR α or β lacking T-cell mutants by reappearance of the surface CD3/Ti complex or following expression of both chimeric genes as an intact receptor. Analysis of cells for surface expression of the c*TCR* can be accomplished by using either anti-CD3 antibodies (in the case of the single-chain-into-mutant strategy) or by the binding of anti-idiotypic antibodies or antigen (when available). The latter requires the proper association of the molecular heterodimer and the antibody V regions to conform the correct idiotope and antigen binding site. Using fluorescent ligands and analysis by FACS (fluorescence activated cell sorter) allows the screening of a large number of cell-lines in a short time. In addition, it is a sensitive technique which enables the detection of as few as 10^3 molecules per cell, provides information as to the heterogeneity of the cells, and allows the specific sorting and separation of the desired population.

An additional method to verify the surface expression of the c*TCR* is by specific immunoprecipitation of surface ^{125}I-labelled molecules. Although this method is not as simple as immunofluorescence, it provides information on the size, structure and composition of the cTCR/CD3 complex.

ii. Detection of cTCR protein

The use of mild detergent lysis of cells allows recovery of non-denatured proteins, which may then be checked for the presence of the specific cTCR chains. These can be found as a cytoplasmic or membranal complex with the CD3 chains either non-covalently bound or bound through a disulphide bond with the complementary TCR chain. For fast screening of large numbers of samples, the cell lysates may be blotted directly onto nitrocellulose filters then stained with the appropriate antibody. Negative (parental cells) and positive (the antibody used for the cTCR construction) controls should be included. To further evaluate the results, positive lysates can be studied by Western analysis. Because of possible sensitivity of many idiotopes to denaturating agents such as the SDS and reducing agents used for SDS-PAGE, care has to be exercized in treatment of samples. We found it useful to include protease inhibitors in the lysis buffer, to reduce concentration of SDS and omit the reducing agents in the sample buffer, and to avoid heating prior to polyacrylamide gel electrophoresis and electroblotting on to the filter (see *Protocol* 5).

Protocol 5. Detection of cTCR in cell lysates

A. *Cell lysis*

1. Harvest cells, count, and wash twice in cold PBS.
2. Transfer cells into an Eppendorf tube and spin them down at 1000*g* for 2 min.
3. Gently re-suspend the cells at 10^8/ml in ice-cold lysis buffer composed of 0.14 M NaCl, 20 mM Tris pH 8.0, 10 mM EDTA, 1% NP-40, 1 mM PMSF, 10 μg/ml Aprotinin, and 10 μg/ml leupeptin (Protease inhibitors, Sigma).

4. Leave the tubes for 30 min on ice, spin down nuclei in a refrigerated centrifuge at 12 000*g* for 10 min.
5. Keep supernatant. Aliquot and freeze at −70°C until use.

B. *Immuno dot-blot analysis*

This is a simple, fast and sensitive method to detect cTCR molecules in lysates. The procedure below was adopted for use in the Minifold II Slot-Blotter of Schleicher & Schuell.

1. Assemble the slot-blotter device using water-soaked nitrocellulose filter.
2. Load 25 μl of the lysate and 1:5 and 1:25 dilutions in lysis buffer into each row of slots. Include lysates of parental cell for controls, the idiotypic MAb (and unrelated one) if anti-id antibodies are used, or lysates of T cells containing the TCR if anti-TCR antibodies are used.
3. Leave for 10 min then apply a vacuum until the slots are emptied.
4. Air-dry the filter.
5. Soak it in blocking solution containing 10% skimmed milk in PBS + 0.05% NaN_3, by overnight rocking at 4°C.
6. Transfer the filter into the first antibody (anti-id or anti-TCR) diluted in 0.1% BSA in PBS + 0.05% Tween-20 (use approximately 10 ml of diluted antibody). Rock for 2 h at room temperature.
7. Wash filter three times in PBS–Tween (by rocking for 15 min each wash).
8. Add 10 ml of peroxidase-labelled anti-Ig (or Protein A) as the second antibody, diluted as recommended by the supplier in 0.1% BSA in PBS–Tween. Rock for 2 h at room temperature.
9. Wash filter three times in PBS–Tween (by rocking for 15 min each wash).
10. Develop blots using chemiluminescence kit, such as ECL (Amersham), by removing buffer and adding substrate (mixed 1:1, for 60 sec at room temperature for ECL kit), remove excess substrate, and wrap in Saran wrap.
11. Expose to film (Hyperfilm, Amersham) for several periods of time to obtain the optimal intensity.

Comments

- Avoid using azide in all wash solutions and antibody diluents, because it might interfere with the peroxidase activity.
- The proper dilutions of first and second antibodies must be pre-determined. Use higher dilutions of the second antibody to decrease background.
- This method can be quantitative using a densitometer if known amounts of idiotypic MAb are used as standards.

Protocol 5. *Continued*

C. *Soluble receptor—ELISA*

Quantitative analysis for active cTCR can be done using a solid-phase immunoassay which takes advantage of the ability of the receptor to bind antigen in antibody affinity and specificity on one end, and presence of the TCR epitopes on the other end.

1. Coat the wells of 96 multititre immunoplate with protein antigen by adding 100 μl of solution of 5–50 μg/ml of antigen in PBS, and incubate it overnight at 4°C.
2. Aspirate antigen, wash plate with PBS–Tween and leave for at least 2 h at room temperature, in blocking solution composed of 1% BSA in PBS–azide.
3. Wash with PBS–Tween.
4. Add 100 μl of serial dilutions of cell lysates diluted in lysis buffer and incubate for 2 h at 4°C.
5. Aspirate and wash three times with Tween–PBS.
6. Add 100 μl of anti-id or anti-TCR antibodies, diluted in 0.1% BSA–PBS to a pre-determined concentration and incubate for 2 h at 4°C.
7. Aspirate and wash three times with Tween–PBS.
8. Add 100 μl of anti-Ig peroxidase-labelled second antibody, diluted in 0.1% BSA–PBS to a pre-determined concentration and incubate for 2 h at 4°C.
9. Aspirate and wash three times with Tween–PBS.
10. Add 100 μl peroxidase substrate: *o*-phenylenediamine (OPD) in 0.05 M phosphate–citrate buffer pH 5.0 containing 0.03% H_2O_2 (Sigma products P6787 and P9305).
11. Leave for 10–30 min in the dark for colour development.
12. Stop the reaction by adding 50 μl of 2 M sulphuric acid and read the absorbance in an automatic ELISA reader at 450 nm.

4.2 Functional analysis of transfectants

4.2.1 Re-expression of CD3 in TCR-loss mutants

The availability of TCR chain-loss mutants provides a way to identify the expression of a single chain of the chimeric receptor. Since the surface expression of CD3 is dependent on the presence of the TCR chains, these mutants are CD3− and cannot respond to CD3/Ti-specific stimuli. The introduction of the missing chain in the form of a chimeric receptor allows the re-expression of CD3, which can be detected by measuring T-cell activation and cytokine secretion in response to mitogens such as ConA or PHA, or to immobilized anti-CD3 MAbs. These cells may then be analysed for antigen binding if transfected with both chains, or may be used as a cell population for transfection of the complementary chimeric TCR chain.

4.2.2 Specific stimulation with antigen

The ultimate test of the proper expression of the c*TCR* is the ability to respond to the antigen for which the antibody is specific. This response should be MHC non-restricted and trigger the T cell to execute the effector function it has been programmed to, such as cytokine production and/or cytotoxic activity. Both early or late receptor-activated functions have been reported following stimulation with the cTCR and these can be also applied for the initial screening phase. Ca^{2+} uptake (1) is an easy measure of early events and IL-2 secretion is a convenient assay for late events that follow TCR-mediated T-cell triggering. The T-cell hybridoma MD45, used by us, offers the advantage of having both cytotoxic effects as well as secreting large amounts of IL-2 upon stimulation (2). Previous studies have demonstrated the need for immobilization of antigen for optimal triggering of T cells through the CD3/Ti complex. In fact, we have demonstrated that soluble antigen effectively inhibits T-cell stimulation via the cTCR.

For specific stimulation, transfected cells are cultured with antigen either presented in a cellular form or immobilized on to a solid support such as the plastic of the tissue-culture well. Immobilized anti-idiotypic antibody can also serve as a specific means of stimulation. The supernatant of these cell cultures may then be tested for the presence of cytokine using either biologic assay or by ELISA (methods for T-cell stimulation are also discussed in Chapters 7 and 19).

4.2.3 Antibody or soluble antigen blocking studies

The inhibitory effects of soluble antigen offers a way to further document the specificity of the response of T cells bearing the c*TCR*. The addition of soluble antigen to such T-cells diminishes their response to immobilized antigen in a competitive fashion. Similarly, soluble anti-idiotypic antibodies, which bind the Fv, compete with the binding of antigen to the cTCR, and thereby inhibit the stimulation. Adding varying concentrations of soluble antigen allows an assessment of the affinity of the cTCR. This may be of particular importance when soluble antigen is expected within a system, as is found with a variety of tumour antigens.

Protocol 6. IL-2 production assay

cTCR transfected cells can be stimulated by target cells (in suspension or monolayer) and by immobilized antigen or antibodies. It should be noted that the conditions given in this protocol are those which we have found to be optimal in our systems. Conditions for stimulation must be optimized for each cell used (see also Chapter 11).

Protocol 6. *Continued*

1. (a) For immobilizing antigen or antibody—coat 96-well flat-bottom plates with an appropriate antigen or stimulatory antibody. For stimulation through the CD3 molecule, use 100 μl of 1 μg/ml purified anti-murine CD3 Mab No. 2C11 or anti-human CD3 MAb No. OKT3. Antibodies are diluted in 0.05 M carbonate–bicarbonate buffer, pH 9.5. Anti-idiotypic antibodies should be used in a similar way, but their effective concentration has to be determined.

   (b) For cellular antigens—in the case of adherent stimulators—grow cells in monolayers; for non-adherent cells add 100 μl of irradiated stimulator cells (the optimal number should be pre-determined for each system).
2. Harvest the transfectants, count, wash, and re-suspend each at a concentration of 1×10^6/ml in RPMI or DMEM medium containing 10% FCS, 10 mM Hepes and 5×10^{-5} M of β-mercaptoethanol.
3. Aspirate the solution from the antigen- or antibody-coated plates. For plates with cells, take special care not to disrupt the monolayer.
4. Add 100 μl of medium to the wells. For stimulation with cellular antigens, anti-idiotype, and OKT3, the addition of a final concentration of 10 ng/ml TPA (12-*o*-tetradecanoylphorbol 13-acetate, Sigma) enhances stimulation. It is mandatory for Jurkat cells.
5. Include negative controls of medium ± TPA. Combination of the Ca^{2+} ionophore Ionomycin (Sigma) at 200 ng/ml and 10 ng/ml TPA by-passes the CD3/TCR-mediated T-cell activation and represents an adequate control for the ability of the cell to respond.
6. Add 100 μl of cells to each of the wells (including the non-transfected parental cells), and incubate for 24–48 h at 37 °C.
7. Remove 50–100 μl supernatant for IL-2 determination.

Determination of IL-2 production

- For IL-2 bioassay, such as those using the IL-2-dependent CTL-L, the culture supernatant must be completely free of viable cells. A way to ensure this is to freeze–thaw the supernatant prior to assay. Standardization of bioassays and data analysis are described in Chapter 11.
- For ELISA assay, 50–100 μl of supernatant is transferred to the appropriate plate as stated by the manufacturer. We have used a murine IL-2 ELISA kit available from Becton–Dickinson, and a human IL-2 ELISA kit manufactured by R&D systems.

Acknowledgement

The studies reported here were supported in part by The US–Israel Binational Foundation for Basic Science. Z.E. is incumbent of Marshall and Rnette Ezralow Chair in Chemical and Cellular Immunology.

References

1. Kuwana, Y., Asakura, Y., Utsunomiya, N., Nakonishi, M., Arata, Y., Itoh, S., *et al.* (1987). *Biochem. Biophys. Res. Commun.*, **149,** 960.
2. Gross, G., Gorochov, G., Waks, T., and Eshhar, Z. (1989). *Transplantation Proc.*, **21,** 127.
3. Gross, G., Waks, T., and Eshhar, Z. (1989). *Proc. Natl. Acad. Sci. USA*, **86,** 10024.
4. Eshhar, Z. and Gross. G. (1990). *Br. J. Cancer*, **62,** suppl. X, 27.
5. Gorochov, G., Gross, G., Waks, T., and Eshhar, Z. (1990). *Cellular Immunity and the Immunotherapy of Cancer, UCLA Symposia on Molecular and Cellular Biology, New Series* (ed. M. T. Lotz and O. J. Finn), pp. 97–101. Wiley-Liss, New York.
6. Becker, M. L. B., Near, R., Mudget-Hunter, M., Margolies, M. N., Kubo, R. T., Kaye, J. *et al.* (1989). *Cell*, **58**, 911.
7. Goverman, J., Goimez, S. M., Segesman, K. D., Hunkapillerk, T., Lang, W. E., and Hood, L. (1990). *Cell*, **60,** 929.
8. Sambrook, J., Fritsch, E. F., and Maniatis, T. (1989). *Molecular Cloning: A Laboratory Manual* (2nd edn). Cold Spring Harbor Laboratory Press, Plainview, NY.
9. Kriegler, M. (1990). *Gene Transfer and Expression: A Laboratory Manual*. Stockton Press, New York.
10. Mulligan, R. C. and Berg, P. (1981). *Proc. Natl. Acad. Sci USA*, **78,** 2072.
11. Southern, P. J. and Berg, P. (1982). *J. Mol. Appl. Gen.*, **1,** 327.
12. Mason, J. O., Williams, K. G., and Neuberger, M. S. (1985). *Cell*, **41,** 479.
13. Zaller, D. M., Yu, H., and Eckhardt, L. A. (1988). *Mol. Cell. Biol.*, **8,** 1932.
14. Gross, G., Waks, T., Levy, S., Levy, R., and Eshhar, Z. (In preparation.)
15. Morey, Y. Y., Keshet, E., Ram, D., and Kaminchik, Y. (1980). *Mol. Biol. Rep.*, **6,** 203.
16. Kabat, E. A., Wu, T. T., Reid Muller, M., Perry, H. M., and Grottesman, U. S. (1987). *Sequences of Proteins of Immunological Interest* (4th edn). Department of Health and Human Services, Washington, DC.
17. Orlandi, R., Gussow, D. H., Jones, P. T., and Winter, G. (1989). *Proc. Natl. Acad. Sci. USA*, **86**, 3833.
18. Maloney, D. G., Kaminski, M. S., Burowski, D., Haimovich, J., and Levy, R. (1985). *Hybridoma*, **4,** 191.
19. Innis, M. A., Gelfand, D. H., Sninsky, J. J., and White, T. J. (1990). *PCR Protocols: A Guide to Methods and Applications*. Academic, San Diego, CA.
20. Culver, K., Cornetta, K., Morgan, R., Morecki, S., Aebersold, P., Kasid, A., *et al.* (1988). *Proc. Natl. Acad. Sci. USA*, **88,** 3155.
21. Kaufmann, Y., Berke, G., and Eshhar, Z. (1981). *Proc. Natl. Acad. Sci. USA*, **78**, 2502.

22. Ohashi, P. S., Mak, T. W., Van den Elsen, P., Yanagi, Y., Yoshikai, Y., Calmen, E., *et al.* (1985). *Nature*, **315,** 606.
23. Potter, H. (1988). *Anal. Biochem.*, **174,** 361.
24. Felgner, P. L. Gadek, T. R., Holm, M., Roman, R., Chan, H. W., Wenz, M., *et al.* (1987). *Proc. Natl. Acad. Sci. USA*, **84,** 7413.
25. Chomczynski, P. and Sacchi, N. (1987). *Anal. Biochem.*, **162,** 156.
26. Kubo, R. T., Born, W., Kappler, J. W., Marrack, P., and Pigeon, M. (1989). *J. Immunol.*, **142,** 2736.
27. Henry, L., Tian, W., Ritterhaus, C., Ko, J., Marsh, H. C. jnr, and Ip, S. H. (1989). *Hybridoma*, **8,** 577.
28. Brenner, M. B., McLean, J., Scheft, H., Warnke, R. A., Jones, N., and Strominger, J. L. (1987). *J. Immunol.*, **138,** 1502.

22

The use of pre-clinical rodent models for cancer immunotherapy

ROBERT H. WILTROUT

1. Introduction

Most scientists agree that pre-clinical rodent tumour models provide some information that is useful to the design of immunotherapeutic approaches for human cancers (1). There is, however, some disagreement as to the types of pre-clinical information that can be extrapolated to humans and the extent to which this information will be predictive for responses (2, 3). The types of information derived from rodent tumour models include the detection of anti-tumour activity of a test agent (e.g. actual tumour regression), the regimen (e.g. doses, routes, and timing) by which optimal anti-tumour effects are achieved, and the cellular and molecular mechanism(s) responsible for the observed tumour regression. Given the great diversity of rodent tumour models, it is not surprising that different tumour models may provide more or less of this information than do others and some may relate more closely to certain kinds of human cancers than do others. Thus, the choice of a pre-clinical tumour model is in large part predicated on the scientific hypothesis to be tested. Different tumour models vary greatly with regard to their complexity and expense, a factor which must be considered if the model is to be used for extensive screening for simple anti-tumour activity. In this case confirmation of activity and more detailed questions must be addressed in secondary, and sometimes more complex, models. This chapter will briefly outline the various applications and types of pre-clinical rodent tumour models, and then discuss in detail the practical use of a transplantable murine renal carcinoma (Renca). It will also provide a brief overview of other available models.

2. General types of rodent tumour models

Tumour models differ greatly with regard to their complexity and suitability for testing various hypotheses. The general types of models are outlined below and discussed in detail in Chapter 2.

2.1 Transplantable primary tumours

In most cases, transplantable syngeneic tumours are the easiest and least expensive models to utilize. In theory, they are identical in antigen display to normal tissue of the host strain from which they were derived, with the exception that they may also express additional tumour-associated antigens. Limitations of these types of models can include genetic drift of the tumour line after an increasing number of passages, rapid growth (that may be uncharacteristic of most human neoplasms), and the fact that the host is relatively healthy until the late stages of tumour growth. However, some immunotherapeutic agents that have initially been detected using these models have shown activity in more stringent rodent models and in human clinical trials. These models are relatively easy to use and monitor, because the tumour cells are usually injected by the subcutaneous or intradermal routes from where it is easy to monitor their progress. Intraperitoneal injection is often used in situations where the endpoint is a change in survival time.

2.2 Transplantable metastatic tumours

The most challenging aspect of cancer treatment is the need to treat disseminated disease (4). The ability of tumour cells to metastasize to different anatomical locations greatly increases the complexity of cancer treatment. Thus, pre-clinical models that allow the development of treatment strategies relevant to metastatic disease are of critical importance. This is particularly true for the development of immunotherapeutic protocols since the various sites of metastasis formation (e.g. lymph nodes, lung, liver) differ considerably in the composition of resident leukocyte populations, which may result in qualitatively or quantitatively different immune responses in those locations. Many transplantable tumours are amenable to the study of at least some aspects of the treatment of metastases. These models are divided into two general categories, experimentally established metastases versus those that derive spontaneously from established primary tumours.

2.2.1 Experimental metastasis models

As the name implies, these are models in which the metastatic nodules are artifically established by circumventing many of the early stages of the metastatic process. The process of spontaneous metastasis is quite complex, involving many genetic, biochemical, and host factors (4). Therefore, it is also highly variable and often requires extended periods of tumour growth. For these reasons methodology has been developed to rapidly establish consistent numbers of metastases in the lung and liver, which are often targets for tumour metastasis during the progression of human cancer. Reproducible numbers of pulmonary metastases can be rapidly established by the intravenous injection of a single-cell suspension of tumour cells. These established tumour foci can then be treated by various immunotherapeutic agents at stages of growth ranging from micrometastatic to advanced. Likewise, metastases can be preferentially established in the liver by the injection of a single-cell suspension of tumour cells into the spleen from where they efficiently seed the liver via the portal venous circulation. In both of these techniques the establishment of metastases in a specific organ is not absolutely exclusive, but can be almost so for some tumours.

2.2.2 Spontaneous metastasis models

As the name implies, the development of metastases in this setting occurs spontaneously from an established primary tumour. The primary tumour can be implanted in a variety of anatomical locations including the skin or dermis, the kidneys, or in the footpad of a limb. Depending on the biology of the tumour, the metastatic process proceeds at varying rates and efficiency. In particular there is great variability in the kinetics, organ tropism, and efficiency of metastasis formation from one tumour to another. There can also be considerable variability in metastasis formation by an individual tumour within and between experiments. This generally results from the fact that the metastatic process is a complex cascade of events and the disruption of any of these events may significantly alter the ability of tumour cells to successfully metastasize. For example, variability in the immune status of the host rodent due to infection, age, or stress may impact on this process. Alternatively, any variability in the preparation or location of the tumour cell inoculum may also induce some variability. Another potential disadvantage is the relatively long-term nature of the experiments. On the other hand, a major advantage of this type of model is that it is very therapeutically challenging in that successful approaches depend on being able to treat an established primary tumour and metastases in different anatomical locations. Of course, this situation is much more analogous to the human clinical picture where the primary tumour may be treatable by surgery, radiation, or chemotherapy while the residual disease is refractory to these approaches. Another similarity of this model to human cancer is that the host is 'conditioned' by a considerable tumour burden before therapy is initiated. This type of model is generally used as a second-generation test of agents that previously demonstrated anti-tumour effects in transplantable primary or experimental metastasis experiments.

2.3 Primary autochthonous tumours

The most challenging models for the evaluation of immunotherapeutic protocols are those in which tumours actually arise in their hosts. Not surprisingly, these models are usually quite difficult to work with for several reasons. First, there is rodent-to-rodent variability in the amount of time required to generate tumours. This variability occurs to some extent regardless of whether the oncogenic stimulus is genetic predisposition, a chemical or physical (e.g. UV light) carcinogen, or a tumourigenic virus. The biological complexity associated with oncogenesis, tumour development, and tumour metastasis all contribute to this variability. Thus, numerous rodents need to be put on study to assure that adequate numbers of tumour-bearers with malignancies of similar stage are available for statistically sound experiments. This requires the use of increased numbers of rodents at the initiation of experimentation to compensate for the probability that tumours will not grow equally or at all, in every rodent. A further problem is that there can be a relatively long time lag from the time of oncogenesis until the tumours have progressed to the point that they are clinically advanced. Thus, the costs of animal maintenance for these types of studies can be quite high. One possible additional disadvantage (for at least some of these models) is the fact that many of the oncogenic stimuli, including viruses, UV light, and chemical carcinogens, induce highly immunogenic tumours. Since most human tumours are currently considered to be poorly immunogenic, it is somewhat questionable whether the same mechanisms operative against highly immunogenic tumours are effective against poorly immunogenic cancers. The advantages of these models include the fact that the tumour has been newly formed from the tissue of the host in which it grows. This excludes genetic drift as a factor in expression of antigens distinct from the host. Further, the host is subjected to the as yet not well understood processes associated with oncogenesis and tumour progression. These processes may well induce undefined stresses and problems for the host that would most closely mimic the situation for a patient in the response to his or her own tumour. Such a situation may well provide the most stringent test of immunotherapeutic approaches to cancer treatment. However, because of their complexity and expense, the use of autochthonous tumour models is usually reserved for a stringent test of immunotherapeutic approaches detected in other models. Alternatively, these models may be used to study some specific aspect of the tumour–host interaction, such as the immune suppression induced by UV light (5).

2.4 Xenografts of human tumours in athymic mice

Because rodent tumours may differ from human tumours in some aspects of their basic biology, many investigators have chosen to study some facets of immunotherapy against human tumour transplants in athymic mice (6). Athymic mice exhibit a pronounced, but not absolute, suppression in T-lymphocyte-mediated immunity by virtue of an impaired ability to form mature T cells. This defect in T-cell-mediated function permits the progressive growth of some human tumours, although additional immunosuppressive pre-treatments with radiation or chemotherapeutic drugs may be required in some situations. The major advantage of these xenograft models is obvious, in that the treatment modality to be tested can actually be evaluated directly against human neoplastic tissue.

Xenograft models are particularly useful for evaluating biological agents that may have direct anti-tumour activity, such as monoclonal antibody–toxin conjugates. These immunotoxins bind directly to tumour cells and kill through the disruption of vital biochemical pathways. Xenograft models are much less useful for evaluating the anti-tumour potential of immunostimulators, since the effector-to-target interaction would become a non-physiological xenogeneic response; for example, cytokines such as interferons or interleukins could stimulate rodent natural killer cells or macrophages to recognize and kill human tumours. The relevance of such effects to cancer treatment in a human is probably quite limited and therefore of little obvious value. Overall, there is a distinct niche for the use of human tumour xenograft models, but it is limited.

3. Application and description of a transplantable murine renal cancer model

As outlined in Section 2 above, there are a variety of approaches to the use of pre-clinical rodent models for the design and evaluation of immunotherapy. All have inherent strengths and weaknesses. Within each class of tumour model there are many individual tumours that have been studied. Each specific experimental tumour has its own unique properties and some have considerable limitations. For the sake of simplicity, I have chosen one model for a detailed description of practical methodology. Many of the principles and details of this model are easily extrapolated to other experimental tumour models with only minor modification. The model I will discuss is one of murine renal cancer (Renca) which offers a number of advantages for the development and evaluation of immunotherapeutic strategies. I wish to clearly state that the remaining portion of this chapter is predicated on my belief that the major relevance of pre-clinical models lies in the elucidation of basic mechanisms by which the immune system can be induced to recognize and reject tumours. So, I do not proceed from the perspective that doses and schedules of biological response modifiers that have activity in rodents will extrapolate directly to treatment of cancer in humans. Nor do I believe that immunotherapeutic protocols developed against a particular tumour histotype in the rodent are necessarily limited to, or specific for, the same tumour type in humans. Rather, the accumulated evidence suggests that pre-clinical models are useful in detecting prototype approaches for cancer treatment. These general approaches must then be broadly evaluated in clinical trials in order to maximize efficacy.

3.1 Intrarenal Renca as a model for treatment of a primary tumour

The Renca renal adenocarcinoma arose spontaneously in a BALB/c mouse and was originally isolated by Dr Sarah Stewart at the National Cancer

Institute. Subsequently, Murphy and Hrushesky (7) and Williams *et al.* (8) characterized the growth of this tumour in syngeneic mice. This tumour can be injected in the orthotopic site (kidney) and from there it invades locally and metastasizes to the regional lymph nodes, lungs, and liver. The immunogenicity of Renca has been reported to be low to moderate (9).

In our hands, the Renca tumour behaves as previously described, with progressive metastases developing in the lymph nodes, lungs, and liver following the injection of 1×10^5 viable tumour cells under the capsule of the left kidney (10). Tumour-bearing mice will routinely die in 35–45 days. Because the Renca tumour becomes highly vascularized as it develops (7) and grows progressively from the orthotopic site in a manner similar to that described for human renal cell cancer (11), we speculated that it would be a good model for the evaluation of immunotherapeutic approaches to cancer treatment. In the following sections I will provide the methodological details for the various ways in which we have used this model.

Renca can be transplanted into a variety of sites, depending on the type of immunotherapeutic approach to be studied. In our studies we have actually studied Renca primary tumours after subcutaneous (sc), intradermal (id), intraperitoneal (ip), and intrarenal (ir) implantation. In general, the growth rates of this tumour are similar regardless of which of these sites is used, with the exception that implantation ip results in a slightly shorter survival time (about 28–32 days). I will describe the detailed methodology for the ip passage and the ir injections because they are the procedures that we have most routinely used.

Protocol 1. Intraperitoneal passage of Renca

- The tumour cells to be used are obtained from an ip passage in normal mice, or from a tissue-culture line. If the tumour is derived from an *in vivo* passage, it is sterilely excised, and dissociated by compression with the flat side of a 50 ml syringe plunger.[a]

1. Pipette the dissociated tissue into a 50 ml tube and re-suspend it in 50 ml of culture medium.
2. Allow the suspended material to sediment for 3–5 min.
3. Remove the supernatant, spin out the cells, and count the viable cells with the aid of trypan blue.
4. Re-suspend the cells to 2×10^5/ml and then inject 0.5 ml ($\times 10^5$) into BALB/c mice.
5. Harvest the tumour from humanely euthanased animals 10–14 days later.

[a] The dissociation procedure can be varied such that the tumour can also be minced into small pieces and gently forced through a mesh screen and filtered through gauze prior to suspension in 50 ml of medium. Alternatively, some tumours are too dense to be dissociated by simple physical means, and may require mincing followed by enzymatic dissociation with proteases and DNase. A more complete discussion of tissue dissociation is found in Chapter 1.

Protocol 2. Intrarenal injection of Renca

- The tumour cells to be used are usually obtained from an ip passage in control BALB/c mice, as described in *Protocol 1*.

1. Anaesthetize mice using a recognized inhalable anaesthetic such as Metafane (300 litres/min of oxygen) in a Plexiglass box with a vented hood. Alternatively, an injectable anaesthetic can be used; consult your institution's animal welfare officer.
2. Upon induction of level III, stage 2–3 anaesthesia, make a lateral incision 0.5 inches below the spine on the mouse's left flank. The incision should be approximately 1 inch in length.
3. Apply gentle pressure to the abdomen until the left kidney is clearly visible against the peritoneal membrane.
4. Use a 27-gauge needle and a syringe to *carefully* inject 1×10^5 cells, in 0.1 ml, under the capsule of the left kidney.
5. Close the incision with autoclips.
6. Carefully monitor the mice for safe recovery from the surgery.
7. Begin the required therapeutic approaches 7 or more days after injection of the tumour.

In some experiments, mice are treated with the primary tumour in place. Generally, the tumour begins to invade locally by day 7 and metastases begin to form by day 11. Thus, in some experiments the primary tumour may be resected prior to the use of immunotherapy and/or chemotherapy to treat the residual disseminated disease. The location of the primary tumour in the kidney (a paired organ system) makes its resection relatively simple, and closely mimics the clinical situation in which a patient's tumour-bearing kidney is often removed prior to the treatment of metastatic disease. Thus, *Protocol 3* details our procedure for nephrectomy of the tumour-bearing kidney.

Protocol 3. Nephrectomy of Renca-bearing kidney[a]

1. Anaesthetize the tumour-bearing mice as described in *Protocol 2* until level III, stage 2–3 anaesthesia has been achieved.
2. Remove the autoclips over the initial incision and make a larger incision, over the first one.
3. Make a small incision in the exposed peritoneal membrane, and apply gentle pressure to the abdomen to expose the tumour-bearing kidney.
4. Gently pull the kidney through the peritoneal membrane with sterile

Protocol 3. *Continued*

forceps and clamp a pair of haemostats around the artery; tie the artery off with a surgical knot below the haemostat, using 3/0 gut.

5. Resect the kidney above the haemostat, remove the haemostat and insert the ligature back into the peritoneum.
6. Pull the skin together and secure it with autoclips.
7. Place the animals on a paper towel in a cage, in a warm draft-free area until they are fully awake. The mice are allowed a further 3–4 h of recovery before immunotherapy or chemotherapy is initiated.

[a] Beginning at about day 11, it becomes more difficult to resect the tumour-bearing kidney safely. At this point, the tumour is relatively large, with an extensive blood supply and considerable local growth. Some mortality must be expected and this incidence of mortality increases as a function of time after day 11.

A major advantage of this model, where the primary tumour grows in the kidney and then spontaneously disseminates to other organs, is its flexibility. Different therapeutic approaches can be evaluated against progressively more advanced disease, and disease located in different organs. However, the model is relatively complex when the tumour is implanted in the kidney and good surgical skills are required. An alternative to this approach is to implant the tumour sc and treat the disease at various times thereafter. The Renca tumour will metastasize well from this site, although surgical removal of an advanced sc tumour is difficult, which can limit this approach somewhat. The endpoint of this variation of the Renca model is when the mice become moribund. Thus, the anti-tumour effects obtained with different treatments are measured largely by extensions in survival time, or by outright cure. The time to these endpoints can be 2–4 months, depending on the effectiveness of the immunotherapy being tested, which results in relatively slow accumulation of data. For this reason, as well as other considerations about the mechanisms of anti-tumour activity, we often employ two variants of this approach that use experimentally established metastases as the target for treatment.

3.2 The use of Renca for the formation of experimental pulmonary metastases

The major advantages of experimental metastasis models for the evaluation of immunotherapeutic strategies are reproducibility of tumour burden, and the relatively short duration of the experiment. The principal disadvantage is that the host rodent is relatively healthy at the time therapy is initiated, generally 3 to 10 days after the injection of the tumour. The easiest type of experimental model to employ is one where the tumour injection is made via the intravenous (iv) route, as outlined in *Protocol 4*.

Protocol 4. Establishment of Renca pulmonary metastases

1. Gently warm normal BALB/c mice under a lamp for a brief period of time to dilate their tail veins.
2. Carefully restrain the mouse, with the tail exposed.
3. Inject 1–2 × 10^5 viable Renca cells into the lateral tail vein in 0.25 to 0.5 ml HBSS, using a 25- or 26-gauge needle.[a]
4. Carefully remove the needle and hold the penetration point briefly with a tissue paper between thumb and forefinger, to minimize bleeding.
5. Treatments are generally initiated 3 to 10 days thereafter. Since the serum half-life of most cytokines is short, they are routinely delivered by the ip route, often several times per day.
6. All mice are routinely euthanased about 14 to 17 days after tumour injection, and grossly visible metastases are enumerated.
7. Some pigmented tumours (such as melanomas) can be easily enumerated directly under a dissecting microscope. However, other tumours do not differ significantly in colour from normal lung tissue. Such unpigmented tumours can be enumerated 24 h after the lungs are fixed in Bouin's solution.
8. An even better approach (if the tumour-bearing lungs are to be photographed) is to use India ink. Briefly, a 50% solution of India ink is injected, via the trachea for lung metastases (−4 ml) or the portal vein for liver metastases (−15 ml). The organs are then suspended in Fekete's solution (300 ml 70% ethanol + 30 ml formalin + 15 ml glacial acetic acid) for 6 h. The metastases show up as white nodules on a black background.

[a] The goal of these studies is to achieve a high, but quantifiable, number of metastases on the lung, usually 200 to 250 metastases are optimal. This is achieved by performing preliminary dose–response and time-course experiments to ascertain the appropriate parameters for the specific tumour under study. Such studies are critical because the colonizing efficiency of experimental tumours varies greatly!

The experimental pulmonary metastasis model described above is well-suited to use with the Renca tumour, since Renca spontaneously metastasizes to the lung from an ir implant, and the lung is a major site of metastasis in human renal cancer.

3.3 The use of Renca for the formation of experimental hepatic metastases

Because the liver is often a site of metastasis formation during the progression of human cancers (e.g. colon cancer), and the architecture and leukocyte components of the liver and lung differs markedly, models of experimental hepatic metastases are often studied. This model is useful for application to the Renca tumour because metastases spontaneously form in the liver during progressive growth from an ir implant. The principal disadvantages of this approach are the same as those outlined above for the experimental lung metastasis model. In addition, the establishment of hepatic metastases involves a minor surgical procedure, and some tumour metastases are formed with great frequency in the lungs as well as the liver. The major advantages are speed of data acquisition and the ability to study the effects of immunotherapy in an organ where metastases often form in human cancer patients.

Protocol 5. Establishment of Renca hepatic metastases[a]

1. Use the same anaesthesia protocols as before.
2. Make a lateral incision of about 1 inch in the left flank as before, and an additional incision in the peritoneal membrane.
3. Gently massage the spleen, with its blood supply intact, through the peritoneal incision.
4. A 0.5 ml volume of HBSS containing about 5×10^5 Renca cells is then *slowly* injected, via a 27-gauge needle.
5. Wait for about 1 min to allow the tumour suspension to clear from the spleen, then clamp and ligate the blood supply, and remove the spleen.
6. Close the incision with autoclips and allow the mice recover as before.

[a] The same types of preliminary studies as those described in *Protocol 4* should be performed for this model, in order to optimize the establishment of metastases.

3.4 Summary of pre-clinical immunotherapy results obtained using the Renca tumour model

The most successful immunotherapeutic protocols identified during our studies with the Renca model have been those that included interleukin-2 (IL-2). Our approach has been to use relatively nontoxic regimens of IL-2 (e.g. 5 to 10 μg given one to three times per day) in combination with other forms of immunotherapy or chemotherapy. Under these conditions, IL-2 alone has had relatively little effect on the growth of either ir, sc, or ip primary tumours, although the use of IL-2 in combination with adoptively transferred IL-2-activated lymphocytes did significantly extend the survival of mice bearing even advanced, disseminated Renca (12–14). In contrast, IL-2 alone has proved to be quite effective in reducing the number of pulmonary Renca metastases by up to 95% and the number of hepatic Renca metastases by up to about 75%. The effectiveness of IL-2 has been increased by its use in combination with other cytokines (notably IFNα and IFNγ) or with cytokine inducers such as the investigational drug flavone acetic acid (FAA). Specifically, we have noted that the combination of IL-2 plus FAA can cure many mice with advanced Renca (15), and the substitution of IFNα + IFNγ (both of which are induced by FAA) for FAA results in about 25 to 30% long-term survivors. Furthermore, the combination of IFNα + IFNγ has enhanced direct antitumour effects *in vivo* on Renca and significantly extends the survival of mice that have minimal ip tumour burdens (16). More recently, we have noted that interleukin-7 (IL-7) also has anti-metastatic effects whereby the number of Renca metastases in the lung or liver is reduced by about 50 to 75%.

Thus, the predictions from the pre-clinical Renca model would be that IL-2 and IFNs, or combinations thereof, would induce anti-tumour effects in humans, and that these would be mostly partial. Furthermore, the combination of FAA + IL-2 might be expected to be even more active.

As a general point, it is important to emphasize that the site of tumour growth is often important when one considers the routes by which treatment is to be administered. For example, successful treatment of murine renal cancer that has disseminated from an intrarenal implant requires the treatment of localized peritoneal disease as well as distant visceral metastases. In general, the treatment of pulmonary and hepatic metastases is effectively accomplished by injection of effector cells or chemotherapy via the iv route. However, the treatment of intraperitoneal tumour is most effective when adoptively transferred cells are injected via the ip route because intravenously injected lymphocytes do not localize well to the peritoneal cavity (14). Thus, in the instance of adoptive immunotherapy, as well as in some cases for chemotherapy, there can be advantages to delivering these treatments by both the iv and ip routes (14). In general, because of their pharmacokinetic profiles, cytokines are usually administered via the ip route and repeated daily injection is usually required.

3.5 Relationship between clinical results and pre-clinical predictions

The two most active cytokines identified in the Renca pre-clinical model, as well as in a variety of other models, are IL-2 and IFNα. It is interesting that to date these are also the most active cytokines yet identified for the treatment of human renal cancer and both have higher response rates than conventional chemotherapy (17–19). Furthermore, the combination of IL-2 + IFNα may be even more active than either cytokine alone (20), as is the combination of IFNα + IFNγ (21). Although multicentre studies will be required to verify these results, they do provide some encouragement that the use of pre-clinical rodent models can identify active therapeutic regimens. While the magnitude of IL2- or IFN-induced anti-tumour effects in rodents seems greater than in humans, it is important to note that most of the responses in mice are actually only analogous to partial responses in humans.

The clinical results with FAA + IL-2 have been more difficult to reconcile with the results obtained in pre-clinical studies. While the pre-clinical model predicted potent anti-tumour activity of this combination, the results obtained from clinical trials were negative. Subsequent additional pre-clinical evaluations revealed that FAA did not stimulate cytokine gene expression or cytokine production from human leukocytes *in vitro*, in contrast to strong cytokine induction from mouse leukocytes (22). Therefore, although the mouse and human immune system are similarly stimulated by some cytokines such as IL-2 and IFNα, they are not necessarily stimulated equally by all biological agents. In the case of FAA, the pre-clinical model may still be useful to establish the cellular and molecular mechanisms of action with the hope that similar mechanisms can be stimulated in humans by other agents. In addition, these results point out that there is a role for combining pre-clinical animal model studies with *in vitro* experiments on human leukocytes as part of a total pre-clinical evaluation.

4. General survey of widely used pre-clinical rodent models

Although a detailed review of the advantages and disadvantages of the many available rodent tumour models is beyond the scope of this chapter, I will provide a brief overview of some of the most widely used models. This is done more as a point of reference for those entering the field of tumour immunology than as a resource for those already established in this area. In the interest of brevity, this information is presented in *Table 1*, and includes specific references which can be used to obtain the practical details unique to the use of each model. The reader should bear in mind that this is not an all-inclusive list of available models, nor does it reflect the belief that these models are inherently better than others that were not included. These are simply some of the most widely used pre-clinical tumour models available.

5. Implications of biological variability that exists between rodent tumour models

The reader should be careful to bear in mind that while all of the pre-clinical tumours shown in *Table 1* share the basic property that they are tumourigenic, they can differ markedly from each other in many ways. For example, experimental tumours differ substantially with regard to immunogenicity, growth rate, propensity for spontaneous metastasis, induction of host immune suppression, susceptibility to the various lytic mechanisms utilized by different effector leukocytes, and in their basic structure. The methodology that I have described above for the Renca model is generally applicable to many of the tumours listed in *Table 1*, with the caveat that some differences in

Table 1. Characteristics of widely used transplantable tumours

Species	Tumour model	Tumour histotype	Strain	Immunogenicity	References
Mouse	FBL-3	Leukaemia	C57BL/6	High	23
	MCA-102	Fibrosarcoma	C57BL/6	Poor	24, 25
	MCA-105	Fibrosarcoma	C57BL/6	Weak	24, 25
	MCA-106	Fibrosarcoma	C57BL/6	Weak	24, 25
	MCA-38	Colon adenocarcinoma	C57BL/6	Moderate	24, 25
	B16	Melanoma	C57BL/6	Weak	26
	UV-2237	Fibrosarcoma	C3H/HeN	Moderate	26, 27
	SA-1	Sarcoma	A/J	Moderate	28
	L5178Y	Lymphoma	DBA/2	Moderate	28
	P815	Mastocytoma	DBA/2	Weak	28
	Renca	Renal adenocarcinoma	BALB/c	Moderate	7, 10
Rat	MADB106	Mammary adenocarcinoma	F344	Moderate	29
Human	HT-29	Colon carcinoma	Athymic mouse	N/A	30
	A375	Melanoma	Athymic mouse	N/A	30
	Ovcar 3	Ovarian carcinoma	Athymic mouse	N/A	31

appropriate sites of tumour growth, tumour preparation, inoculum dose, and time to desired growth state may vary. Therefore, it is critical that all of these factors be optimized for each tumour, in each laboratory. In addition, since considerable heterogeneity exists between these tumours, and between the rodent strains or patients from which they were derived, one should not necessarily expect identical responses to a specific type of immunotherapy.

6. Summary

Given these constraints, pre-clinical tumour models are valuable tools for identifying immunotherapeutic approaches that may be useful to treat cancer in humans. Pre-clinical models are particularly valuable for elucidating the complex immunological mechanisms by which various biological response modifiers induce anti-tumour effects *in vivo*. In particular, it is important to note that there are many similarities between the human and mouse immune systems that cause such mechanistic conclusions to be consistent in both species. Most general conclusions derived about immunoregulation in the mouse are analogous to the subsequent results obtained in humans. However, when evaluating the biological effects of cytokines in rodents one needs to consider possible variation in the degree to which various mouse and human cytokines react with mouse tissue. Some cytokines of human origin, e.g. IL-2, appear to be completely reactive on mouse tissue, while others such as IL-6 and TNFs are largely but not completely cross-reactive. Some cytokines such as the IFNs exhibit very high species restriction. Where possible, parallel comparative studies should be performed at some point with rodent versus human cytokines, before assuming that the biological effects of human cytokines on rodent cells are quantitatively or qualitatively complete. However, the ultimate test of these agents, and regimens for their use, remains carefully performed clinical trials.

References

1. Kelly, S. A., Malik, S. T. A., and Balkwill, F. R. (1989). *Cancer Surveys*, **8,** 741.
2. Herberman, R. B. (1983). *J. Biol. Resp. Modif.*, **2,** 217.
3. Balch, C. M., Bleyer, W. A., Krakoff, I. H., and Peters, L. J. (1990). *Cancer Bull.*, **42,** 266.
4. Fidler, I. J. (1990). *Cancer Res.*, **50,** 6130.
5. Kripke, M. L. (1990). *J. Natl Cancer Inst.*, **82,** 392.
6. Houghton, J. A. and Houghton, P. J. (1987). In *Rodent Tumour Models In Experimental Cancer Therapy*, (ed. R. F. Kallman), pp. 199–204. Pergamon, New York.
7. Murphy, G. P. and Hrushesky, W. J. (1980). *J. Natl. Cancer Inst.*, **50,** 1013.
8. Williams, P. D., Pontes, E. J., and Murphy, G. P. (1981). *Res. Commun. Chem. Pathol. Pharmacol.*, **34,** 345.
9. Hrushesky, W. J. and Murphy, G. P. (1973). *J. Surg. Res.*, **15,** 327.

10. Salup, R., Herberman, R. B., and Wiltrout, R. H. (1985). *J. Urol.*, **134,** 1236.
11. Bassil, B., Dosoretz, D. E., and Prout, G. R., jnr (1985). *J. Urol.*, **134,** 450.
12. Salup, R. R. and Wiltrout, R. H. (1986). *Cancer Immunol. Immunother.*, **22,** 31.
13. Salup, R. R. and Wiltrout, R. H. (1986). *Cancer Res.*, **46,** 3358.
14. Salup, R. R., Back, T. A., and Wiltrout, R. H. (1987). *J. Immunol.*, **138,** 641.
15. Wiltrout, R. H., Boyd, M. R., Back, T. C., Salup, R. R., Arthur, J. A., and Hornung, R. L. (1988). *J. Immunol.*, **140,** 3261.
16. Sayers, T. J., Wiltrout, T. A., McCormick, K., Husted, C., and Wiltrout, R. H. (1990). *Cancer Res.*, **50,** 5414.
17. Horoszewicz, J. S. and Murphy, G. P. (1989). *J. Urol.*, **142,** 1173.
18. Rosenberg, S. A., Lotze, M. T., Yang, J. C., Aebersold, P. M., Linehan, W. M., Seipp, C. A., *et al.* (1989). *Ann. Surg.*, **210,** 474.
19. West, W. H. (1989). *Cancer Treat. Rev.*, **16,** Suppl. A, 83.
20. Rosenberg, S. A., Lotze, M. T., Yang, J. C., Linehan, W. M., Seipp, C., Calabro, S., *et al.* (1989). *J. Clin. Oncol.*, **7,** 1863.
21. Ernstoff, M. S., Nair, S., Bohnson, R. P., Miketic, L. M., Banner, B., Gooding, W., *et al.* (1990). *J. Clin. Oncol.*, **8,** 1637.
22. Futami, H., Eader, L. A., Komschlies, K. L., Bull, R., Gruys, M. E., Ortaldo, J. R., *et al.* (1991). *Cancer Res*, **51,** 6596.
23. Cheever, M. A., Thompson, D. B., Klarnet, J. P., and Greenberg, P. D. (1986). *J. Exp. Med.*, **163,** 1100.
24. Ettinghausen, S. E. and Rosenberg, S. A. (1986). *Immunopathol.*, **9,** 51.
25. Rosenberg, S. A. (1986). In *Important Advances in Oncology*, (ed. V. T. DeVita, jnr, S. Hellman, and S. A. Rosenberg), pp. 55–91. Lippincott, Philadelphia.
26. Fidler, I. J. (1978). *Cancer Res.*, **38,** 2651.
27. Kripke, M. L. (1977). *Cancer Res.*, **37,** 1395.
28. North, R. J., Neubauer, R. H., Huang, J. J. H., Neuton, R. C., and Loveless, S. E. (1988). *J. Exp. Med.*, **168,** 2031.
29. Sone, S. and Fidler, I. J. (1982). *Cancer Immunol. Immunother.*, **12,** 203.
30. Kozlowski, J. M., Fidler, I. J., Campbell, D., Xu, Z.-L., Kaighn, M. E., and Hart, I. R. (1984). *Cancer Res.*, vol. number, 3522.
31. Hamilton, T. C., Young, R. C., McKoy, W. M., Grotzinger, K. R., Green J. A., Chu, E. W., *et al.* (1984). *Cancer Res.*, **43,** 5379.

23

Use of the tumour spheroid model in immunotherapy

IRMA E. GARCIA DE PALAZZO, MICHELE HOLMES, KATHERINE ALPAUGH, and LOUIS M. WEINER

1. Introduction

Progress in solid tumour cellular therapy research has been hampered by the lack of appropriate *in vitro* models to assist in the study of effector cell infiltration, penetration, and tumour lysis. Multicellular human tumour spheroids (MHTS) have addressed several of the deficiencies inherent in monolayer cell-culture systems. Although MHTS lack stroma and vasculature, they provide model systems of intermediate complexity, in which three-dimensional growth enhances cell–cell interactions to create physiologically relevant microenvironments. MHTS formation has been achieved with a variety of cell types including gliomas, sarcomas, adenocarcinomas, melanomas, and neuroblastomas. MHTS have been used extensively in the past decade as *in vitro* models to characterize the effects of radiation on organized tumours possessing poorly oxygenated, necrotic cores. More recently, spheroids have been used to characterize radiolabelled antibody penetration and binding.

Only recently have MHTS been employed to study therapeutic modalities centred around cellular interactions. The use of MHTS targets has provided valuable insights into the cytotoxic potential and mechanisms by which interleukin-2 (IL-2) activated cells (LAK cells) bind to, and induce necrosis of, cells growing in organized tumours (1–3). The advantage of this system over conventional label-release assays lies in requiring the effectors to disrupt organized tumours and exhibit infiltrative potential.

In this chapter we will present our experience with bispecific antibody targeting of activated effector cells to MHTS. Lymphocytes activated in IL-2 acquire the ability (LAK activity) to lyse fresh autologous and allogenic tumours. This tumour lysis can be augmented by appropriate monoclonal antibodies with tumour specificity. The bulk of this LAK cell property, antibody-dependent cellular cytotoxicity (ADCC), is primarily promoted by large granular lymphocytes (LGLs). To improve the efficacy of tumour-specific monoclonal antibody therapy, bispecific antibodies, which monovalently bind effectors and tumour targets, have been developed and characterized. Such molecules have been prepared as chemically linked antibody heteroconjugates or as bispecific monoclonal antibodies derived by somatic cell hybridization of two existing hybridomas. Diverse tumour antigens have been targeted, while the effector cell targets usually have been elements of the T-cell receptor/CD3 complex. Fcγ receptor epitopes outside the immunoglobulin Fcγ binding domain also are attractive effector cell targets, since cytotoxicity may be triggered by binding to these epitopes. Bispecific antibodies targeting tumours and the high-affinity Fcγ receptor expressed by polymorphonuclear leukocytes and mononuclear phagocytes (FcγRI) have been prepared and shown to be potent inducers of relevant tumour lysis (4).

This laboratory has focused on the production and characterization of bispecific monoclonal antibodies which target tumours and FcγRIII, aiming to exploit the potent tumouricidal properties of LGLs, which express this Fc receptor. Significant tumour lysis potentiation by these antibodies has been demonstrated by standard *in vitro* ^{51}Cr release assay utilizing tumour monolayers (5). Although this standard cytotoxicity assay, which measures radioactive release, assesses the general tumour-lytic capability of effectors, it does not address the ability of the effector cells to infiltrate and mediate solid tumour destruction. The MHTS model has been shown, in our experience, to be an appropriate *in vitro* model to study effector–target cell interactions; this system permits demonstration of the ability of bispecific antibody to augment tumour infiltration and lysis, by the specific targeting of effector populations.

2. Methods and experimental design

2.1 MHTS generation and growth

Multiple techniques have been employed by other researchers to generate MHTS (6). Successful MHTS growth has been accomplished in our laboratory with several tumour cell-lines. One of these lines, SW948, a colon adenocarcinoma cell-line, was obtained from the American Tissue Culture Collection (ATCC, Rockville, Maryland), and maintained in monolayer culture in Leibovitz (L-15) medium (Gibco, Grand Island, New York) supplemented with 10% foetal calf serum and 50 U/ml penicillin–streptomycin (Pen-Strep), prior to trypsinization and harvest. The harvested single-cell suspensions ($(0.5–1) \times 10^7$ cells) were returned to a 1% agarose-coated flask in 30 ml of medium (75 cm^2 NUNC, Denmark). The agarose coating prevents the cells from re-attaching to the plastic surface and, as a result of the high cell density, cells begin to attach to one another. Cultures were incubated in a humidified chamber at 37°C in 5% CO_2 for seven days. At this time, one-third of the medium was removed and replaced with 10 ml fresh medium. Cultures were maintained with weekly medium exchange until the MHTS reached sizes of 200–400 μm in diameter. We have found that 75 cm^2 flasks are preferred to smaller flasks, since a greater number of MHTS can be grown with fewer medium changes.

SW948 MHTS reached 400 μm diameter in 7–10 days. MHTS harvested from the early phases of growth were generally more homogeneous in size and morphology. At excess cell seeding densities ($>1 \times 10^7$ cells) the size distribution of the spheroids became more heterogeneous, especially with the SW948 cell-line. Spheroids of approximately equal size were manually selected with Pasteur pipettes and expanded for experimental use.

Protocol 1. Generation of SW948 MHTS

1. Grow the cells to confluence in T-175 flasks (Nunc) in L-15 medium (Gibco) + 10% FCS, 50 U/ml Pen-Strep.
2. Trypsinize the cells and obtain single-cell suspensions.
3. Suspend 1×10^7 cells in 30 ml medium in T-75 flasks (Nunc), pre-coated with 1% agarose, with the flasks lying flat.
4. Incubate the cells in a humidified chamber at 37°C in 5% CO_2 for seven days.
5. Remove one-third of the medium and replace it with 10 ml fresh medium.
6. Maintain the cultures until MHTS reach an average size of 200–400 μm.

2.2 Preparation of IL-2-activated lymphocytes

In our laboratory, peripheral blood mononuclear cells are isolated from healthy volunteers. Briefly, heparinized venous samples are separated on Ficoll–Hypaque and the monocytes adhered out on gelatin-plasma coated flasks (37°C for 60 min). The remaining peripheral blood lymphocytes are placed in culture for 3–5 days in 1000 units recombinant IL-2/ml (IL-2 is added on days 1, 3, 5) (7). LAK cells are tested for their cytotoxic capability with and without bispecific antibodies using single-cell suspensions of SW948 as the target cells in a standard 4 h ^{51}Cr release assay (5).

2.3 Antibodies

The bispecific monoclonal antibody CL158 was used in the MHTS experiments. Briefly, CL158 was prepared by somatic cell fusion of two hybridoma lines, one secreting antibody to CA19-9 and the other to FcRIII, the Fcγ receptor for aggregated immunoglobulin expressed by large granular lymphocytes (8). Standard techniques of limiting dilution and ELISA screening identified clones exhibiting bispecific antibody activity. This antibody has been shown to be a potent promoter of lysis of an allogeneic CA19-9 expressing human tumour cell-line (SW948) by IL-2-activated large granular lymphocytes, even in the presence of excess human immunoglobulin (8). In this series of experiments, supernatants of CL158 were employed. CL158 has been partially purified by ion exchange chromatography. The supernatants and partially purified antibody possess similar properties of cytotoxicity potentiation.

2.4 Co-culture of MHTS with LAK cells and antibodies

MHTS with diameters of 200–400 μm were selected for use in these studies. MHTS were cultured with LAK cells alone, or with LAK cells in the presence of various antibodies. LAK cells were resuspended to 2×10^6 cells/ml in L-15 medium containing 1000 U rIL-2/ml. LAK cells (250 μl) (5×10^5) were added to each 17×100 mm polystyrene tube containing a suspension of MHTS equivalent to a packed volume of 100 μl (approximately 10^6 tumour cells) in the same medium. 100 μl of a 1:100 dilution of CL158 culture supernatant was added to SW948 MHTS-containing tubes, yielding a final bispecific antibody concentration of 7 ng/ml. In experiments using IL-2-activated whole blood, a similar volume of SW948 MHTS and antibody concentration was maintained in tubes containing a volume of whole blood which had an equivalent number of effector cells. Tubes were placed on a rocker platform for 24 h at 37°C. Samples were then harvested and analysed by morphology and immunohistochemistry as described below.

Protocol 2. Assay for SW948 MHTS infiltration by human LAK cells

1. Using a sterile Pasteur pipette, visually remove MHTS from the T-75 flask and aliquot equal packed volumes of MHTS (about 100 μl) into 17×100 mm sterile polystyrene tubes, suspended in complete L-15 medium supplemented with 1000 U/ml recombinant IL-2. Set up at least four tubes.
2. Save one tube as a control.
3. To the other tubes, add varying numbers of effector cells, in the presence or absence of anti-tumour antibodies.
4. Place tubes on a rocker platform (Red Rotor, Hoefer Scientific Instruments, San Francisco, California) and rotate secured, capped tubes, sealed with parafilm, gently for 24 h at 37°C.

2.5 Histology and immunohistochemistry

Spheroids were washed in PBS, pelleted, fixed in 2.5% glutaraldehyde for 30 min, and embedded in 3% agar. Some pellets were dehydrated in graded alcohols and embedded in paraffin. Sections (5 μm) were cut and stained with haematoxylin and eosin for histological examination. CA19-9 antigen expression in the multicellular spheroids was studied by immunoperoxidase staining using the Vectastain ABC kit as described (9). Lymphocyte infiltration was studied with mouse antibodies PD7/26/16 directed against human leukocyte common antigen (Anti-LCA, DAKO Corporation, Carpinteria, California). The slides were developed with diaminobenzidine and counterstained with haematoxylin and examined.

Protocol 3. Preparation for histological and immunohistological analysis

1. Centrifuge the tubes containing MHTS at 400*g* for 5 min at room temperature.
2. Wash cell pellets with PBS and gently re-suspend.
3. Repeat step **1**.
4. Immerse cell pellets in 2.5% glutaraldehyde for 30 min.
5. Embed glutaraldehyde-fixed pellets in warmed 3% agarose solution. Allow it to cool.
6. Alternatively, the PBS-washed, fixed pellets can be dehydrated in graded alcohols and embedded in paraffin.

Histological evaluation was performed by studying a minimum of 12 spheroids per experimental group. Grading of histological damage was evaluated by determining the percentage of each examined MHTS demonstrating necrosis. The average percentage of necrosis in the examined spheroids in a given experimental group was determined and reported as follows: 76–100% as Grade 4, 51–75% as Grade 3, 26–50% as Grade 2, 1–25% as Grade 1, and no damage as Grade 0. All samples were read by at least two independent observers in blinded fashion. Immunofluorescence was used to evaluate specific lymphocyte sub-set infiltration into SW948 MHTS by labelling LAK cells with Leu 19-PE (anti-CD56 phycoerythrin conjugate, Becton-Dickinson, Mountain View, California) for 30 min, removing unconjugated antibody by washing, then co-incubating the labelled LAK cells with SW948 MHTS for 4 h. Samples were washed to remove unconjugated effectors and slide preparations were analysed by fluorescent microscopy using a Nikon UFX-II instrument (10).

3. Results

3.1 Morphology and differentiation characteristics of SW948

SW948 MHTS exhibited morphological evidence of adenocarcinoma differentiation. Gland-like structures consisting of a lumen surrounded by closely apposed cells with basally oriented nuclei were present in SW948 MHTS (*Figure 1*). Histological sections of SW948 spheroids grown to sizes greater

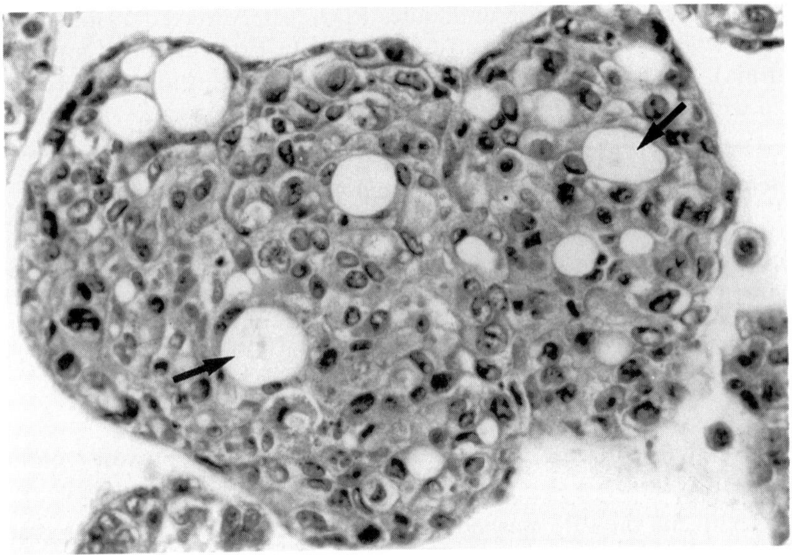

Figure 1. Microscopic features of SW948 spheroids. Arrow denotes the gland-like structures consisting of lumens surrounded by closely apposed cells. No central necrosis of the tumour is observed because this represents an early stage of development (approximate size of this MHTS: 200 μm). Hematoxylin–eosin stained section × 100.

than 400 μm showed necrotic cells in the centres, surrounded by shells of viable cells (*Figure 2*). Ultrastructurally, SW948 MHTS possessed typically adenocarcinoma features. Microvillous projections extending from the apical surface facing the lumen, could be demonstrated. Ultrastructural features of SW948 spheroids and xenografts grown in immunodeficient mice were essentially identical (*Figure 3*). Microvillous projections extending from the luminal surface and an abundance of junctional complexes, including desmosomes, could be found in SW948 MHTS by transmission electron microscopy (*Figure 4*). SW948 MHTS were found to have uniform cell surface expression of CA19-9 antigen by immunohistochemical analysis.

3.2 Histological and immunohistochemical characterization of LAK cell infiltration of MHTS

Histological examination of SW948 spheroids for evidence of necrosis and destruction of the spheroid integrity revealed minimal damage when spheroids were incubated with LAK cells alone. In contrast, the addition of bispecific antibody to LAK cells resulted in cell damage at the periphery of the MHTS at 4 h. After 24 h of incubation, the spheroids were 75 to 85% necrotic, with necrosis distributed throughout the spheroids.

Immunohistochemical assessment for lymphocyte infiltration revealed that

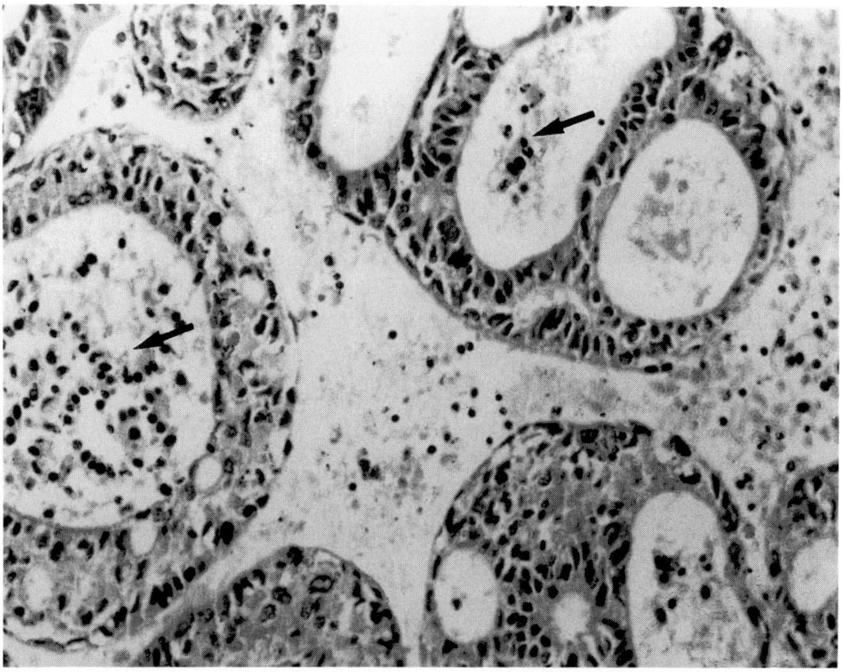

Figure 2. Histological section of SW948 MHTS grown to sizes between 300 and 400 μm. Arrows identify necrotic cells in the centres, surrounded by shells of viable cells. Haematoxylin–eosin × 40.

the co-culture of LAK cells with SW948 MHTS resulted in minimal infiltration of lymphocytes after 24 h (*Figure 5* A). When SW948 MHTS were incubated with LAK cells and 7 ng/ml CL158, superficial cellular infiltrates were demonstrated within 4 h of incubation, while spheroid penetration with lymphocyte infiltrates was evident after 24 h (*Figure 5* B). Immunofluorescent microscopy for evidence of labelled LAKs infiltrating SW948 MHTS in the presence of CL158 demonstrated that CD56+ expressing cells were the components of the infiltrating lymphocyte population.

Although it has proven difficult to purify large quantities of the CA19-9 × 3G8 bispecific antibody (CL158), clonal supernatants and partially purified antibodies have been shown to be equally effective in promoting SW948 MHTS destruction by human LAK cells. To study the specificity of the enhancement effect of CL158 bispecific antibody when LAK cells were co-cultured with SW948 spheroids, other antibodies were tested under identical culture conditions. These included the parent antibodies of the CL158 hybrid hybridoma, CA19-9 and 3G8, both are of the IgG1 isotype. These IgG1 isotypic antibodies do not promote ADCC. An IgG2a class switch mutant of CA19-9, which mediates ADCC of SW948 cells in monolayers by LAK cells,

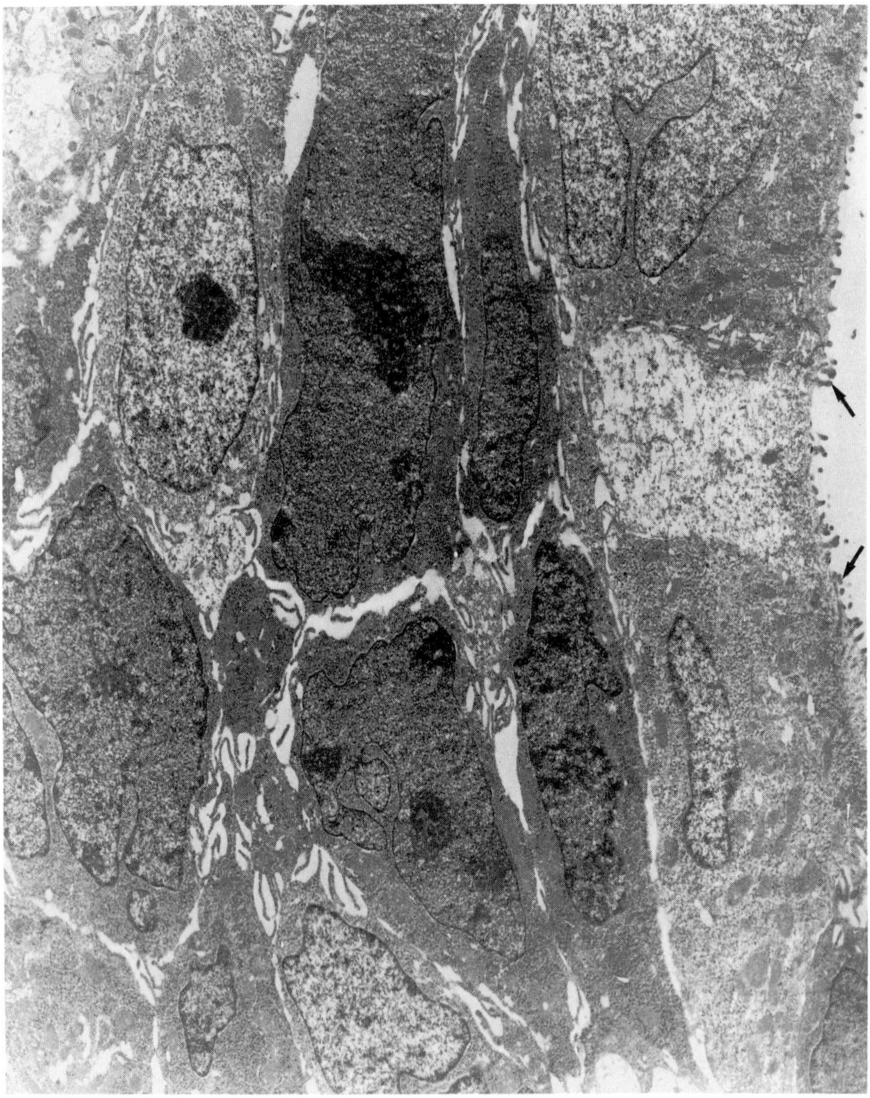

Figure 3. Ultrastructural features of SW948 xenograft. Arrows denote microvillous projections extending from the apical surface facing the lumen (× 1800, transmission electron microscopy).

was used as a positive control. When SW948 MHTS were incubated with LAK cells and CA19-9 or 3G8, fewer than 25% of the cells showed morphological changes suggesting histological damage (pyknotic nuclei, interruption of the cytoplasmic membrane, vacuolization of the cytoplasm, etc.). Incubation of SW948 MHTS with LAK cells and the IgG2a variant of the monoclonal

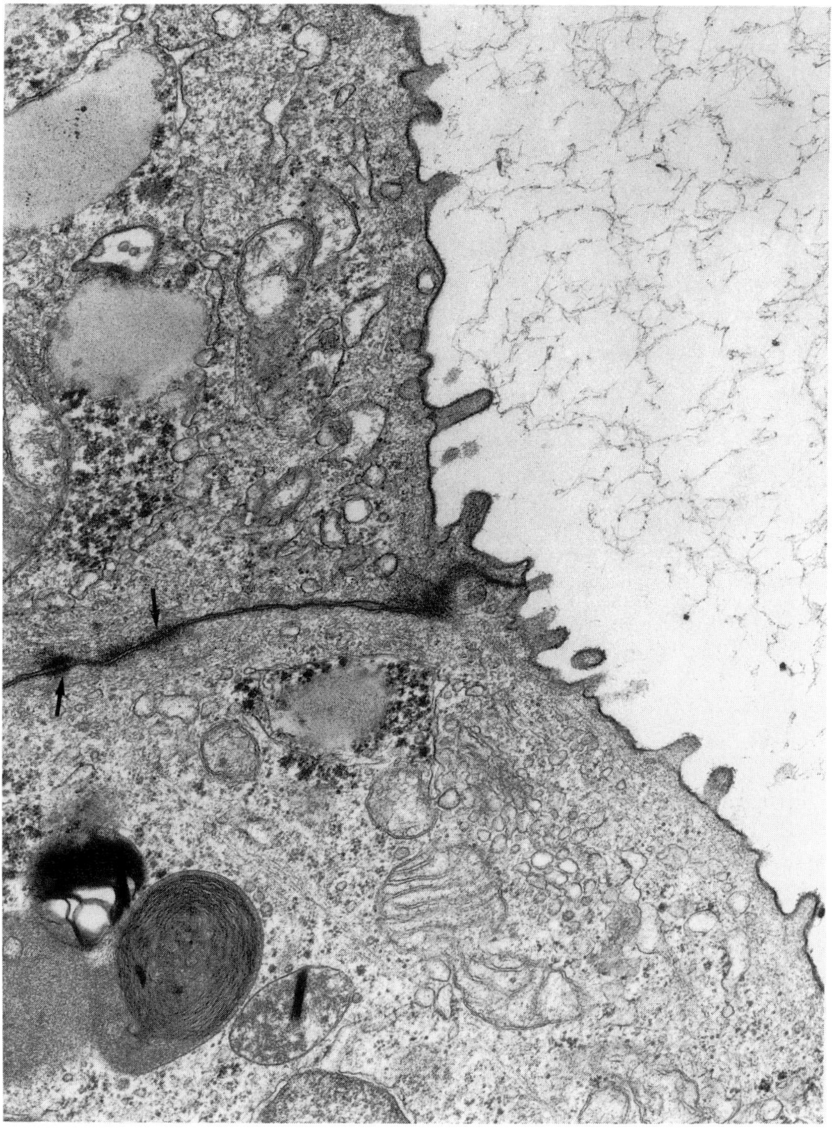

Figure 4. Ultrastructural features of SW948 MHTS. Microvillous projections extending from the luminal surface. Arrow denotes desmosomes between cells (× 30 000, transmission electron microscopy).

antibody CA19-9 resulted in a slightly higher percentage of cell-damage characterized by the same changes observed above but preservation of the general morphological appearance of the spheroids was maintained. When SW948 MHTS were incubated with bispecific antibody and LAK cells, target

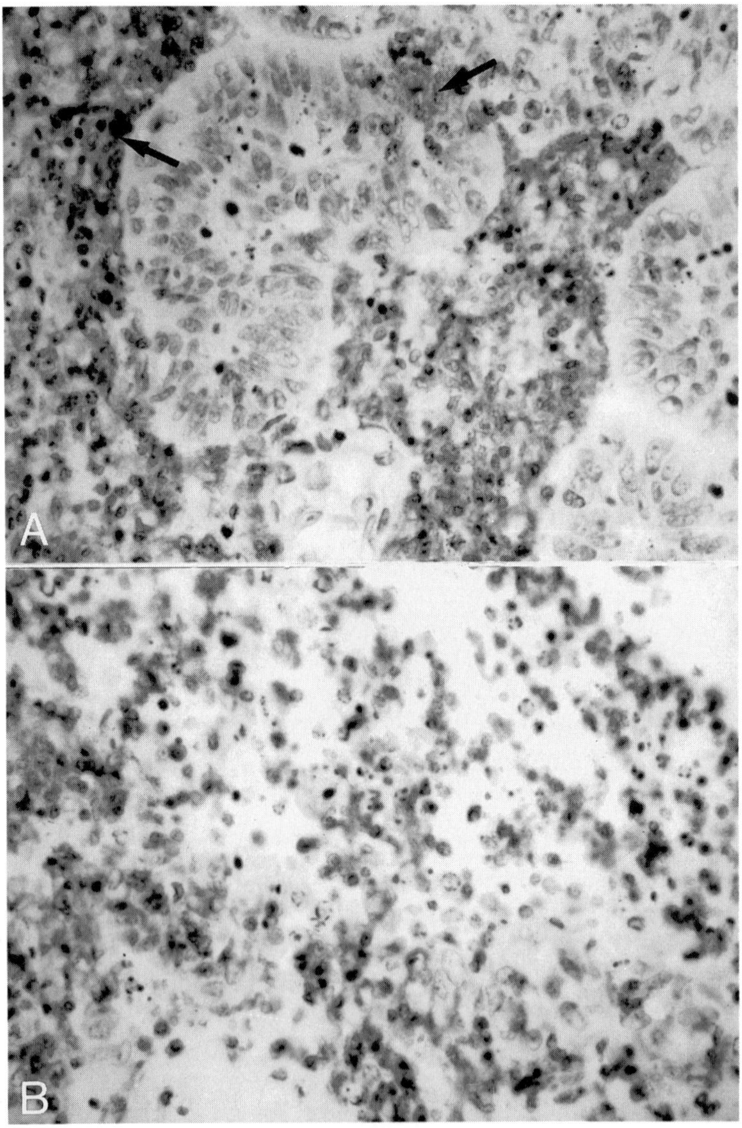

Figure 5. 300–400 μm MHTS, prepared as described in the text, were incubated with 0.5:1 effector (E):target (T) ratios of LAK cells for 24 h, embedded in agarose, and analysed by immunoperoxidase reaction with antibody to leukocyte common antigen (LCA) as described in the text. Slides were counterstained with haematoxylin–eosin. LCA-labelled lymphocytes stained brown due to the substrate diaminobenzidine (DAB). A: MHTS exposed to LAK cells at 0.5:1 E:T ratios. Observe how the MHTS are preserved although some lymphocyte infiltration (arrows) can be seen at the periphery of the spheroid. B: MHTS exposed to LAK cell at 0.5:1 E:T ratio and CL158 bispecific antibody (7 ng/ml final assay concentration). Note how the MHTS are disintegrated. Only small clusters of cells remain, with no structural preservation.

cells displayed a variety of degenerative and disintegrative changes characterized by the frequent presence of 'ghost cells' or completely destroyed cells. An increased number of effector cells were observed infiltrating these MHTS when compared with the controls. It is noteworthy that neither of the changes described above were observed when tumours were incubated with CL158 in the absence of LAK cells. Extensive damage to SW948 MHTS was also observed when they were co-cultured with LAK cells and CL158 in the presence of human serum (15% v/v). When the SW948 MHTS were incubated with heparinized, IL-2-activated whole blood, lysis augmentation was also preserved.

4. Concluding remarks

When tumour cells are cultured as MTHS, they show the ability to reconstitute tissue structures that, in many aspects, resemble the architecture of the corresponding *in vivo* tumours. They also behave similarly to cells in solid tumours. The cells situated at the periphery of the tumour close to the nutrient source remain viable and active; the cells in the core of the spheroid stop cycling and eventually die as the spheroids enlarge.

We have used the MHTS model as a system of intermediate complexity to study cell–cell interactions in the presence of bispecific monoclonal antibody, hoping to increase the ability of the effector cells to infiltrate and kill the tumour, and have shown that bispecific antibodies augment the lysis of organized tumour by LAK cells. Histological evidence of leukocyte infiltration and necrosis far exceeded that seen with LAK cells alone. Using this model, the IgG2a isotype variant of CA19-9 had relatively few effects on spheroid activity, even though it can mediate ADCC by LAK cells growing in a monolayer culture. In contrast, CL158, a bispecific antibody with identical tumour specificity, was an extremely potent enhancer of tumour lysis, leukocyte infiltration, and spheroid destruction. CL158 bispecific antibody binds to CA19-9 antigen and FcγRIII at an epitope on the receptor that is distinct from the immunoglobulin Fc binding domain. As its promotion of tumour killing is preserved in the presence of human immunoglobulins and whole blood, its mechanism of action is not classic ADCC, and the Fc domain of this antibody is not required for its expression of biological activity. More importantly, the lack of competition by human immunoglobulin may confer a therapeutic advantage for bispecific antibodies designed to target LGLs or other cytotoxic effector cells to tumour sites. Since bivalent antibodies that target FcγRIII can trigger LGL cytotoxicity via this receptor, the binding of bispecific antibodies to tumours and LGLs may provide a cross-linking (and hence activating) signal that efficiently couples appropriate binding to expression of cytotoxic potential. This possibility is also suggested by the extremely low concentrations of bispecific CL158, compared with CA19-9 IgG2a, required to achieve lysis of SW948 cells in a single-cell suspension.

It has been shown by other investigators (2) that LAK cells infiltrate into spheroids derived from human glioma cell-lines. However, infiltration varied according to the glioma cell-line that was used with evidence of tumour cell damage at sites that were distant from the infiltrating peripheral lymphocytes. Other investigators (1) have performed similar studies using a different human glioma spheroid model. They demonstrated substantial cytotoxicity after 24 h. In contrast, peripheral blood lymphocytes did not affect spheroid growth.

The effects of LAK cells alone on SW948 MHTS were less striking in that there was minimal leukocyte infiltration or tumour cell necrosis after 24 h of incubation. Since SW948 MHTS possess typical adenocarcinoma morphology and contain numerous desmosomes and other junctions, it is possible that the infiltration of leukocytes into SW948 MHTS is more restricted than in the glioma spheroids. Experiments to further correlate leukocyte infiltration with expression of junctional complexes by the spheroids are required to address this possibility. Longer periods of incubation may be required to see equivalent degrees of leukocyte infiltration, tumour cell lysis, and destruction of MHTS when LAK cells are used alone. Further studies of the mechanisms of tumour resistance to bispecific antibody-mediated lysis will address the relationship of tumour antigen expression to sensitivity to lysis. Greater understanding of the phenotypic characteristics of LGLs, which promote invasion of MHTS, coupled with identification of effective modulation strategies, will facilitate therapeutic application of these antibodies.

In view of the potential therapeutic applications of LAK cells and antibodies, many other aspects need to be investigated. The inefficiency of spheroid lysis by the LAK and ADCC mechanisms may provide valuable information regarding the obstacles to clinical exploitation of these *in vitro* phenomena. Thus, use of this model of cell-mediated tumour lysis may lead to the identification of new therapeutic strategies with the potential to effect cellular cytotoxicity.

References

1. Iwasaki, K., Kikuchi, H., Miyatake, S., Aoki, T., Yamasaki, T., and Oda, Y. (1990). *Cancer Res.*, **50,** 2429–36.
2. Jääskeläinen, J., Kalliomäki, P., Paetau, A., and Timonen T. (1989). *J. Immunol.*, **142,** 1036–45.
3. Jääskeläinen, J., Lehtonen, E., Heikkilä, P., Kalliomäki, P., and Timonen, T. (1990). *J. Natl. Cancer Inst.*, **82,** 497–502.
4. Shen, L., Guyre, P. M., Anderson, C. L., and Fanger, M. W. (1986). *J. Immunol.*, **137,** 3378–82.
5. Weiner, L. M., Zarou, C., O'Brien, J., and Ring, D. (1989). *J. Biol. Resp. Mod.*, **8,** 227–37.
6. Acker, H., Carlssons, J., Durand, R., and Sutherland, R. M. (ed.) (1984). *Spheroids in Cancer Research: Methods and Perspectives*. Springer, Berlin.

7. Rosenberg, S. A. (1986). In *Important Advances in Oncology*, (ed. V. T. DeVita, S. Hellman, and S. A. Rosenberg), pp. 55–91. Lippincott, New York.
8. Garcia de Palazzo, I. E., Gercel-Taylor, C., Kitson, J., and Weiner, L. M. (1990). *Cancer Res.*, **50,** 7123–8.
9. Hsu, S. M., Raine, L., and Fanger, H. (1981). *Am. J. Clin. Pathol.*, **75,** 816–21.
10. Landay, A., Gartland, G. L., Abo, T., and Cooper, M. D. (1983). *J. Immunol. Methods*, **58,** 337–47.

24

Characterization of metastatic tumour cells

U. P. THORGEIRSSON and A. R. MACKAY

1. Introduction

The metastatic process involves dissemination of tumour cells from a primary site to one or more distant organs. In order to successfully complete all the metastatic steps the tumour cells must leave the primary site, invade surrounding tissues, gain access to lymphatics and/or blood vessels, survive in the circulation, arrest in the microvascular bed of an alternative site, proliferate, extravasate, and finally colonize the target organ (1, 2). The success rate of this complex process is dependent upon multiple cellular and host factors, many of which have been extensively studied in different experimental animal and *in vitro* models.

During metastatic development the tumour cells come in contact with immune cells, such as T lymphocytes (3), natural killer (NK) cells (4), macrophages (5), and natural cytotoxic cells (6). The relative importance of immune cells in metastatic animal model systems is often dependent on the types of tumours involved (7, 8). Immune suppression has been associated with increased metastatic rates in some animal models (9), while in other models no effect, or decrease in metastatic incidence was observed (10).

To study the role of the immune system in metastasis it is necessary to apply a large variety of *in vivo* and *in vitro* immunological and metastasis techniques. This brief review is limited to the more commonly used systems to study tumour invasion and metastasis, *in vitro* and *in vivo*.

2. Animal models

The prerequisite for the understanding of cellular and host events that lead to metastasis, is the availability of experimental animal models. Tumour cell variants of high and low metastatic capacity have been developed in syngeneic animal models (*Table 1*). Studies of human heterotransplants are carried out in immunodeficient or immunosuppressed animals (*Table 2*). Immunosuppression can be accomplished through treatment with cyclophosphamide,

Table 1. Syngeneic tumour metastasis models

Animal	Tumour type	Reference
DBA/2 mice	Methylcholanthrene-induced lymphoma *lymphoma*	Schirrmacher[a]
C57 BL/6 mice	Spontaneous lung carcinoma (Lewis *lung carcinoma*)	Sugiura,[b] Spreafico,[b] Schechter[d]
C57 BL/6 mice	*Melanoma* cells (B16)	Fidler[e]
C3Hf mice	*Reticulum cell sarcoma*	Parks[f]
BALB/c mice	RAW 117H10 *lymphosarcoma*	Brunson[g]
F344 rats	*Mammary carcinoma*	Neri[h]
	Friend leukaemia cells	Bolardeli[i]
	Oncogene/marker gene transfected rat liver epithelial cells	Bisgaardi[a]

[a] Schirrmacher, V. (1979). *Int. J. Cancer*, **23,** 233.
[b] Sugiura, K. (1955). *Cancer Res.*, **15,** 38.
[c] Spreafico, F. (1975). *Eur. J. Cancer*, **11,** 555.
[d] Schechter, B. (1977). *Int. J. Cancer*, **20,** 239.
[e] Fidler, I. J. (1973). *Nature, New Biol.*, **242,** 148.
[f] Parks, R. C. (1974). *J. Natl. Cancer Inst.*, **52,** 971.
[g] Brunson, R. W. (1978). *J. Natl. Cancer Inst.*, **61,** 1499.
[h] Neri, A. (1982). *J. Natl. Cancer Inst.*, **68,** 507.
[i] Bolardeli, F. (1984). *Int. J. Cancer*, **34,** 389.
[j] Bisgaard, H. C. (1991). *AACR Proceedings*, No. 399.

Table 2. Immunodeficient animal models

Animal	Reference
Athymic nude mice	Flanagan,[a] Pantelouris,[b] Giovanelli,[c] Sordat[d]
SCID mouse	Bosma[e]
Athymic nude rats	Eccles,[f] Festing[g]
Immunosuppressed mice	Steel[h]

[a] Flanagan, S. P. (1966). *Genetic Res.*, **8,** 295.
[b] Pantelouris, E. M. (1968). *Nature*, **217,** 370.
[c] Giovanelli, B. C. (1985). *Adv. Cancer Res.*, **44,** 69.
[d] Sordat, B. C. M. (1982). In: *The Nude Mouse in Experimental and Clinical Research*, (ed. J. Fogh and B. C. Giovanelli), p. 95. Academic, New York.
[e] Bosma, G. C. (1983). *Nature*, **301,** 527.
[f] Eccles, S. A. (1980). In: *Immunodeficient Animals for Cancer Research*, (ed. S. Sparrow), p. 167. Academic, New York.
[g] Festing, N. W. (1978). *Nature*, **274,** 365.
[h] Steel, G. G. (1982). In: *The Nude Mouse in Experimental and Clinical Research*, (ed. J. Fogh and B. C. Giovanelli), p. 207.

glucocorticoids, irradiation, or by injecting antisera specific for B lymphocytes, T lymphocytes, or macrophages.

3. *In vivo* metastasis assays

3.1 Tumour cell preparation

When using cultured tumour cells it is important to use only cell preparations with more than 85% cell viability for injections. Trypsinization should be limited to 1 min if possible, since longer exposure to trypsin may shorten the cell survival *in vivo* (11). To avoid clumping, tumour cells must be washed free of serum and injected in Ca^{2+}- and Mg^{2+}-free Hank's balanced salt solution (HBSS). Passing the cells through a 27-gauge needle will also help break up clumps (see also Chapter 1).

Protocol 1. Collagenase dissociation of tumours

1. Dissect out the tumour, remove capsule, necrotic areas, and blood clots, if necessary.
2. Rinse the tumour in HBSS and cut into 1–2 mm pieces with scissors or surgical blades. Place the pieces in a sterile flask containing a magnetic stirrer. Add 0.14% collagenase (Type I) and 0.03% deoxyribonuclease I dissolved in serum-free medium and allow to stir in a 37°C water bath for 30 min.
3. Allow the larger tumour fragments to settle, then decant the single-cell suspension and repeat the process three times.
4. Spin down the cells after each harvesting, wash once in HBSS, and store on ice until the three rounds have been completed.
5. Filter the cells through a 100-mesh stainless steel sieve and centrifuge at 200*g* for 5 min.
6. Suspend the pellet in HBSS and determine the number of viable cells by trypan blue exclusion (12). Use only preparations of more than 85% viable cells for injections (see also Chapter 1).

3.2 Routes of injection

Tumour cells are inoculated into experimental animals by various routes in order to assess their metastatic capability. Experimental or intravenous metastasis demonstrate only that the tumour cells can seed and grow in a distant organ after they have been introduced into the systemic circulation. Spontaneous metastases from a subcutaneous site reflects the more complex capability of tumour cells to complete all the steps of the metastatic process.

Protocol 2. Intravenous injection

In mice and rats, a lateral tail vein is the most commonly used route for intravenous inoculation.

1. Dilate the vein by dipping the tail into warm water, or place the animal under a lamp (150W light bulb) at a distance of 8 inches for 5 min. The time interval between the tumour cell preparation and the injections should be as short as possible.
2. Prepare a single-cell suspension in HBSS without Ca^{2+} or Mg^{2+} at a concentration of 10^6 to 10^7 cells per ml and keep on ice. At the time of inoculation agitate the test tube containing the tumour cells and draw up to 0.2 ml of the cell suspension into a tuberculin syringe with a 26-gauge ¾-inch needle.
3. Wipe the tail with 70% ethanol and push the needle into the vein at a slight angle. It is an indication that the needle is outside the vein if a resistance is felt upon injection.
4. Inject between 0.1 and 0.2 μl of cell suspension and withdraw the needle.

Protocol 3. Subcutaneous injection

Use a tuberculin syringe and a 25-gauge ½-inch needle.

1. Prepare the tumour cells as described in *Protocol 1* and adjust the cell density to 10^6 to 10^7/ml.
2. Direct the needle into the inguinal region and inject subcutaneously 0.1–0.2 ml of the tumour cell suspension. Pinch the needle track to avoid a retroflux of the tumour cells. The interscapular area can also be used for subcutaneous injections. Co-injection of tumour cells and Matrigel has been demonstrated to enhance tumour growth in athymic nude mice (13).
3. Measure tumour size (diameter and depth) weekly with vernier calipers.

In the case of **spontaneous metastasis** assays, the observation period can be prolonged by removing the subcutaneous tumour under light anaesthesia. The following modified techniques can be used with footpad, intraperitoneal, intrasplenic and intradermal injections:

- For *footpad injection*, use a 0.25 cm^3 syringe and a 27-gauge ⅜-inch needle. Tumour cells are adjusted to 5×10^6–5×10^7 cells/ml and injected in a volume of 0.05 ml. The needle is inserted into the posterior footpad (the proximal side of the central pad).
- For *intraperitoneal injection*, use a tuberculin or a 3 cm^3 syringe (up to 2 ml

can be injected into the abdominal cavity of a mouse). Insert a 25-gauge, ½-inch needle into the abdomen (not deeper than 6 mm), just lateral to the umbilicus and inject the tumour cells.

- *Intrasplenic implantation* of human colorectal carcinoma cells has been demonstrated to be a successful method to produce liver metastasis in nude mice (14). Mice are anaesthetized and the peritoneal cavity is opened aseptically to expose the spleen (see also Chapter 22). Inject tumour cells (up to 10^6 cells/0.05 ml of HBSS without Ca^{2+} or Mg^{2+}) under the capsule of the spleen. Close the abdominal wall with sutures and the skin with metal wound clips.
- *For intradermal injection*, use a 0.25 cm^3 syringe and a 27-gauge, ½-inch needle. Adjust the tumour cell count to 5×10^7 cells/ml. Inject 0.05 ml (no more) into the skin which will blanch and swell from the inoculum. Compress the skin as the needle is withdrawn.

Protocol 4. Quantitative assessment of metastasis in mice

The period from the time of injection to sacrifice of the animals varies depending upon the site of inoculation, tumour growth rate, and general health of the animals. For quantitation of experimental metastasis, the animals are commonly sacrificed 3–6 weeks following intravenous injections, and 8–12 weeks following subcutaneous injections.

1. Kill the mouse by administering an overdose of pentobarbitol or by other acceptable methods of euthanasia.
2. Pin the mouse on to a board and wash with 70% ethanol.
3. Use blunt scissors to remove the skin and expose peritoneum, thorax, and neck.
4. Open the abdominal cavity and remove the sternum and anterior portions of the ribs.
5. For enumeration of pulmonary metastasis, inflate the lungs *in situ* with Bouin's fixative (glacial acetic acid (1 part); 37% formaldehyde (5 parts); saturated picric acid (15 parts)). Expose the trachea, insert a needle through the trachea at the level of the cricoid cartilage. Inject the Bouin's solution until the lungs fill the thoracic cavity. Before withdrawing the needle clamp the trachea to avoid retroflux of the fixative. Remove the heart, lungs, and thymus as a block and fix in Bouin's solution for 4–18 h. Remove abdominal organs and examine for metastasis. Look specifically for lymph-node involvement.
6. Remove the primary tumour. Measure its size using vernier calipers, or weigh the tumour after removal of attached soft tissues.
7. Enumerate pulmonary metastases under a dissecting microscope.

---

4. *In vitro* assays to study the metastatic phenotype

4.1 Tumour invasion assays

Numerous *in vitro* models have been developed to evaluate different parameters involved in tumour invasion. These methods assess tumour cell confrontation with a variety of host tissues, such as embryonic organs, chorioallantoic membrane, cartilage, bone, mesentery, urinary, bladder, amnion, and basement membrane matrix. In *Table 3*, representative

Table 3. *In vitro* invasion models

Host tissue	Reference
Chick embryo heart	Mareel[a]
Chick embryo mesonephros	Barski[b]
Chick embryo lung, intestine, gonad, skin	Wolff[c]
Chick embryo stomach	de Ridder[d]
Rat embryo yolk sac	Maignan[e]
Chick chorioallantoic membrane	Easty,[f] Hart,[g] Chambers[h]
Cartilage	Pauli[i]
Rat mesentery	Strauli[j]
Human decidua	Schleich[k]
Endothelial matrix	Jones[l]
Canine vein	Poste[m]
Mouse urinary bladder	Poste[m], Verschueren[n]
Rat hepatocytes	Roos[o]
Collagen gels	Schor[p]
Human amnion	Thorgeirsson[q]
Basement membrane matrix (Matrigel)	Albini[r]

[a] Mareel, M. M. (1979). *Virch. Arch. B. Cell Pathol.*, **30,** 95.
[b] Barski, G. (1965). *J. Natl. Cancer Inst.*, **34,** 495.
[c] Wolff, E. (1957). *Arch. Anat. Microsc. Morphol. Exp.* **46,** 173.
[d] de Ridder, L. (1977). *Arch. Geschwulstforsch.*, **47,** 7.
[e] Maignan, M. F. (1979). *Biol. Cell*, **35,** 229.
[f] Easty, D. M. (1974). *Br. J. Cancer*, **29,** 36.
[g] Hart, I. R. (1978). *Cancer Res.*, **38,** 3218.
[h] Chambers, A. F. (1982). *Cancer Res.*, **42,** 4018.
[i] Pauli, B. U. (1981). *Cancer Res.*, **41,** 2084.
[j] Strauli, P. (1981). *Virch. Arch. (Cell Pathol.)*, **35,** 93.
[k] Schleich, A. B. (1976). *J. Natl. Cancer Inst.*, **56** 221.
[l] Jones, P. A. (1980). *Cancer Res.*, **40,** 3222.
[m] Poste, G. (1980). *Cancer Res.*, **40,** 1636.
[n] Verschueren, H. (1987). *Invas. Metast.*, **7,** 1.
[o] Roos, E. (1981). *J. Cell Sci.*, **47,** 385.
[p] Schor, S. L. (1980). *J. Cell Sci.*, **46,** 171.
[q] Thorgeirsson, U. P. (1982). *J. Natl. Cancer Inst.*, **69,** 1049.
[r] Albini, A. (1987). *Cancer Res.*, **47,** 3239.

examples of different assay systems are listed and referenced. Protocols are given for two assays which permit quantitative assessment of invasive tumour cells, using either intact basement membrane (amnion) or basement membrane matrix (matrigel) as an invasion barrier.

4.2 Amnion invasion assay

Human amnion is composed of a single layer of epithelium attached to a continuous basement membrane overlying a dense, non-vascular stroma. For invasion assays, the amnion is separated aseptically from the chorion of a term placenta within 24 h of delivery. It is rinsed three times in PBS containing 50 μg/ml each of penicillin and streptomycin. The amnion is incubated in 0.1 M ammonium hydroxide at room temperature for 30 min. The epithelial layer is then gently wiped off with sterile gauze, followed by washing in HBSS until the pH is neutralized. The de-epithelialized amnion can be refrigerated and stored for at least three weeks in minimum essential medium, in the presence of antibiotics as described above.

The invasion chambers are composed of two Lucite rings. The upper ring measures 1.0 cm in height and the lower ring 0.2 cm in height. The outside diameter of the rings measures 3.2 cm and the inside diameter 1.2 cm (other types of invasion chambers may be used). The amnion is stretched over the bottom side of the upper rings, with the stromal side facing up. Millipore filters (5 or 8 μm pore size) are placed on the amnion over the rings. Care must be taken to avoid air bubbles in order to get good contact between amnion and filter, which are then fixed tightly between the two rings, with four screws.

The amnion is cut at the periphery of the rings and the chambers placed in a 6-well tissue-culture dish containing approximately 2.5 ml of medium per well. It is important to avoid air bubbles between the medium and the Millipore filter. Assays are done in triplicate. The tumour cells are added to the basement membrane side of the amnion at a concentration of 5×10^5 to 1×10^6 in 1.5 ml of medium which is either serum-free, or contains 2% Nu-serum. The invasion assays are carried out at 37°C (5% CO_2, 95% air) for variable lengths of time (1–7 days), dependent upon the invasiveness of the tumour cell types under study. The filter and attached amnion are fixed in 70% ethanol overnight, stained with haematoxylin and eosin, dehydrated in ethanol, and cleared in xylene. Lastly, the filter is peeled away from the amnion and both mounted on a microscope slide. The total number of cells that have penetrated the entire thickness of the amnion and on to the Millipore filter are counted at 400 × magnification. For the enumeration of tumour cells attached to the amnion, 10 representative fields are counted and the total number of cells on the 0.76 cm^2 basement membrane surface calculated. Radiolabelled tumour cells can also be used in the assay.

Protocol 5. Matrigel chemoinvasion assay

Matrigel consists of a basement membrane matrix extracted from Engelbreth Holm Swarm mouse tumour.

1. Dilute the Matrigel to 10 mg/ml in cold, sterile distilled water. Polycarbonate filters (polyvinyl-pyrrolidone-free), measuring 13 mm in diameter and 8 μm pore size, are placed in Boyden chemotaxis chambers. The filters are coated with Matrigel (25–30 μg/filter), and allowed to dry in a laminar airflow hood.
2. Rehydrate the Matrigel-coated filters in serum-free medium. Tumour cells ((2–3) $\times$ 10^5 cells/ml) are suspended in serum-free medium containing 0.1% BSA and added to the upper chamber in a volume of 0.8 ml.
3. Place 0.2 ml of conditioned serum-free medium from NIH/3T3 cells as a chemoattractant in the lower chamber.
4. Incubate in a humidified CO_2 incubator at 37°C for 5 h.
5. Remove the tumour cells on the upper surface of the filter mechanically using a cotton swab. Then fix the filter in methanol and stain with haematoxylin and eosin. The cells that invaded to the lower surface of the filter are quantitated by an image analyser (Optomax 4).

Note: for description of routine chemotaxis assays see (15).

5. Proteolytic activity

Increase in tumour cell enzymatic activity has been correlated with metastatic potential in some experimental tumour models. Three classes of proteinases will be mentioned here (matrix metalloproteinases, plasminogen activators, and cathepsins), although a number of other types of proteinases have been associated with metastasis. Matrix metalloproteinases (MMP) implicated in malignancy include type-I (mammalian) collagenase (MMP-1), 72 kd type-IV collagenase/gelatinase (MMP-2), 92 kd type-IV collagenase/gelatinase (MMP-9), stromelysin (MMP-3), and Pump-1. The substrate specificity and the significance of each of these enzymes in tumour invasion *in vivo* has not yet been clearly defined. However, metalloproteinases have been implicated as active participants in tumour invasion in an *in vitro* model (16). Plasminogen activators (PA) have also been described as playing an important role in tumour invasion (17, 18). Similarly, lysosomal enzymes, such as cathepsin B have been reported to facilitate invasion and metastasis (19).

Proteolytic activity in cultured cells and tissues can be assessed by zymography, using different types of substrates that are either co-polymerized with acrylamide in SDS-PAGE (20), or used in an overlay gel (21).

For studies of MMP and PA, the following substrates are incorporated into SDS-PAGE: type-I collagen for the MMP-1, gelatin for the MMP-2 and MMP-9, casein for MMP-3, and casein and plasminogen for PA. For studies of tissue inhibitors of metalloproteinases (TIMP), plasminogen activator inhibitors (PAI), and serine proteinase inhibitors the appropriate proteinases are incorporated into the gels. The bands that are resistant to proteinase digestion represent the inhibitor activity.

Protocol 6. Zymograms for proteinases (20)

1. Prepare gels and running buffer as for regular SDS-PAGE, except for the incorporation of 0.1% gelatin, 0.1% type-I collagen, 0.04% type-IV collagen, 0.1% casein, or 0.1% casein + plasminogen (12 μg/ml) into the separating gel.
2. Electrophorese the samples under non-reduced conditions at 9 mA. Minigel electrophoresis can be performed at room temperature, but larger gels should be run at 4°C. Samples are analysed either directly or concentrated. For gelatin zymograms, use tumour cell supernatants without concentration, or a minimum of 2 μg of protein per sample. For the other types of substrate gels, use up to 20 μg of protein.
3. Following electrophoresis: wash the gels three times in 50 mM Tris–HCl (pH 7.4) containing 2% Triton X-100 for 30 min (minigels 15 min) with shaking at room temperature, followed by three washes in 50 mM Tris (pH 7.4) for 5 min. Then incubate the gels in a buffer containing 50 mM Tris, 0.2 M NaCl, 5 mM $CaCl_2$, 1% Triton X-100, 0.02% NaN_3, pH 7.4 at 37°C. The incubation time is usually 16 h, but can be varied, depending on the intensity of the proteolytic activity.
4. Stain the gels in 0.1% Coomassie blue dissolved in a mixture of acetic acid:methanol:water (1:3:6) for 1 h (minigel 30 min) at room temperature and destain in the same mixture without the dye. Proteolytic activity is seen as clear bands in the stained gels.

Protocol 7. Reverse zymograms for metalloproteinase inhibitors (22)

1. Prepare gels and running buffer as for regular 14% SDS-PAGE except for incorporation into the separating gel of 0.1% casein and 30% v/v serum-free culture supernatants from a cell-line expressing high MMP-3 activity (the human breast carcinoma cell-line, MDA-MB-231, can be used for this purpose). Use concentrated culture supernatants, or cell lysates, containing 10–20 μg of protein.
2. Electrophorese the gels and process as described above, except for 72 h incubation in the collagenase buffer.

Protocol 7. *Continued*

3. In parallel to the reverse zymograms, the samples are also analysed by regular 14% SDS-PAGE. Inhibitor bands are visualized as darker staining areas when compared to the regular SDS-PAGE.

Protocol 8. Soluble type I collagenolytic assay (23)

1. Incubate serum-free culture supernants (100 μl) with 10 μl of trypsin (1 mg/ml) at 37°C for 10 min, followed by addition of 10 μl of soybean trypsin inhibitor (5BTI, 5 mg/ml).

2. Neutralize [^{3}H]-type-I collagen in 0.1 M acetic acid (specific activity 1.5×10^6 c.p.m./mg) with 1 M Tris (pH 7.4). The substrate is diluted to contain 10000 c.p.m. per assay with a buffer (Tris–HCl, pH 7.4, 0.15 M NaCl, 4 mM $CaCl_4$) containing 0.5 mM N-ethylmaleimide (NEM) and 0.1 mM phenylmethylsulphonyl fluoride (PMSF).

3. Inoculate the radiolabelled substrate with the culture supernatant in a final volume of 250 μl at 25°C for 18 h. Each assay is performed in triplicate, with and without 25 mM EDTA. Stop the reaction by adding 20 μl of 0.25 M EDTA and incubate at 39°C for 10 min. Then, precipitate undegraded collagen with ethanol (final concentration of 18%) and incubate at room temperature for 30 min.

4. Centrifuge the mixture at 6000*g* at 4°C for 30 min and count for radioactivity in a beta scintillation counter.

The assay is performed with and without trypsin activation to measure the amount of active collagenase. One unit of MMP-1 is defined as the amount of enzyme degrading 1 μg of native collagen at 25°C.

Protocol 9. Soluble type-IV collagenolytic assay (24)

1. Incubate serum-free culture supernatants (400 μl with or without concentration) with 50 μl of trypsin (0.2 mg/ml), followed by the addition of 10 μl of SBTI (5 mg/ml). Place on ice for 10 min. Instead of trypsin, 1–2 mM *p*-aminophenylmercuric acetate (APMA) can be used to activate collagenase(s).

2. Neutralize [^{3}H]proline-labelled type-IV collagen, as described above for MMP-1 and add to the supernatant in a buffer (50 mM Tris-HCl, pH 7.4, 0.2 M NaCl, 5 mM CaCl) containing 3.8 mM NEM, and 1000 kallikrein inhibiting units of aprotinin. Samples are assayed in triplicate, with or without 10 mM EDTA. For measurements of active enzyme(s), samples are tested with and without trypsin or APMA.

3. Incubate the tubes at 35–37°C for 16 h, and terminate the reaction by adding 10 mM EDTA and 70 μl of a mixture of 10% trichloracetic acid (TCA) and 0.5% tannic acid. The final volume of each sample should be 700 μl
4. After 30 min incubation on ice centrifuge the samples at 17000*g* for 15 min and count 650 μl of the supernatant for radioactivity in a beta scintillation counter.

Determination of serum and tissue-culture levels of the urokinase type of plasminogen activator (u-PA), tissue type plasminogen activator (t-PA), and plasminogen activator inhibitor, type 1 (PAI-1) can be done by the use of ELISA (25–27). For details of assays for cathepsin and cysteine proteinase inhibitors see (28–30).

6. Tumour cell surface

Some of the cell surface components which have been shown to be modified in metastatic cells are listed below in *Table 4*.

Table 4. Cell surface molecules associated with metastasis

Surface components	**Reference**
Gangliosides	Merritt,[a] Minor[b]
Gangliosides and sialylglycoproteins	Yogeeswaran[c]
Carbohydrates	Finne,[d] Imimura[e]
Glycoproteins	Steck[f]
Sialylglycoproteins	Murayama[g]
Major histocompatibility complex (MHC)	Gopas[h]

[a] Merritt, W. D. (1978). *J. Natl. Cancer Inst.*, **60**, 1313.
[b] Minor, K. M. (1982). *Cancer Res.*, **42**, 4631.
[c] Yogeeswaran, G. (1978). *Cancer Res.*, **38**, 1336.
[d] Finne, J. (1980). *Cancer Res.*, **40**, 2580.
[e] Imimura, T. (1984). *Cancer Res.*, **44**, 791.
[f] Steck, P. A. (1983). *Exp. Cell Res.*, **147**, 255.
[g] Murayama, K. (1986). *Cancer Res.*, **46**, 1395.
[h] Gopas, J. (1989). *Adv. Cancer Res.*, **53**, 89.

References

1. Fidler, I. J., Gersten, D. M., and Hart, I. R. (1978). *Adv. Cancer Res.*, **28**, 149.
2. Schirrmacher, V. (1985). *Adv. Cancer Res.*, **43**, 1.
3. Zoller, M. (1985). *Immunol. Immunother.*, **19**, 189.
4. Hanna, N. (1982). *Cancer Metastasis Rev.*, **1**, 45.
5. Fidler, I. J. and Poste, G. (1982). *Springer Seminars of Immunopathology*, vol. 5, p. 161. Springer, Berlin.

6. Stutman, O., Paige, C. J., and Figarella, E. F. (1978). *J. Immunol.*, **121**, 1819.
7. Schirrmacher, V., von Hoegen, P., Heicappel, R., and Altevogt, P., (1987). In *Immune Responses to Metastases*, (ed. R. B. Herberman, R. H. Wiltrout, and E. Gorelik), vol. II, p. 1.
8. Fogler, W. E. and Fidler, I. J. (1987). In *Immune Response to Metastases*, (ed. R. B. Herberman, R. H. Wiltrout, and E. Gorelik), vol. II, p. 43.
9. Kim, U., Baumler, A., Carruthers, C., and Bielat, K. (1975). *Proc. Natl. Acad. Sci. USA*, **72,** 1012.
10. Fidler, I. J., Gersten, D. M., and Riggs, C. (1977). *Cancer*, **40,** 46.
11. Fidler, I. S. (1978). *Methods Cancer Res.*, **115,** 399.
12. Tennert, J. R. (1964). *Transplantation*, **2,** 685.
13. Fridman, R., Kibbey, M. C., Royce, L. S., Zain, M., Sweeney, T. M., Jicha, D. L., *et al.* (1991). *J. Natl. Cancer Inst.*, **83,** 769.
14. Giavazzi, R., Jessup, J. M., Campbell, D. E., Walker, S. M., and Fidler, I. J. (1986). *Cancer Res.*, **46,** 1928.
15. Gauss-Muller, V., Kleinman, H. K., Martin, G. R., and Schiffmann, E. (1980). *J. Lab. Clin. Med.*, **96,** 1071.
16. Thorgeirsson, U. P., Liotta, L. A., Kalebic, T., Margulies, I. M., Thomas, K., Rios-Candelore, M., *et al.* (1982). *J. Natl. Cancer Inst.*, **69,** 1049.
17. Dano, K., Andreasen, P. A., and Grondhal-Hansen, J. (1985). *Adv. Cancer Res.*, **44,** 170.
18. Axelrod, J., Reich, H., and Miskin, R. (1989). *Mol. Cell. Biol.*, **9,** 2133.
19. Sloane, B. F., Rozkin, J., Johnson, K., Taylor, H., Crissman, J. D., and Honn, K. V. (1986). *Proc. Nat. Acad. Sci. USA*, **83,** 2483.
20. Mackay, A. R., Hartzler, J. L., Pelina, M. D., and Thorgeirsson, U. P. (1990). *J. Biol. Chem.*, **265,** 2129.
21. Birkedal-Hansen, H. and Taylor, R. E. (1982). *Biochem. Biophys. Res. Commun.*, **107,** 1173.
22. Mackay, A. R., Ballin, M., Pelina, M. D., Farina, A. R., Nason, A. M., Hartzler, J. L., *et al.* (1992). *Invasion and Metastasis*. (In press.)
23. Emonard, H., Christiane, Y., Smet, M., Grimaud, J. A., and Foidart, J. M. (1990). *Invasion and Metastasis*, **10,** 170.
24. Salo, T., Liotta, L. A., and Tryggvason, K. (1983). *J. Biol. Chem.*, **258,** 3058.
25. Binnema, D. J., van Iersel, J. L., and Dooijeward, G. (1986). *Thrombosis Res.*, **43,** 569.
26. Woijta, J., Binder, B. R., Huber, K., and Hoover, R. L. (1989). *Thrombosis and Haemostasis*, **61,** 289.
27. Resch, I., Krutisch, G., Geiger, M., and Binder, B. R. (1989). *Thrombosis and Haemostasis*, **62**, 299.
28. Green, G. D. J., Kembhavi, A. A., Davies, M. E., and Barrett, A. J., (1984). *Biochem. J.*, **218,** 939.
29. Rozhin, J., Robinson, D., Stevens, M. M., Lah, T. T., Honn, K. V., Ryan, R. E., *et al.* (1987). *Cancer Res.*, **47,** 6620.
30. Rozhin, J., Gomez, A. P., Ziegler, H. H., Nelson, K. K., Chang, Y. S., Fong, D., *et al.* (1990). *Cancer Res.* **50,** 6278.

Index

antibodies, *see* bispecific antibodies, immunoglobulin engineering, human monoclonal antibodies, *and* radiolabelling of immunoglobulins

B-cells, *see* human monoclonal antibodies
bispecific antibodies 225
  Fab conjugates 225, 226, 233, 237
    bispecific F(ab)2 conjugates 237
    chemical flow-diagrams 235, 236
    preparation of F(ab)2 fragments 231, 232
    trispecific F(ab)3 conjugates 239
  general reagents and equipment 226–9
    HPLC analysis of conjugates 240, 241
  IgG conjugates 225
  linking agents 225, 226
  removing contaminants 242, 243
  targeting of LAK-cells 388

cell engineering
  cytokine secretion 293
    by tumour cells: examples and references 294; secretion levels 301; tumourigenicity 300
    packaging cells 295; construction, care, etc. 296–9
    viral vectors 294; assaying secretion levels 298; infection of target cells 299, 300
  expression of novel T-cell receptors 345
    applications 348
    designing constructs: antibody selection 349; cloning of Ig V-region genes 352; expression vectors 350; TCR gene structure 350
    examples and references 347
    functional analysis of transfectants: cell-surface expression 361; immunochemical 362; mRNA expression 360; response to specific antigen 365
    general strategy 346
    target cells: choice of 355; transfection, electroporation 357; transfection, protoplast fusion 358
    transfectant selection 358
  immortalization 321
    autocrine growth factor loops 323
    general strategy 324
    of lymphocytes 326; cell purification 336; cell stimulation 337; choice of constructs 328; establishment of cell-lines 341; viral infection 338
    oncogenes 322
  see also viral transfection
cytokines
  bioassays
    IL-1 181, 182
    IL-2 182, 302, 365
    IL-4 302
    IL-6 182
    IL-8 185
    tumour necrosis factors 183
  mRNA analysis 159
    see also ribonucleic acid
  quantitative bioassay
    theoretical considerations 179; curve fitting 187, 188; raw data 186; standardization 189
  secretion by tumour cells 293
    see also cell engineering
cryopreservation
  monocytes
  T-cells 124
  T-cell clones 137
  tumour cell-lines 12
cytotoxicity assays
  for LAK-cells 318
  for monocytes 109
  for NK-cells 87, 88
  for T-cells 127

ELISA *This technique is used widely in the various protocols described in the book. Please see the appropriate chapters for more details.*
enzymatic dissociation of tumour tissue
  common enzymes 35
  to prepare tumour cells 401
  to prepare tumour cell-lines *see also* tumour cell-lines 6
  to prepare T-cells 122
  to prepare T-cell clones 134

enzymatic dissociation of tumour tissue (*cont.*)
to prepare tumour-infiltrating leukocytes 309
for fluorescence analysis 34
expression of recombinant DNA
cells
Cos cells 248
tumour cells 293
plasmids
cytokine secretion 294
humanizing rodent Ig specificities 269, 273
Ig-fusion proteins 249, 259
single-chain Fv proteins 287
T-cell receptor constructs 351

flow cytometry
cell staining
direct 30
effect of chemical fixation 42
effect of enzymes 35
indirect 31
lymphoid tumours—common markers 47
monocytes 106, 107, 108
staining in association with DNA markers 44, 48
DNA analysis
aneuploid and diploid populations 37, 40, 44
dissociation of wax-embedded specimens 37
effect of chemical fixation 43
extraction of nuclei 38, 40
proliferation: BrdU 55; Ki67 52; PCNA 52
staining in association with cell-surface markers 44, 48
solid tumours 49
sample preparation
bone marrow 33
brush specimens 39
lymph-node 39
needle biopsies 39
peripheral blood 30
peritoneal washings 33
tumour tissue 34
standardization and controls
calibration 46
controls 45
false positives 32

human monoclonal antibodies 191
Epstein–Barr virus (EBV) 192
EBV; source (B95-8) 196
EBV; transformation 200
EBV transformants;
fusion 205
maintenance 202
heterohybridomas 192
heteromyelomas 192
human B-cells
purification 193
selection of IgG positives 195
in vitro sensitization 196; secondary challenge 197; primary challenge 198; CD40 activation 199; screening for specific antibody 201
humanized monoclonal antibodies, *see* immunoglobulin engineering
transfectomas 275

immunoglobulin engineering 245
antibody fusions 257–60
by homologous recombination 259
humanizing rodent Ig specificities 263
CDR grafting 266; by site-directed mutagenesis 268; by *de novo* gene synthesis 272
general strategy 264
V-region cloning by PCR 265, 266
Ig fusion protein possibilities 247
immunoligands 245–8
characterization, detection, purification 252–6
stable expression 251
transient expression 248
maintenance of reading frame 248
Plasmids used in, *see* expression of recombinant DNA
single-chain Fv proteins 279
design considerations 279, 290
expression and purification 285, 287
linker design 280, 282, 283
PCR-based construction 281, 284
site-directed mutagenesis-based construction 284, 286
immunohistochemistry 225, 246

lymphokine activated killer cells
activation with IL-2
continuous 311, 387
inclusion of anti-CD3 315
pulsed 316
adherent LAK cells 314
general characteristics 306

metastasis
characteristics of metastatic cells

assays of invasive capability: amnion invasion 405; references and examples 404
assays of metastatic capability: intravenous 402; subcutaneous 402
assays of proteolytic activity 406; collagenases 408; soluble metaloproteinases 408; zymograms 407
quantitation of metastatic capability 403
tumour cell surface 409
models of metastasis
examples 400
in vivo: hepatic 378; pulmonary 377
multicellular tumour spheroids: growth 386; infiltration by LAK-cells 388, 390; histology 388; morphology 389
spontaneous 371
monocytes
characterization of human
functional: antibody-dependent killing 111; antigen presentation 116; chemotaxis 113; cytokine production 116; phagocytosis 114; production of radicles 112; spontaneous killing 109
phenotypic 99; cell markers 101; monoclonal antibodies 103–8
isolation of human
adherence 95
counterflow centrifugal elutriation 97
density techniques: Ficoll 93; Nycoprep 94; Sepracell MN 93
magnetic beads 98
reagents required 91
from solid tumours 99

natural killer cells
assays of NK-cell function
in human systems 87
in murine systems 88
general characteristics
morphology 82
phenotype 83
response to cytokines 87
preparation of human NK-cells
on density gradients 84, 85
by depletion of non-LGLs 86

polymerase chain reaction *This technique is used widely in the various protocols described in the book. Please see the appropriate chapters for more details.*

radiolabelling of immunoglobulins 209
isotopes of iodine, indium, technecium 209, 211, 213
legal requirements 211
linking isotopes and antibodies 213
Bolton–Hunter reagent 216
Chloramine-T 215
DTPA 218
Iodogen 214
Schwarz method 220
poor labelling 216, 220, 222
ribonucleic acid
dot- and slot-blotting 168
half-life in cytoplasm 177
in situ hybridization 172
Northern blotting
electrophoresis and blotting 164
probing with cDNA: detection 167; hybridization 167; labelling probe 166
PCR analysis of 170
preparation of
cellular RNA: with acid guanidinium 163; with guanidinium and caesium chloride 162; with lithium chloride and urea 161; with SDS and urea 146
messenger RNA 163
RNase protection analysis of 169
transcription rate analysis of
preparation of nuclei 174
preparation of probe 175
transport to cytoplasm 176

SCID mice 199

T-cells
characterization
alloreactive T-cells 145
killing 127
mixed lymphocyte cultures 135, 145
proliferation 126
cloning
activation, prior to 134
assessment of monoclonality 139
generalized cloning protocol 136
medium and growth factors 132
starting material 134
cryopreservation, *see* cryopreservation
isolation
medium and serum 119
purification: by density 123; by magnetic beads 124

starting material: blood 121; lymphoid tissue 121; peritoneal washings 121; tumour tissue 121
T-cell receptor
PCR analysis of: preparation of RNA 146; primer selection 153; primers used in Vβ analysis 150; reproducibility 155; semiquantitative Vβ analysis 148, 151; synthesis of cDNA 147; theoretical considerations 152, 153, 154
Southern blotting of 139
tumour antigens
antibodies against 61
assay and identification 63
purification 61
storage 61
isolation and characterization
immunoblotting 75
initial material 68
degradation 69
epitope mapping 75
solublization 70
purification
with antibodies 71
with lectins 71
by precipitation 73
radiolabelling 72
tumour cell-lines 1
cell-culture requirements 2, 3
characterization 11, 13
see also flow cytometry
preparation from solid tissue 4
primary cultures 10
removal of stromal cells 9
transfected with cytokines, *see* cell engineering
tumour immunogenicity
antigenicity 18
concomitant immunity 21
effects on *in vivo* growth 20
effects on metastasis 22
immunosuppression 24
tumour infiltrating lymphocytes
activation
with IL-2 312
with tumour cells 313
isolation 309
tumour models
examples 381
extrapolation of results to a clinical setting 379
general description of models 370
immunogenicity, *see* tumour immunogenicity
transplantable renal cell carcinoma model
hepatic metastases 378
intraperitoneal passage 374
intrarenal injection 375
nephrectomy 375
pulmonary metastases 377
xenograft 372
tumour spheroids, *see* metastasis

viral transfection
infecting target cells
adherent cells 299, 334
primary cells 338
suspension cells 300
see also cell engineering
packaging cell-lines 296
construction 296, 329, 332
selection 327, 329
screening: for Helper virus 299, 333; for viral production 298, 330
viral vectors
handling 329
system design 325, 328; HIV-based vectors 335